AF603620

BIOCHEMISTRY AND BIOLOGY OF CORONAVIRUSES

ADVANCES IN EXPERIMENTAL MEDICINE AND BIOLOGY

Recent Volumes in this Series

Volume 134
HAMSTER IMMUNE RESPONSES IN INFECTIOUS AND ONCOLOGIC DISEASES
Edited by J. Wayne Streilein, David A. Hart, Joan Stein-Streilein, William R. Duncan, and Rupert E. Billingham

Volume 135
DIET AND RESISTANCE TO DISEASE
Edited by Marshall Phillips and Albert Baetz

Volume 136
BIOLOGICAL REACTIVE INTERMEDIATES II: Chemical Mechanisms and Biological Effects
Edited by Robert Snyder, Dennis V. Parke, James J. Kocsis, David J. Jollow, G. Gordon Gibson, and Charlotte M. Wintmer

Volume 137
THE RUMINANT IMMUNE SYSTEM
Edited by John E. Butler

Volume 138
HORMONES AND CANCER
Edited by Wendell W. Leavitt

Volume 139
TAURINE IN NUTRITION AND NEUROLOGY
Edited by Ryan Huxtable and Herminia Pasantes-Morales

Volume 140
COMPOSITION AND FUNCTION OF CELL MEMBRANES: Application to the Pathophysiology of Muscle Diseases
Edited by Stewart Wolf and Allen K. Murray

Volume 141
BIOCHEMISTRY AND FUNCTION OF PHAGOCYTES
Edited by F. Rossi and P. Patriarca

Volume 142
BIOCHEMISTRY AND BIOLOGY OF CORONAVIRUSES
Edited by V. ter Meulen, S. Siddell, and H. Wege

BIOCHEMISTRY AND BIOLOGY OF CORONAVIRUSES

Edited by
V. ter Meulen,
S. Siddell, and H. Wege
University of Würzburg
Würzburg, Federal Republic of Germany

SPRINGER SCIENCE+BUSINESS MEDIA, LLC

Library of Congress Cataloging in Publication Data

Main entry under title:

Biochemistry and biology of coronaviruses.

"Proceedings of an International Symposium held in October 1980 at the Institute of Virology and Immuno-biology of the University of Würzburg, FRG"–T.p. verso.
Bibliography: p.
Includes index.
1. Coronaviruses–Congresses. I. Meulen, Volker ter. II. Siddell, S. III. Wege, H. [DNLM: 1. Coronaviridae–Congresses. 2. Coronavirus infections–Pathology–Congresses. QW 168.5.C8 B615 1980]
QR399.B56 616'.0194 81-15856
AACR2

DOI 10.1007/978-1-4757-0456-3

Proceedings of an International Symposium held in October 1980 at the
Institute of Virology and Immunobiology of the University of Würzburg, FRG

PREFACE

This book is the result of an international symposium held at the Institute of Virology and Immunobiology of the University of Würzburg, Germany, in October 1980. The intent of this symposium was to provide an opportunity to compare the data on coronavirus structure and replication as well as to discuss mechanisms of pathogenesis. For over a decade coronaviruses have been recognized as an important group of viruses which are responsible for a variety of diseases of clinical importance in animals and man. Recently new and interesting data on the molecular biology and pathogenesis of coronaviruses have become available and this led us to organize this meeting. The uniformity and diversity in this virus group was evaluated from a molecular point of view and the replication of coronaviruses appears to involve aspects which may be unique for this virus group. Additionally, in contrast to other positive strand RNA viruses it became clear that coronaviruses readily establish persistent infections in the host, a phenomenon which may lead to the different subacute or chronic disorders manifested during coronavirus infection.

This volume presents a series of articles based upon the scientific presentation given at the symposium. In addition, there are two articles by B.W.J. Mahy and D.A.J. Tyrrell which summarize the current state of art concerning the biochemistry and biology of coronaviruses, respectively. We believe this book will be of interest to all virologists and particularly to both established workers and newcomers to this field.

V. ter Meulen
S. Siddell
H. Wege

CONTENTS

STRUCTURE AND REPLICATION

THE STRUCTURE AND BEHAVIOR OF CORONAVIRUS A59 GLYCOPROTEINS

Lawrence S. Sturman

Virus Laboratories, Division of Laboratories and Research
New York State Department of Health
Albany, New York 12201

INTRODUCTION

Coronavirus A59 contains three structural proteins. The location of these proteins in relation to the viral envelope and RNA are illustrated in the model shown in Figure 1. A nucleocapsid protein, N, (mw ≃ 50k) forms the nucleocapsid together with the RNA genome. Surrounding the nucleocapsid is a lipoprotein membrane which contains the envelope glycoproteins El (mw ≃ 23k) and E2 (mw ≃180k and 90k). El is an integral membrane protein, the bulk of which lies within the viral membrane and probably spans the lipid bilayer. E2 is a peripheral glycoprotein which forms the characteristic peplomers that are associated with this virion.

In this report I will describe some features of the behavior of these viral glycoproteins and propose models for the structure of El and E2.

CHARACTERIZATION OF E1 AND E2 BASED ON INCORPORATION OF DIFFERENT RADIOLABELED PRECURSORS

Inasmuch as these studies depended on the use of radiolabeled compounds, I would like to first review the relative incorporation of several radiolabeled precursors into El and E2. This information is summarized in Table 1.

Methionine is incorporated into El to a greater relative extent than into the other structural proteins, compared with other labeled amino acids such as valine, leucine, arginine, glutamic acid and mixtures of amino acids. Seventy percent of the radiolabeled methionine incorporated into A59 virus was found in El and only approximately 10% in E2. In contrast, when A59 virus was labeled, with valine, only 40% of the label in the virus was incorporated into El and 20% into E2. E2 was highly labeled by both

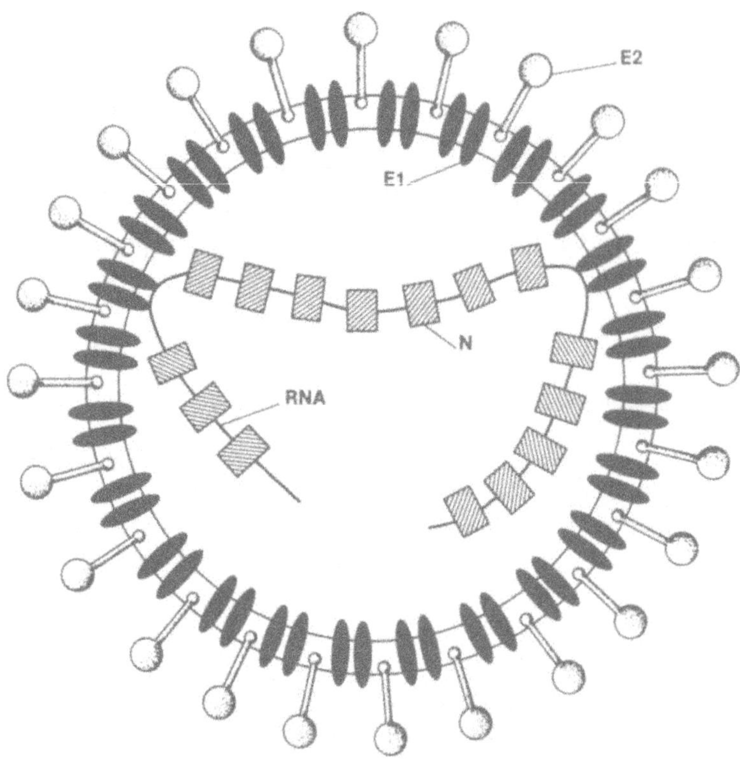

Fig. 1. A schematic model of coronavirus A59 (Sturman et al., 1980)

radiolabeled fucose and glucosamine, whereas El was not labeled by fucose and only to a small extent by glucosamine. The ratio of incorporation of glucosamine relative to valine in El was about one tenth of that in E2. Thus El is the principal viral structural protein which becomes labeled with methionine, whereas E2 is the principal glycoprotein which can be labeled with glucosamine and the only one which can be labeled with fucose. These

Table 1. Radiolabeling Characteristics of Coronavirus A59 Glycoproteins

Designation	Relative extent of labeling with		
	Methionine	Fucose	Glucosamine
E1	++++	-	+
E2	+	++++	++++

differences have been used in following the behavior of E1 and E2 in the virus and after solubilization with SDS or NP40.

CONFORMATIONAL TRANSITION AND AGGREGATION OF THE PEPLOMERIC GLYCOPROTEIN

Several investigators have shown that the thermal lability of coronavirus infectivity is pH dependent. Pocock and Garwes (1975) reported that transmissible gastroenteritis virus infectivity was most stable at pH 6.5 at 37°C and least stable at pH 8. Alexander and Collins (1975) obtained similar results in their study of the effect of pH on the infectivity of avian infectious bronchitis virus.

I will describe the results of experiments with A59 virus which provide evidence that pH dependent thermal lability of coronavirus infectivity is associated with a conformational change in E2 and aggregation of the peplomeric glycoprotein.

In Figure 2, the pH dependence of A59 virus infectivity at 37°C is illustrated. Virus infectivity was measured after 24 hours incubation over a pH range from 4.0 to 8.0 at 4°C and 37°C. Incubation was carried out in a buffer prepared from boric acid, citric acid, diethylbarbituric acid and phosphoric acid (Johnson and Lindsey, 1939). The ionic strength was adjusted to approximate that of physiological saline and fetal bovine serum was added to a final concentration of 10%. At 4°C virus infectivity was stable over much of this pH range, but at 37°C the virus was markedly inactivated above pH 6.5 and below pH 5.0. At 37°C virus infectivity was most stable between pH 6.0 and 6.5.

Analysis of the kinetics of thermal inactivation at 37°C revealed that at pH 8.0 there was a 50% loss in A59 virus infectivity in less than 1 hour. In contrast at pH 6.0 the half life of virus infectivity was 24 hours.

The effect of thermal inactivation at pH 8.0 on the structural proteins of the virus was analyzed by SDS-polyacrylamide gel electrophoresis. A marked change in the electrophoretic mobility of E2 was observed. A typical gel profile is shown in Figure 3. In this experiment, [^{3}H] glucosamine-labeled A59 virus was held at pH 6.0, while [^{14}C] glucosamine-labeled virus was inactivated at pH 8.0 at 37°C for 2 hours. Then the samples were mixed, solubilized in SDS at 25°, and coelectrophoresed.

In the virion at pH 6.0, E2 is found in two forms, as 180k (GP180) and 90k (GP90) dalton species which produce identical tryptic peptide patterns (Sturman and Holmes, 1977). GP90 can be produced from GP180 by treatment of virions with trypsin without significant loss of infectivity.

The control pattern in Figure 3 shows both 90k and 180k molecular weight forms of E2 as well as a small amount of aggregate which did not enter the resolving gel. The electrophoretic mobility of E2 from virions

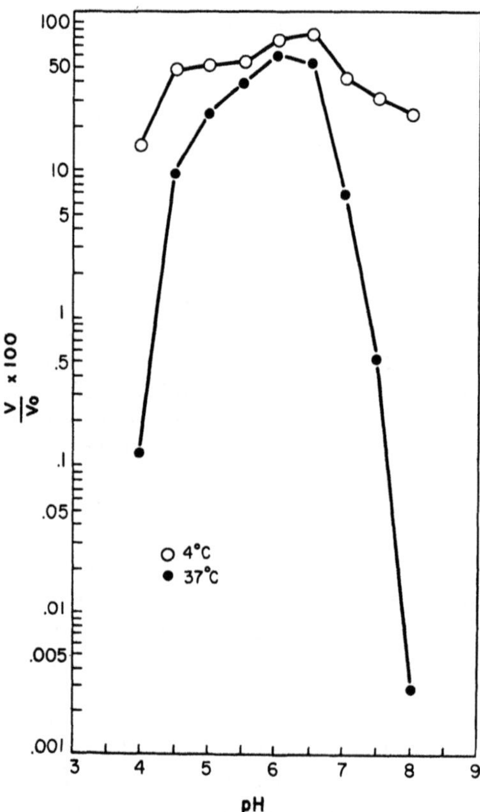

Fig. 2. Survival of A59 virus infectivity after 24 hrs at 4°C or 37°C as a function of pH.

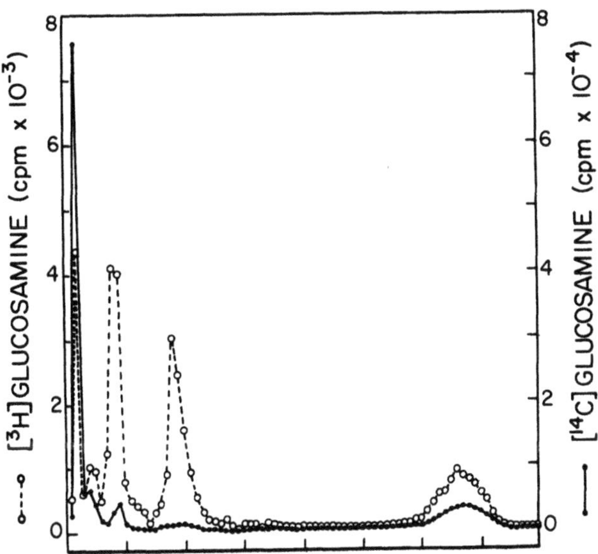

Fig. 3. Co-electrophoresis of the glycoproteins of [^{3}H] glucosamine-labeled, control (pH 6.0, 25°C, O—O) and [^{14}C] glucosamine-labeled, inactivated (pH 8.0, 37°C, 2 hrs, ●—●) A59 virions.

inactivated at pH 8.0 at 37°C was quite different. Very little of this glycoprotein comigrated with the 90k and 180k molecular weight forms from native virions. Most of the E2 from pH 8.0 inactivated virus formed aggregates which remained at the top of the gel.

The other structural proteins, N and E1 were not affected. E1 from pH 6.0 and pH 8.0 treated virus comigrated as a single peak, and in other experiments, the electrophoretic mobility of amino acid labeled nucleocapsid protein was found to be unaltered after pH 8.0 inactivation of virus.

The distribution of E2 between monomeric forms and aggregates after incubation of virus at pH 6.0 and 8.0 at 4°C and 37°C is shown in Table 2.

About 80% of E2 remained as monomers when virus was held at 4°C at either pH 6.0 or pH 8.0, or at 37°C at pH 6.0. In contrast, after incubation of virus at 37°C at pH 8.0 for 2 hours, more than 80% of this glycoprotein was recovered in the form of aggregates at the top of the gel.

Table 2. Aggregation of Virion-Associated E2

Condition[a] pH	°C	GP 180/90 (%)[b]	Aggregate (%)[b]
6	4°	82	18
	37°	88	12
8	4°	80	20
	37°	17	83

[a] Virions incubated for 120 min in 100mM NaCl, 1 mM EDTA, 50 mM Tris Maleate at the indicated pH and temperature.
[b] SDS gel electrophoretic distribution of [^{14}C] glucosamine-labeled E2.

E2 appears to contain both intramolecular disulfide bonds and free sulfhydryl groups (Sturman, L. S. and Holmes, K. V., in preparation). Both must be retained to maintain the native configuration of the peplomeric glycoprotein. As shown in Table 3 the sulfhydryl blocking reagent, p-chloromercuribenzoate (PMB), enhanced E2 aggregation. Incubation of virus in the presence of PMB (10 mM) for 30 minutes at 37°C at pH 8.0 caused 91% of the peplomeric glycoprotein to become aggregated, compared with 34% in controls.

Coronavirus structural proteins can be isolated by disruption of purified virus with the nonionic detergent NP40 at 4°, and the solubilized envelope glycoproteins and viral nucleocapsid can be separated by sucrose density gradient sedimentation (Sturman et. al., 1980).

As with virion associated E2, aggregate formation could be induced in NP40-solubilized E2 by incubation at pH 8.0 at 37°C (Table 4). Only a small proportion of the isolated solubilized glycoprotein became aggregated at pH 6.0 at 4°C or 37°C or at pH 8.0 at 4°C. However, by 2 hours at pH 8.0 at 37°C a substantial amount of aggregation had taken place. PMB enhanced aggregation of isolated E2 as well.

During inactivation of virus at pH 8.0 a portion of the 90k dalton form of E2 was released from the virus. However, none of the 180k dalton species was detached. Cleavage of GP180 with trypsin prior to inactivation at pH 8.0 resulted in release of increased amounts of GP90. A greater amount of E2 was released also as a consequence of disulfide bond reduction and sulfhydryl group blockage (Sturman and Holmes, in preparation). Recent evidence indicates that the two approximately 90k molecular weight products of proteolytic cleavage of GP180 can be distinguished. Hopefully future studies on these two parts of the peplomeric glycoprotein will provide

Table 3. Enhancement of Aggregation of Virion-Associated E2 by 30 Min Incubation with p-Chloromercuribenzoate (PMB)[a]

PMB (mM)	GP 180/90 (%)[b]	Aggregate (%)[b]
None	66	34
10	9	91

[a] Virus treated at pH 8 for 30 min at 37°C in 100 mM NaCl, 1 mM EDTA, 50 mM Tris Maleate, pH 8 with or without PMB.
[b] SDS gel electrophoretic distribution of [^{14}C] glucosamine-labeled E2.

information about the different functional domains within this large molecule.

A MODEL OF E2

A model of E2 based on these findings and results of our earlier investigations (Sturman, 1977; Sturman and Holmes, 1977; Sturman et al., 1980) is shown in Figure 4. E2 is probably attached to the viral envelope through a short hydrophobic region which penetrates the outer lipid bilayer. Carbohydrate side chains (represented by "lollipops") are present on both parts of the large hydrophilic portion of the molecule. Synthesis of E2 is sensitive to tunicamycin (Holmes, personal communication) and therefore the carbohydrate moieties are most likely N-glycosidically linked to the protein. One trypsin sensitive site is exposed near the middle of the amino acid chain. Proteolytic cleavage produces two species which have similar electrophoretic mobilities on SDS polyacrylamide gels. The portion

Table 4. Aggregation of NP40-Solubilized E2

Condition[a] pH	°C	GP 180/90 (%)[b]	Aggregate (%)[b]
6	4°	89	11
	37°	88	12
8	4°	82	18
		57	43

[a] NP-40 solubilized E2 incubated for 120 min in 100 mM NaCl, 1 mM EDTA, 50 mM Tris Maleate at the indicated pH and temperature.
[b] SDS gel electrophoretic distribution of [^{3}H] fucose-labeled E2.

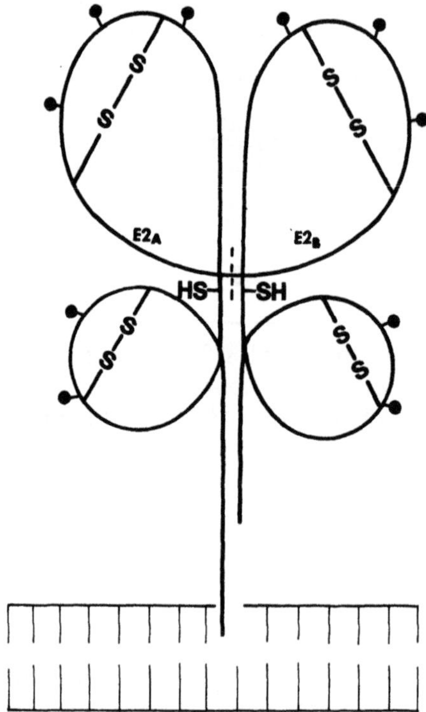

Fig. 4. A model of E2, the peplomeric glycoprotein.

attached to the viral envelope has been designated $E2_A$. The free segment $E2_B$. The condition of disulfide and sulfhydryl groups in E2 appears to be of paramount importance in determining the conformational state of the molecule.

ANOMALOUS BEHAVIOR OF E1 IN SDS-POLYACRYLAMIDE GELS

Let us turn now to the smaller envelope glycoprotein, E1. E1 is substantially different from E2. In the intact virion only a small portion of E1 is susceptible to proteases. Pronase or bromelain treatment of virus results in a decrease in the apparent molecular weight of E1 from 23k to 18k and loss of the carbohydrate containing region (Sturman, 1977; Sturman and Holmes, 1977). Thus most of the E1 molecule is concealed within the viral membrane, except for a small glycosylated portion which extends outside the lipid envelope.

E1 exhibits anomalous behavior on SDS-polyacrylamide gel electrophoresis. After heating to 100°C in SDS, the electrophoretic mobility of E1 is altered and several new forms of lower mobility are produced (Sturman, 1977). β-mercaptoethanol (β-MSH) and dithiothreitol (DTT) exaggerate the effects of heating. These changes in E1 are shown in Figure 5. Figure 5A shows the profile obtained on a 10% cylindrical gel when [^{35}S] methionine-labeled A59 viral proteins were solubilized in SDS at 25°C. E1 migrated as a broad band with an average apparent molecular weight of 23k. The same pattern was obtained when the sample in SDS was treated at 37°C in the presence of 5% β-MSH. However, multiple (three to four) bands of E1 could be resolved in this region when run on slab gels with reducing agent under the same conditions. Heating the sample at 100°C in the absence of reducing agent resulted in the appearance of species with apparent molecular weights of 38k and 60k and a concomitant reduction in the amount of the 23k dalton species. This is shown in Figure 5B. A diffuse increase in the amount of labeled material in the upper region of the gel is also seen. If the sample was heated at 100°C in the presence of reducing agent, the amount of 23k dalton E1 was reduced further and a greater proportion was found near the top of the gel. The pattern obtained thus depended on the conditions employed in preparation of the sample: the temperature and the concentration of reducing agent. However, heating per se was not required to produce changes in the electrophoretic mobility of E1. Freezing also resulted in the appearance of the 38k dalton species. Prolonged treatment of virions with 7M guanidine followed by 9M urea and then 1% SDS all at 25°C in the presence of 1mM β-MSH, resulted in the same changes in electrophoretic mobility of E1 as heating at 100°C in the presence of a high concentration of reducing agent. This suggests that E1 is not completely denatured in SDS at 25°C or 37°C. Heating and reduction of disulfide bonds may promote unfolding of a region of E1 which was incompletely denatured and thus facilitate interactions between hydrophobic domains of the molecule.

INTERACTION OF E1 WITH THE VIRAL NUCLEOCAPSID

Studies with NP40-solubilized E1 illustrates that the conformation of this molecule determines its interaction with viral RNA.

E1 can be solubilized by NP40 at 4°C and separated from E2 and the viral nucleocapsid by sucrose density gradient sedimentation (Sturman et al., 1980). A profile of separated viral components labeled with [^{3}H] fucose and [^{35}S] methionine is shown in the upper panel of Figure 6. The large upper peak consists of [^{35}S] methionine-labeled E1. Below this in the gradient is a peak which contains most of the [^{3}H] fucose label and a small amount of [^{35}S] methionine. This is E2. On the high density cushion is a third peak which contains a large amount of [^{35}S] methionine and a small amount of [^{3}H] fucose. This consists of the nucleocapsid protein N, plus the viral RNA, and a small amount of incompletely solubilized E2. If the mixture of NP40-disrupted virions was incubated at 37°C for 30 minutes before sedimentation, a strikingly different pattern of labeled comonents was obtained. This is shown in the lower panel of Figure 6. The peak of [^{35}S] methionine-labeled E1 was not found at the top of the gradient. A new peak of [^{35}S] label was detected above the high density cushion, and the amount of radiolabeled material on the cushion was markedly decreased. Recovery of the new complex was incomplete due to its adherence to the

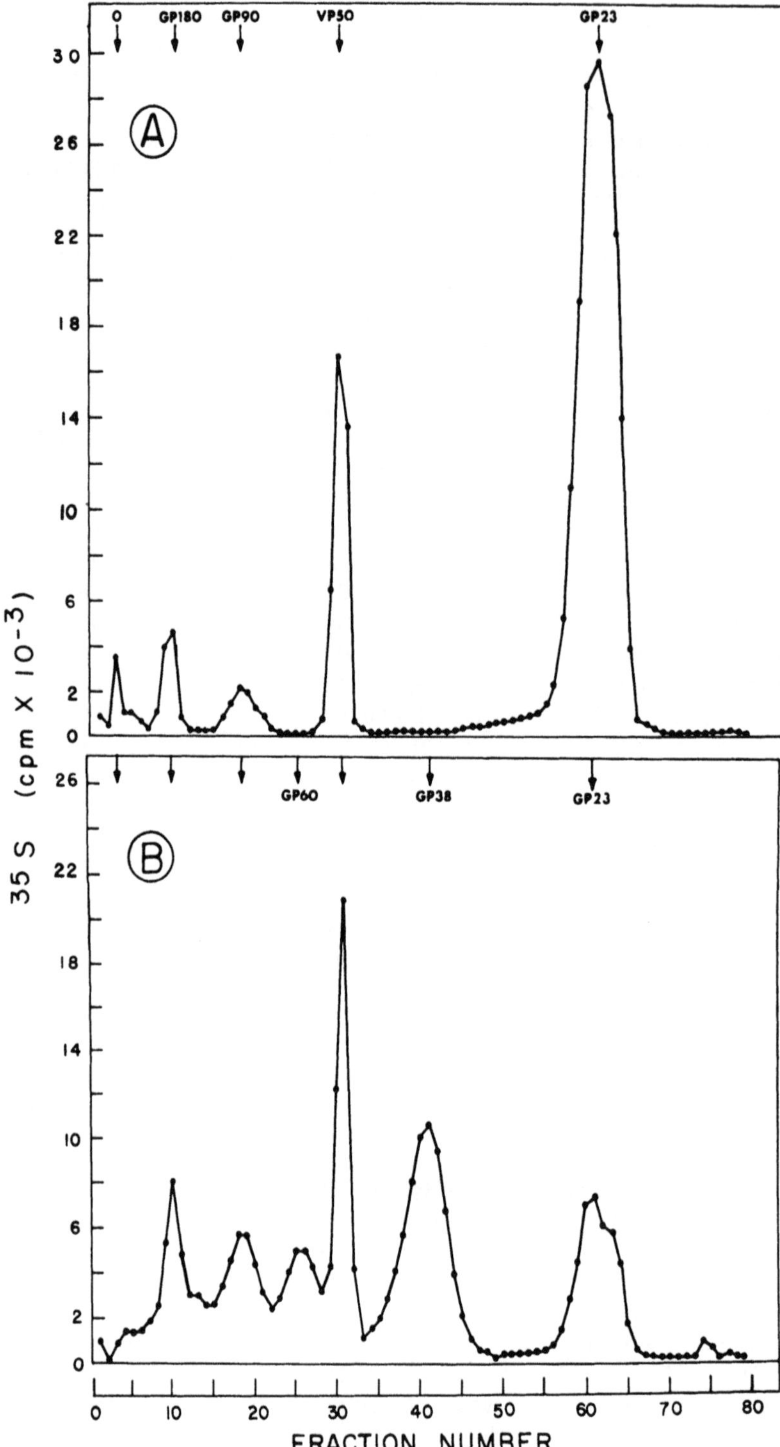

Fig. 5. Effect of boiling on the SDS-PAGE profile of E2. (A)25°C; (B)100°C.

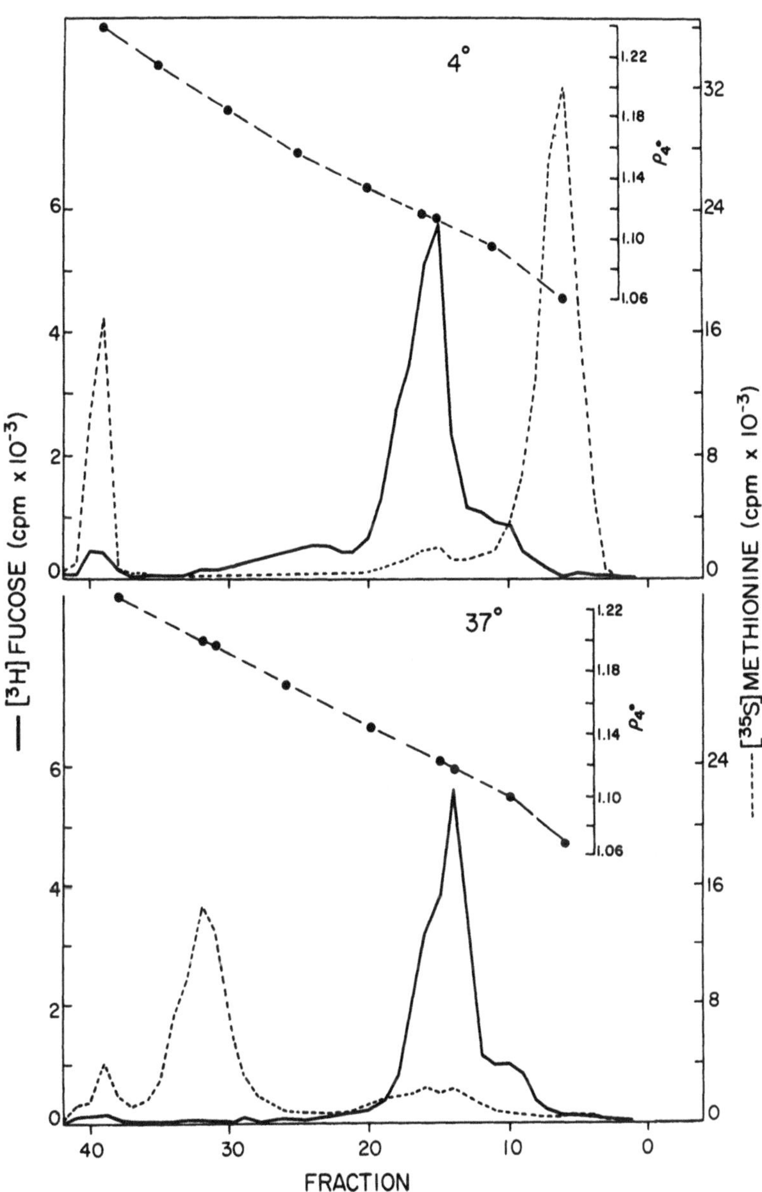

Fig. 6. Sucrose gradient (15-50%) distribution of A59 structural proteins after disruption of the viral envelope with 0.25% NP40 at 4°C and incubation at (upper panel) 4°C; (lower panel) 37°C for 30 min. (Sturman et al., 1980)

centrifuge tube. SDS gel electrophoretic analysis of the new peak revealed that it contained both E1 and N proteins. Experiments with [^{3}H] uridine-labeled virus showed that viral RNA was also present in this complex.

The E1-N-RNA complex could be reconstructed from E1 and viral nucleocapsids which had been isolated separately at 4°C. This is shown in Figure 7. E1 labeled with [^{35}S] methionine and nucleocapsids labeled with [^{3}H] uridine were isolated from virions by treatment with NP40 at 4°C, mixed and incubated at 4°C or 37°C for 30 min. The sedimentation profile obtained after components were mixed at 4°C is shown in Figure 7A and after incubation together at 37°C in Figure 7B.

Further experiments (Sturman et al., 1980) showed that the conformation of NP40-solubilized E1 was altered as the temperature was raised from 4°C to 37°C. At 37°C E1 bound to the RNA in the viral nucleocapsid.

A MODEL OF E1

These studies have led to a provisional model for E1 which is shown in Figure 8. This membrane glycoprotein appears to possess three domains: a small glycosylated hydrophilic region which projects outside the viral envelope, a hydrophobic portion within the membrane, and a third domain which may be associated with the viral RNA in the nucleocapsid inside the viral envelope. Because of the effects of β-MSH and DTT on E1 aggregation, disulfide bonds are placed within the hydrophobic region of the molecule.

DIFFERENCES IN CARBOHYDRATE SIDE CHAINS ON E1 and E2

There are significant differences in the carbohydrate side chains on E1 and E2. E1 and E2 glycopeptides have been analyzed by polyacrylamide gel electrophoresis after borate-ester formation using the method described by Weitzman et al. (1979). Borate ions react with neutral sugars converting them to charged species. The number of borate ions bound to a glycopeptide is a function of the composition, sequence and linkages of the carbohydrates. The electrophoretic patterns of pronase derived glycopeptides from E1 and E2 obtained on tris-borate gels are shown in Figure 9. Borate-glycopeptide complexes of E2 shown in Figure 9A produce a complex pattern of multiple peaks in the upper and middle regions of the gel. At least six components can be resolved by double labeling. The pattern obtained from E1 glycopeptides shown in Figure 9B is quite different. E1 borate-glycopeptide complexes exhibit less variety and are found in the lower third of the gel.

It was mentioned previously that synthesis of E2 is sensitive to tunicamycin. Nevertheless, in the presence of tunicamycin, A59 virus particles are still produced, although reduced in amount. These particles do not possess spikes, but they appear to contain the usual proportions of nucleocapsid and E1. SDS-polyacrylamide gel analysis of such virus is shown in Figure 10. Figure 10A is the profile of control virus labeled with [^{3}H]

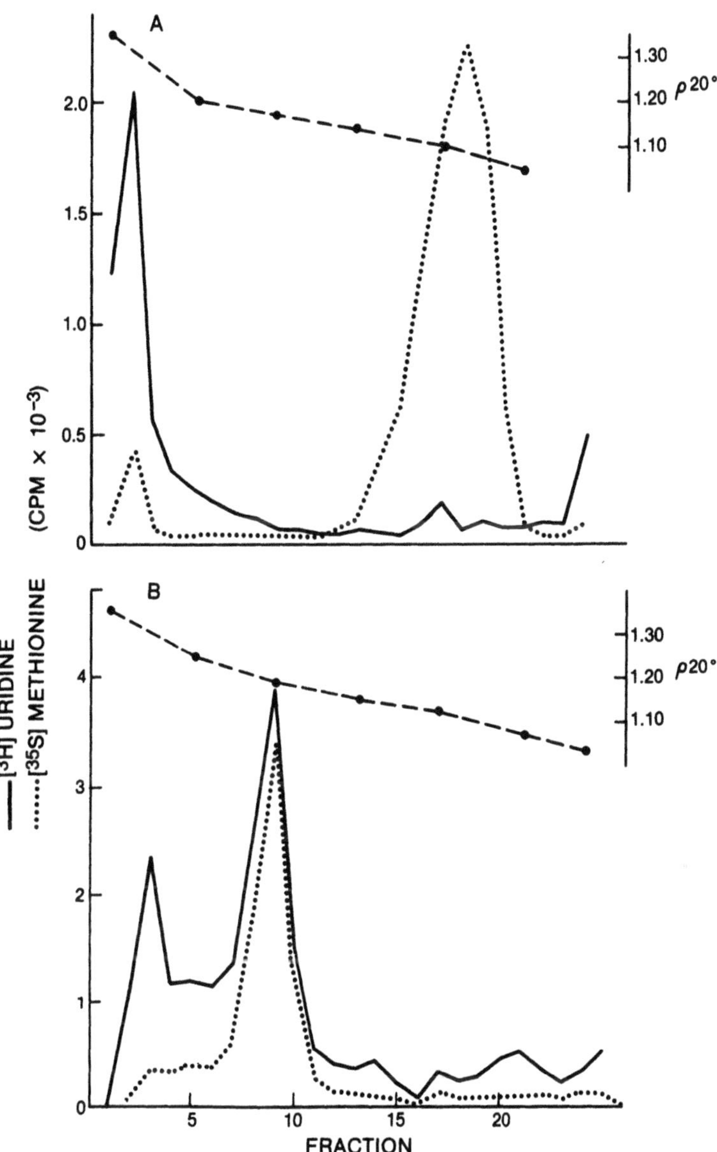

Fig. 7. Temperature-dependent association of isolated E1 and nucleocapsid. [^{35}S] methionine-labeled E1 and [^{3}H] uridine-labeled nucleocapsid were isolated at 4°C, mixed, incubated at (A) 4°C or (B) 37°C for 30 min, and then sedimented into 15 to 50% sucrose gradients (Sturman et al., 1980)

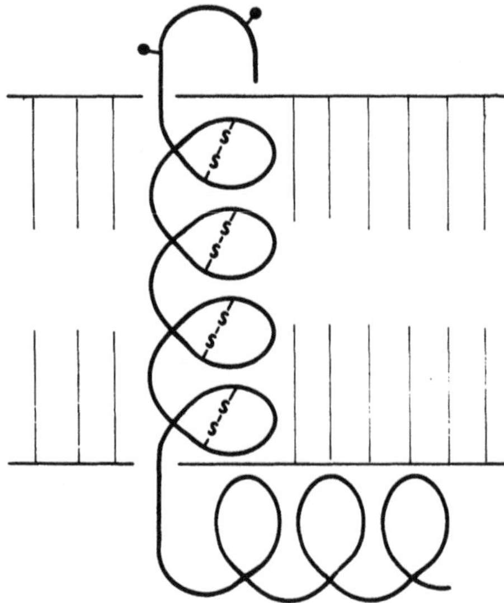

Fig. 8. A model of the membrane glycoprotein, E1.

glucosamine and [^{35}S] methionine. All three structural proteins can be seen: E1, N and E2. Figure 10B is the profile of virions similarly labeled, grown in the presence of 1 μg/ml tunicamycin. There is no E2. E1 and N are found in the same relative proportions as in the control virus. Glycosylation of E1 is not sensitive to tunicamycin. E1 is labeled to the same degree with glucosamine as in the control and has the same apparent molecular weight. The peplomeric glycoprotein, E2, thus appears not to be required for virus maturation. Envelopment of the nucleocapsid may be determined solely by interaction of viral RNA with the reactive domain of the membrane glycoprotein, E1.

Studies by Neimann and Klenk (personal communication) which will be described later at this meeting show that the carbohydrate composition of E1 is different from that of viral glycoproteins with N-glycosidically linked side chains. Their investigations suggest that the carbohydrate linkages in E1 are of O-glycosidic nature. This is consistent with the resistance of E1 glycosylation to tunicamycin.

It should be quite apparent from this report that we are just beginning to learn something about the coronavirus glycoproteins. We need to find out a great deal more about their structure, functional domains, and their dynamic interactions. Our future understanding of the molecular architecture of these viral glycoproteins will undoubtedly add to our comprehension of their roles in infection and disease.

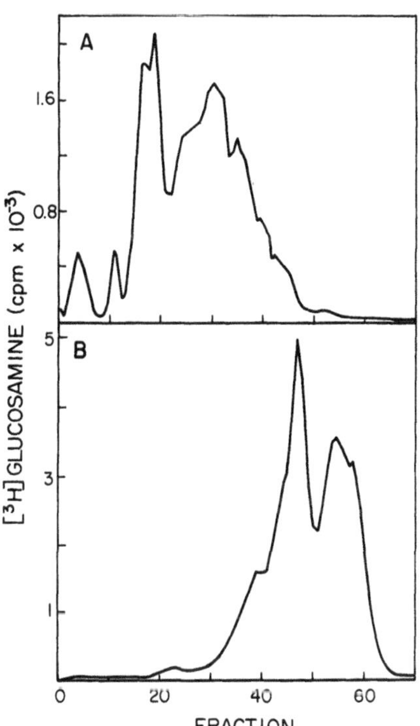

Fig. 9. Tris-borate gel electrophoresis of (A) E 2, (B) E 1 glycopeptides.

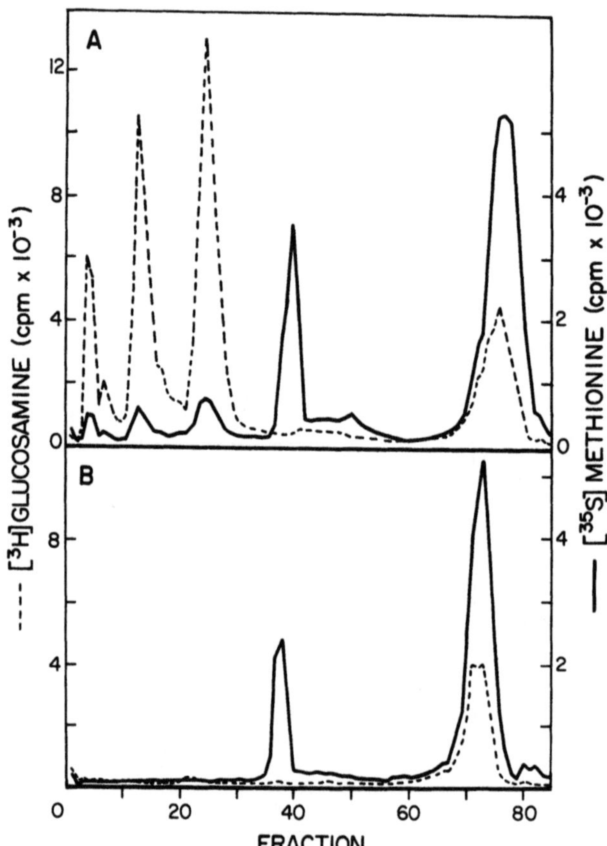

Fig. 10. SDS-polyacrylamide gel electrophoresis profiles of [^{3}H] glucosamine labeled, and [^{35}S] methionine-labeled structural proteins of coronavirus A59. (A) control virus; (B) virus grown in the presence of 1.0 µg/ml tunicamycin.

References

Alexander, D.J., and Collins, M.S., 1975, Effect of pH on the Growth and Cytopathogenicity of Avian Infectious Bronchitis Virus in Chick Kidney Cells, Arch. Virol., 49:339.

Johnson, W.C., and Lindsey, A.J., 1939, An Improved Universal Buffer, Analyst, 64:490.

Pocock, D.H., and Garwes, D.J., 1975, The Influence of pH on the Growth and Stability of Transmissible Gastroenteritis Virus in vitro, Arch. Virol., 49:239.

Sturman, L.S., 1977, Characterization of a Coronavirus I. Structural Proteins: Effects of Preparative Conditions on the Migration of Protein in Polyacrylamide Gels, Virology, 77:637.

Sturman, L.S., and Holmes, K.V., 1977, Characterization of a Coronavirus II. Glycoproteins of the Viral Envelope: Tryptic Peptide Analysis, Virology, 77:650.

Sturman, L.S., Holmes, K.V., and Behnke, J., 1980, Isolation of Coronavirus Envelope Glycoproteins and Interaction with the Viral Nucleocapsid, J. Virol., 33:449.

Weitzman, S., Scott, V., and Keegstra, K., 1979, Analysis of Glycopeptides as Borate Complexes by Polyacrylamide Gel Electrophoresis, Anal. Biochem., 97:438.

STRUCTURAL AND ANTIGENIC RELATIONSHIPS BETWEEN HUMAN, MURINE AND AVIAN CORONAVIRUSES

Malcolm R. Macnaughton

Division of Communicable Diseases
Clinical Research Centre
Harrow, Middlesex HA1 3UJ, UK

INTRODUCTION

There have been numerous reports in the literature describing the morphological and molecular structure of individual coronaviruses and comparing the structure of different strains of the same coronavirus species. However, there have been few attempts to compare the structure of different coronavirus species in the same laboratory. Some work has been done on the antigenic comparison of different coronaviruses, notably by Pederson et al. (17), but there is still considerable dispute about their antigenic relationships. This report is concerned with characterising the structural and antigenic relationships of a number of coronaviruses including various strains of human coronavirus (HCV), mouse hepatitis virus (MHV) and avian infectious bronchitis virus (IBV).

MORPHOLOGY

A previous study (4) has shown that these coronaviruses have similar morphologies. All the coronaviruses were pleomorphic, with a wide range in envelope diameters, although the three IBV strains examined, Massachusetts (Mass), Beaudette (Beau) and Connecticut (Conn) were significantly larger than MHV 3 and HCV 229E (Fig 1). Furthermore, two main types of surface projection were seen, both of about 20 nm in length. One type consisted of typical bulbous coronavirus projections and was seen on most IBV, MHV 3 and HCV 229E particles (Fig 1a). The other type of projection was in the form of a narrow cone and was seen mainly on MHV 3 particles (Fig 1b). We have previously suggested that both

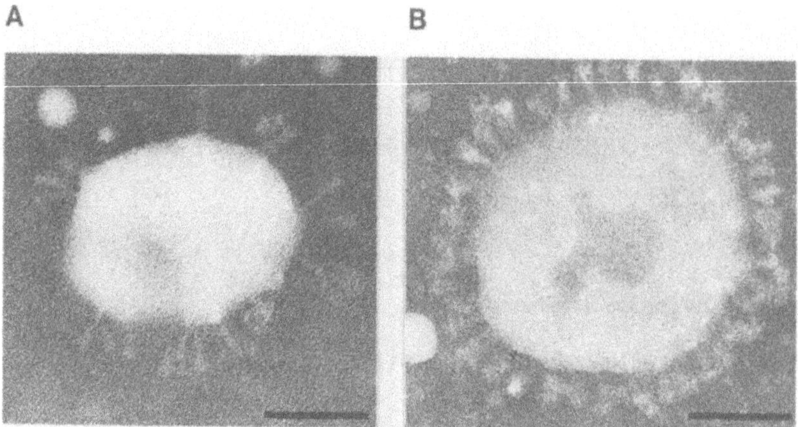

Fig. 1. Purified coronavirus particles negatively stained with 2% potassium phosphotungstate, pH 6.5. a) MHV 3, b) IBV Conn. The bar represents 50 nm.

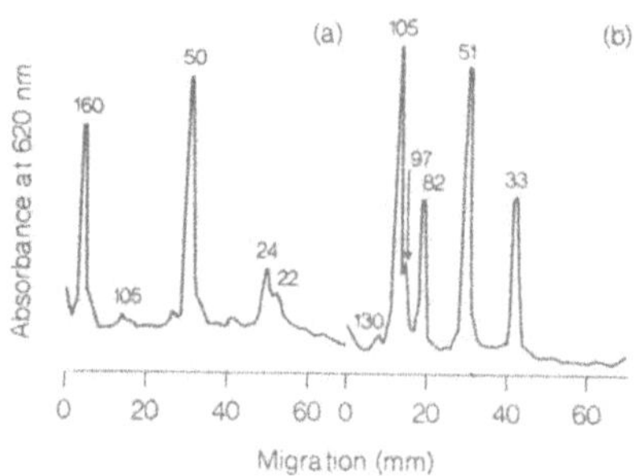

Fig. 2. Densitometer tracings of purified virus polypeptides on 7.5% polyacrylamide gels after staining with Coomassie brilliant blue. a) HCV 229E, b) IBV Conn. The numbers on the graphs represent the mol. wt. x 10^{-3}, and are referred to in the text as VP (virus polypeptide) and VGP (virus glycopolypeptide) followed by the appropriate mol. wt. x 10^{-3}.

projection types are manifestations of the same structures and that the bulbous projections are aggregates of thin cone shaped projections (4).

RNA AND RIBONUCLEOPROTEIN

It is generally accepted that the nucleic acid of coronaviruses consists of a large single stranded RNA molecule of positive polarity. Furthermore, we have shown that the genomes of IBV Beau, MHV 3 and HCV 229E all exist as similar single-stranded RNAs of mol. wt. about 5.8×10^6 with similar lengths of 3'-terminal poly(A) sequences (9).

We have shown that the ribonucleoproteins (RNP) of HCV 229E and MHV 3 can be readily visualised as helical structures by negative staining (12), although no IBV helices could be observed under similar circumstances. However, we have recently observed IBV RNP molecules by shadowing that were generally linear showing only a little helical structure (3). Thus, it appears that the stability of IBV RNP is different from that of HCV 229E and MHV 3, even though they have similar genomes and RNP polypeptides (see below).

PROTEIN COMPOSITION

The polypeptide composition of coronavirus particles is confusing, although most reports now tend to show a relatively simple polypeptide structure which may be common to many coronaviruses. Fig 2a shows a typical polypeptide profile of HCV 229E consisting of four major structural polypeptides. Similar structural polypeptides have been identified for three other HCV strains, HCV PR, HCV TO and HCV OC43, and MHV 3. Fig 2b shows the structural polypeptides of IBV, which are different from those of HCV or MHV. However, two recent reports (1,7) have shown IBV polypeptides more similar to those shown in Fig 2a, although other recent reports show more complex polypeptide patterns (2,16). The reported differences in the polypeptide composition of IBV may be due to contamination with host polypeptides (2) and/or be due to the aggregation of certain of the glycopolypeptides (10).

The position of the structural polypeptides in the virus particles has been studied, and those of HCV 229E (Fig 2a) are described as a typical example. The large mol. wt. glycopolypeptides, VGP 160 and VGP 105 (not resolved in Fig 2a), form the surface projections. This has been shown by digestion of the virus particles with bromelain or other proteolytic enzymes, or by treatment with dithiothreitol or nonidet P40 (10). In all cases VGP 160, and probably VGP 105, were removed from the virus particles along with the surface projections. RNP has been isolated on sucrose density gradients from nonidet P40 treated virus particles and shown to consist of VP 50 and RNA. We have also suggested, by exclusion, that VGP 24 and VP 22 comprise the envelope polypeptides (10). Similar results were obtained with other HCV strains and MHV 3.

The polypeptide composition of the subcomponents of IBV has also been determined, and results broadly similar to those of HCV 229E have been obtained. Large mol. wt. polypeptides form the surface projections, VP 51 corresponding to VP 50 of HCV 229E comprises the RNP, and the small mol. wt. glycopolypeptide VP 33 forms the membrane polypeptide (3,11,13).

ANTIGENIC RELATIONSHIPS

Previous studies on the antigenic relationships of coronaviruses, using a variety of techniques, have produced a confusing pattern of interrelationships (14,19). A recent comprehensive study by Pederson et al (17) has shown that mammalian coronaviruses can be grouped into at least two main antigenic groups by fluorescent antibody studies. Many of these interrelationships have been confirmed and extended by other workers (summarised in 14, 17, 19). The viruses in these two antigenic groups are shown in Table 1. It is interesting to observe that this grouping of viruses cuts through virus groups by the species affected. IBV, the only avian coronavirus to be extensively studied, has been shown to be antigenically unrelated to the mammalian coronaviruses (14,19), and thus apparently forms a separate antigenic group.

The antigenic relationships between coronavirus species and strains within these species have been studied by enzyme-linked immunosorbent assay (ELISA). ELISA has been shown to be highly sensitive and to detect a broad range of antigenic specificity. The ELISA technique used has been described previously (5) using sucrose gradient purified antigens and immune sera to these antigens raised in rabbits (5). Detailed ELISA results for the IBV strains are shown below as examples, while results obtained for the HCV strains and MHV 3 are summarised for convenience.

Table 2 shows that the ELISA reaction is extremely sensitive for IBV Mass, detecting antibody at dilutions of rabbit anti-IBV Mass of 1:102400. Reactions were considered positive for ratios of immune to pre-immune sera absorbance values of 2 or more at the same dilution (5). Similar results were obtained for IBV Beau and IBV Conn against anti-IBV Beau and Conn, respectively. Table 3 shows that no antigenic differences could be detected by ELISA between IBV Mass, Beau and Conn, even though IBV Mass and Beau are not related to IBV Conn by neutralisation and apparently have different glycopolypeptides (2,16) from IBV Conn. Thus the ELISA is

Table 1 Antigenic relationships of selected mammalian coronaviruses[a]

Group 1	Group 2
HCV OC43	HCV 229E
MHV	TGEV
CDCV	FIPV
HEV	CCV
RCV	
SDAV	

[a] Adapted from Pederson et al (17) and incorporating other results summarised by Pederson et al. (17), McIntosh (14) and Tyrrell et al. (19). CDCV, calf diarrheal coronavirus; HEV, haemagglutinating encephalomyelitis virus of swine; RCV, rat coronavirus; SDAV, sialodacryoadenitis virus of rats; TGEV, transmissible gastroenteritis virus of swine; FIPV, feline infectious peritonitis virus; CCV, canine coronavirus.

Table 2 ELISA of IBV Mass against anti-IBV Mass[a]

Serum	Anti-IBV Mass	
Dilution	Pre-immune	Immune
1 : 1600	0.04	0.69
1 : 6400	0.03	0.34
1 : 25600	0.03	0.17
1 : 102400	0.02	0.06
1 : 409600	0.02	0.03

[a] Data are given as absorbance values at 405 nm after 30 minutes. IBV Mass dilution 1 : 400.

Table 3 ELISA of IBV strains Mass, Beau and Conn against anti-IBV Mass, anti-IBV Beau and anti-IBV Conn[a]

IBV strain[b]	Anti-IBV Mass[c]		Anti-IBV Beau[c]		Anti-IBV Conn[c]	
	Pre-immune	Immune	Pre-immune	Immune	Pre-immune	Immune
Mass	0.02	0.79	0.04	0.70	0.03	0.69
Beau	0.02	0.70	0.03	0.71	0.02	0.64
Conn	0.01	0.67	0.02	0.61	0.01	0.52

[a] Data are given as absorbance values at 405 nm after 30 minutes

[b] IBV dilutions 1:400

[c] Anti-IBV dilutions 1:400

highly sensitive and detects no antigenic differences between distinct IBV strains.

Other studies have used sucrose gradient purified MHV 3 and several HCV strains in order to determine their antigenic relatedness by ELISA. Eight HCV isolates were obtained by Dr H.E. Larson at the Clinical Research Centre, Harrow and Dr S.E. Reed and Dr A.D. Macleod at the Common Cold Unit, Salisbury, from volunteers with colds (8, and unpublished data). Three of these isolates, KI, PR and TO, were readily adapted to growth in tissue culture, while the other isolates, AD, HO, GI, PA and RO, could only be grown in human foetal trachea and nasal mucosa organ cultures (8). Only the tissue culture adapted isolates were extensively analysed as only relatively small quantities of the organ culture adapted isolates were available. The morphology and polypeptide structures of PR and TO were shown to be the same as the prototype 229E and OC43 viruses, although PR and TO were shown to be distinct strains by neutralisation (Dr S.E. Reed, unpublished results).

The new isolates were compared with each other and strains 229E and OC43 using immune sera to these viruses prepared from rabbits, and sera from volunteers experimentally infected with HCVs. The HCV strains fell into at least two distinct antigenic groups, the HCV 229E group comprising strains 229E, KI, PR, TO and HCV OC43 (6). The other strains AD, HO, GI, PA and RO have not been completely characterised yet. However, preliminary results show that the strains are related to either the HCV 229E group viruses or HCV OC43. Experiments are in progress to resolve this problem and to identify any common HCV antigenic components. Finally, it is perhaps worth emphasising that the HCV 229E group viruses all readily grew in tissue culture; while HCV OC43 and HCV strains AD, HO, GI, PA and RO, were not readily adaptable to tissue culture, although recent reports have shown that HCV OC43 can be tissue culture adapted (15,18).

No antigenic relationship was observed between HCV 229E group viruses and MHV 3 by ELISA (5), although care had to be taken to remove contaminating serum components that can lead to spurious reactions. On the other hand, antigenic reactions were observed between HCV OC43, grown in suckling mouse brain (obtained from Dr S.E. Reed), and MHV 3 grown in mouse embryonic fibroblasts (12) using immune antisera obtained from rabbits. However, no such recctions have so far been obtained using AD, HO, GI, PA and RO strains grown in human organ culture against MHV 3 antisera from rabbits, or MHV 3 against human sera from volunteers inoculated with these HCVs. These results suggest that MHV 3 and HCV strains AD, HO, GI, PA and RO belong to different antigenic groups. However, the common antigenic components between HCV OC43 and MHV 3 (also described in 14, 17, 19) may be due to mouse antigens, as

Table 4 Antigenic groups of selected coronaviruses by ELISA

Group 1	IBV strains Mass, Beau and Conn
Group 2	HCV strains 229E, PR, KI, and TO
Group 3	HCV strain OC43 and MHV strain 3

The classification of HCV strains AD, HO, GI, PA and RO is unclear at present.

these studies all used HCV OC43 grown in suckling mouse brain. Thus, the coronaviruses studied can be grouped into at least three main antigenic groups by ELISA (Table 4), with the HCV strains AD, HO, GI, PA and RO probably being related to the HCV 229E group or HCV OC43.

CONCLUSIONS

There appear to be at least two main coronavirus groups. One group contains the IBV strains, which show significant morphological, structural and antigenic differences from the mammalian coronaviruses. Mammalian coronaviruses form the other main group, and these viruses are morphologically and structurally similar to one another, although they do seem to fall into different antigenic groups by ELISA. The HCV strains fall into at least two antigenic groups, the HCV 229E group and HCV OC43, with HCV OC43 being antigenically related to MHV 3. The classification of HCV strains AD, HO, GI, PA and RO is unclear at present.

ACKNOWLEDGEMENTS

Thanks are due to Miss M.H. Madge for technical assistance, Mrs H.A. Davies for electron microscopy, Dr C.A. Kraaijeveld for help with ELISA, Dr H.E. Larson and Dr S.E. Reed for HCV isolates and volunteer paired sera, and Dr S.E. Reed for HCV OC43 grown in suckling mouse brain. Dr C.A. Kraaijeveld, Dr S.E. Reed and Dr D.A.J. Tyrrell provided useful discussions during the course of this work.

REFERENCES

1. D. Cavanagh, Personal communication (1980)
2. M.S. Collins and D.J. Alexander, Avian infectious bronchitis virus structural polypeptides: effect of different conditions of disruption and comparison of different strains and isolates, Arch. Virol. 63: 239 (1980)
3. H.A. Davies, R.R. Dourmashkin and M.R. Macnaughton, Ribonucleoprotein of avian infectious bronchitis virus, J. gen. Virol. In press. (1981)
4. H.A. Davies and M.R. Macnaughton, Comparison of the morphology of three coronaviruses, Arch. Virol. 59: 25 (1979)
5. C.A. Kraaijeveld, M.H. Madge and M.R. Macnaughton, Enzyme-linked immunosorbent assay for coronaviruses HCV 229E and MHV 3, J. gen. Virol. 49: 83 (1980)
6. C.A. Kraaijeveld, S.E. Reed and M.R. Macnaughton, Enzyme-linked immunosorbent assay for detection of antibody in volunteers experimentally infected with human coronavirus 229E group viruses, J. clin. Microbiol. In press.
7. J.A. Lanser and C.R. Howard, The polypeptides of infectious bronchitis virus (IBV-41 strain), J. gen. Virol. 46: 349 (1980)
8. H.E. Larson, S.E. Reed and D.A.J. Tyrrell, Isolation of rhinoviruses and coronaviruses from 38 colds in adults, J. med. Virol. 5: 221 (1980)
9. M.R. Macnaughton, The genomes of three coronaviruses, FEBS Letts 94: 191 (1978)
10. M.R. Macnaughton, The polypeptides of human and mouse coronaviruses, Arch. Virol. 63: 75 (1980)
11. M.R. Macnaughton and H.A. Davies, Two particle types of avian infectious bronchitis virus, J. gen. Virol. 47: 365 (1980)
12. M.R. Macnaughton, H.A. Davies and M.V. Nermut, Ribonucleoprotein-like structures from coronavirus particles, J. gen. Virol. 39: 545 (1978)
13. M.R. Macnaughton, M.H. Madge, H.A. Davies and R.R. Dourmashkin, Polypeptides of the surface projections and the ribonucleoprotein of avian infectious bronchitis virus, J. Virol. 24: 821 (1977)
14. K. McIntosh, Coronaviruses: a comparative review, Curr. Tops. Microb. Immunol. 63: 85 (1974)
15. A.S. Monto and L.M. Rhodes, Detection of coronavirus infection of man by immunofluorescence, Proc. Soc. exp. Biol. Med. 155: 143 (1977)
16. E. Nagy and B. Lomniczi, Polypeptide patterns of infectious bronchitis virus serotypes fall into two categories, Arch. Virol. 61: 341 (1979)
17. N.C. Pederson, J. Ward and W.L. Mengeling, Antigenic relationship of the feline infectious peritonitis virus to coronaviruses of other species, Arch. Virol. 58: 45 (1978)

18. O.W. Schmidt, M.K. Cooney and G.E. Kenny, Plaque assay and improved yield of human coronaviruses in a human rhabdomyosarcoma cell line, J. clin. Microbiol. 9: 722 (1979)
19. D.A.J. Tyrrell, D.J. Alexander, J.D. Almeida, C.H. Cunningham, B.C. Easterday, D.J. Garwes, J.C. Hierholzer, A. Kapikian, M.R. Macnaughton and K. McIntosh, Coronaviridae: second report, Intervirology, 10: 321 (1978)

ANTIGENIC RELATIONSHIPS OF CORONAVIRUSES DETECTABLE BY PLAOUE NEUTRALIZATION, COMPETITIVE ENZYME LINKED IMMUNOABSORBENT ASSAY, AND IMMUNOPRECIPITATION

J.C. Gerdes, L.D. Jankovsky, B.L. DeVald, I. Klein
and J.S. Burks

Department of Microbiology and Immunology
Rocky Mountain Multiple Sclerosis Center
University of Colorado Health Sciences Center
4200 East Ninth Avenue
Denver, CO 80262, U.S.A.

ABSTRACT

The antigenic relationships of mouse coronaviruses JHM and A59, human viruses OC43 and 229E, and multiple sclerosis (MS) isolates SD and SK have been investigated by plaque neutralization, competitive enzyme linked immunoabsorbent assay, and immunoprecipitation.

A59, SK, or SD plaques are neutralized by antiserum prepared against homologous as well as heterologous virus. Plaque neutralization also demonstrated weak reactivity between SD or SK and mouse virus JHM but no reactivity with human coronavirus 229E. An antiserum prepared against human virus OC43 neutralized viruses SD and SK but not mouse viruses A59 or JHM.

In a competitive enzyme linked immunoabsorbent assay (cELISA) the binding of antiserum prepared against MS isolate SK to bound SK antigen was inhibited to a comparable degree using OC43, SD, or A59 viral antigens. Coronavirus 229E or uninfected cell antigens did not block the binding of anti-SK serum to bound antigen. However, a cELISA utilizing OC43 as bound antigen and competing an anti-OC43 serum suggests that virus OC43 may be more closely related to SK than A59.

Specific viral polypeptides that share antigenic determinants have been identified by immunoprecipitation of S^{35} methionine labeled viral infected cell extracts. Polypeptides of similar molecular weight were precipitated from A59, SD, or SK infected cell extracts by SD, SK, OC43, or A59 antisera. Our data suggests that the mouse coronavirus A59, human coronavirus OC43, and MS isolates SD and SK contain antigenically related polypeptides of similar molecular weight.

INTRODUCTION

We recently reported the isolation of two coronaviruses from fresh, unfrozen multiple sclerosis (MS) autopsy material (3). One of these viruses (SD) was detected following the intracerebral (IC) inoculation of weanling BALB/c mice. The second isolate (SK) was evident on the twelfth subculture of mouse 3T3 (17Cl-1) cells inoculated with homogenized MS tissue. Chronic or latent infections by murine coronaviruses are frequently encountered in mouse breeding colonies (4,7,18). Therefore, careful evaluation of the human or murine origin of these MS isolates is necessary. In an attempt to identify species specific antigenic markers, we have compared the antigenic properties of human coronaviruses 229E and OC43 and murine coronaviruses JHM and A59 with MS isolates SK and SD. The viruses are compared by plaque neutralization, competitive enzyme linked immunoabsorbent assay (cELISA), and by immunoprecipitation utilizing homologous and heterologous antisera.

MATERIALS AND METHODS

Cells and virus. The source of known human and mouse coronaviruses has been previously described (5). Coronaviruses SD and SK are viruses isolated from multiple sclerosis patients as previously described (3). Mouse viruses, A59 and JHM, and MS isolates, SD and SK, were grown in 17Cl-1 cells and purified from supernatant fluids by polyethylene glycol (PEG) precipitation and sucrose density gradients (14,19). Human virus 229E was grown in WI38 cells. Human virus OC43 was grown in suckling mouse brain utilizing C57 black mice (15). Virus concentrations of OC43 was estimated by hemagglutination of chicken erythrocytes (11).

Antiserum. Antiserum directed against coronaviruses A59, SK, and SD were produced utilizing sucrose gradient purified virus injected into rabbits, guinea pigs, and mice according to protocol previously described (5). Antiserum to human coronaviruses are reference antisera obtained from the Center for Disease Control and kindly supplied by Dr. Harold Kaye. Antisera directed against OC43 virus was titered by hemagglutination inhibition (9).

Plaque neutralization. Coronaviruses SD, SK, A59, and JHM produced plaques on confluent monolayers of DBT cells (8) grown in 60 mm petri dishes. Details of the method will be published elsewhere (5). Human virus 229E was plaque assayed on confluent monolayers of WI38 cells utilizing a similar technique. All antisera used in plaque neutralization studies were heat inactivated at 56°C for 30 minutes. Plaque neutralizations for the various antisera were determined by a comparison of the degree of neutralization of the test antisera compared to control plaque numbers. Control neutralizations utilized fetal calf serum or preimmune serum diluted to a comparable level to that of the test antiserum dilution.

cELISA. The ELISA technique utilized alkaline phosphatase conjugated anti-IgG of the appropriate species according to the methods described by Voller (20). Purified viral antigen was bound to Cooke M29AR (Dynatech Laboratories) microELISA plates overnight at 4°C in a humid chamber. After antigen binding, the plates were washed with phosphate buffered saline pH 7.2 (PBS) containing 0.5% TWEEN-20 for 10 min., then rinsed twice with distilled H_2O to prevent nonspecific binding. Viral antigens utilized as competitors were solubilized in a buffer containing 0.02 M Tris pH 7.4, 0.05 M sodium chloride, 0.5% deoxycholic acid (DOC), and 0.5% NP-40 (lysis buffer). Serial two-fold dilutions of competing antigen were incubated overnight at 4°C with a constant amount of antibody. Absorbed antisera was then reacted for 60 minutes at 37°C with antigen bound to the microELISA plate, washed, and reacted with conjugated anti-IgG and substrate. The colorimetric reaction was read utilizing a Titertek multiskan microELISA reader (Flow Labs).

The competing antigens for viruses SK and A59 were purified by sucrose density gradients prior to disruption with NP40 lysis buffer. Virus OC43 was partially purified from infected suckling mouse brain (20% homogenates) by adsorption and elution from human "O" erythrocytes according to the methods of Kaye et al (10). Control competitors included supernatants or cytoplasmic extracts of uninfected cells.

Immunoprecipitation. A detailed description of procedures for infected cell radiolabeling and immunoprecipitation will be published elsewhere (5). Briefly, uninfected or virus infected monolayers (multiplicity of infection 0.1-1.0 pfu/cell) of 17Cl-1 cells were radiolabeled with S^{35} methionine in the presence of 1 ug/ml of actinomycin D. Sixteen to twenty hours post-infection, cytoplasmic extracts were prepared utilizing the lysis buffer described above and nuclei were removed by centrifugation. Immunoprecipitation of viral specific peptides from these cytoplasmic extracts utilized formalin fixed and washed staphylococcus aureus, Cowan I strain, as described by Kessler (12). Precipitated antigen-antibody-Staph A complexes are washed five times with 1% Tritom-X 100, 1% DOC, and 0.15 M sodium chloride pH 7. The final pellet is resuspended in 50 microliters of sodium dodecyl sulfate (SDS) sample buffer (2% SDS, 10% glycerol, 0.001% bronphenol blue, 62.5 millimolar Tris hydrochloride pH 6.8, 1.2 M Urea, 0.1% Beta mercaptoethanol. The proteins are solubilized at 37°C for 60 minutes and analyzed by SDS polyacrylamide gel electrophoresis (13). Polyacrylamide gels consisted of a 10-20% acrylamide gradient in Tris glycine cross-linked with N,N'-diallyl-tartardiamide (DATD) (6). Gels were impregnated with PPO (2,5-diphenyloxazole) utilizing the methods of Bonner and Laskey (1). Molecular weights were estimated relative to radiolabeled VSV markers (21).

RESULTS

Reciprocal plaque neutralizations. Neutralization of plaque formation using antisera prepared against different coronaviruses is shown in Table I. The degree of homology of the viruses can be measured by a comparison of neutralization values. These are defined as the highest serum dilution capable of 50% neutralization of 60–150 plaques. The results reveal that MS isolates SK and SD are antigenically related to A59 and more distantly to mouse virus JHM. Human coronavirus 229E appears to be distinct from the other viruses. However, antiserum prepared against OC43 neutralizes SD and SK but shows no neutralization at a 1:20 dilution of mouse viruses A59 or JHM. This result can be interpreted to indicate that MS isolates SD and SK are more closely related to the human virus OC43 than are the mouse viruses.

Hemagglutination and hemagglutination inhibition. The human coronavirus OC43 is known to hemagglutinate chicken and human "O" erythrocytes. We, therefore, investigated the ability of viruses SD and SK to hemagglutinate these cells. OC43 was the only virus capable of hemagglutinating erythrocytes. In addition, only antisera directed against OC43 inhibited this hemagglutination. Therefore, although viruses SK and SD are antigenically related to OC43, they differ from this virus in that they do not hemagglutinate erythrocytes and they replicate in mouse cell lines.

RECIPROCAL PLAQUE NEUTRALIZATIONS[1]

Antisera	Mouse		MS Isolates		Human
	JHM	A59	SK	SD	229E
Anti-SK	500	1,200	10,000	10,000	<20
Anti-SD	40	100	2,000	2,000	<20
Anti-OC43[2]	<20	<20	80	160	<20
Anti-229E	<20	<20	<20	<20	1,000
Anti-A59	40	500	320	320	<20

[1]Numbers given are the highest serum dilution causing greater than 50% neutralization of approximately 100 plaques

[2]Hemagglutination inhibition titer for this antiserum utilizing chicken erythrocytes was 1:640

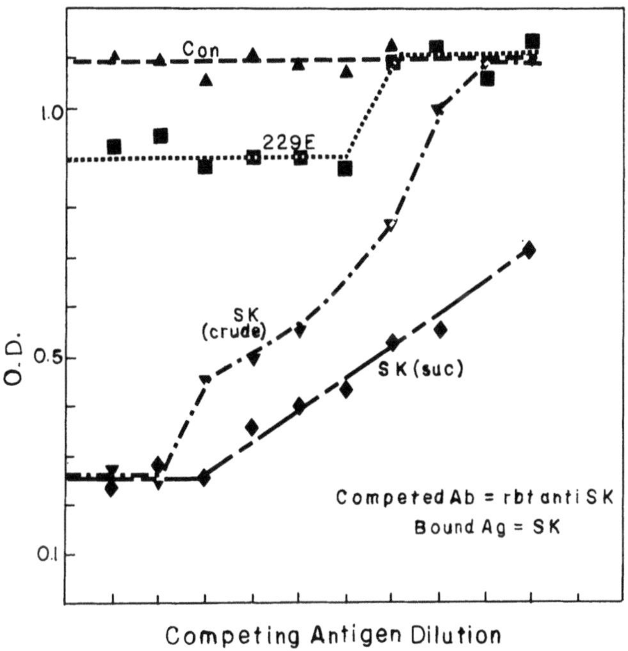

Figure 1: cELISA demonstrating absorption of rabbit antisera directed against coronavirus SK by NP40 extracts of homologous (SK) or heterologous (229E) viral antigen. Purified SK virus is the antigen bound to the microELISA plate. SK (crude) = virus obtained directly from infected 17Cl-1 cell supernatants used as competing antigens. SK (suc) = purified virus used as competing antigen. Con = uninfected cell supernatant as competing antigen.

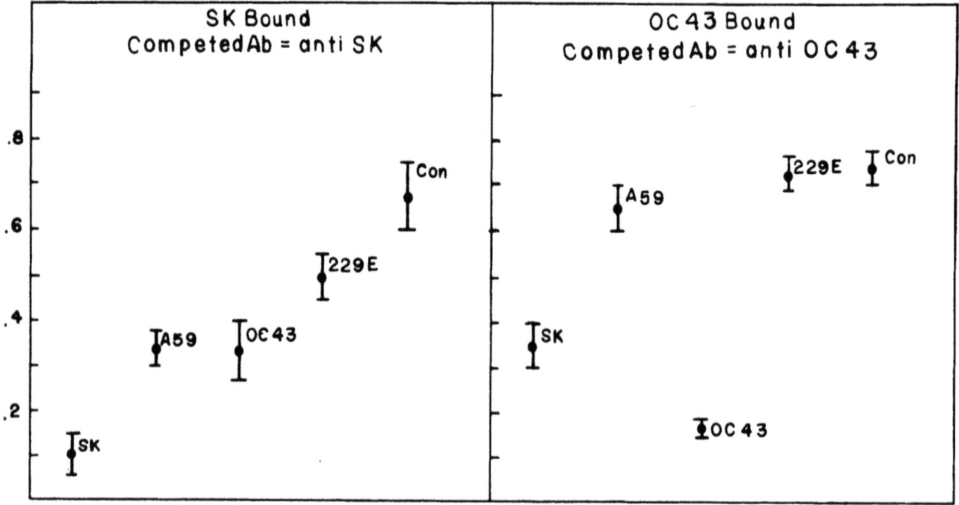

Figure 2: cELSIA using SK bound antigen (left) or OC43 bound antigen (right). Mean absorbance values ± one standard deviation are given for each competitive antigen at saturation.

Competitive enzyme linked immunoabsorbent assay (cELISA). This assay measures the relatedness of different viral antigens by their capacity to block the binding of specific antibody to viral antigen bound on the plastic surface of microELISA plates. For this assay purified viral antigen is bound to plastic using standard ELISA techniques (20). Serial dilutions of NP40 disrupted, competing viral antigens are incubated 10-24 hours at 4°C with a constant amount of antisera. This absorbed antisera is then reacted with the bound antigen. Utilizing homologous virus as the competing antigen results in a nearly complete inhibition of antibody binding to the antigen bound on the plastic (Figure 1). However, heterologous antigen inhibits binding to an extent proportional to the degree of homology. A representative experiment utilizing virus SK as the bound antigen and adsorbing rabbit anti-SK antiserum with the homologous (SK) antigen or heterologous (229E) antigen is shown in Figure 1. A linear relationship is observed for competing antigen concentrations capable of saturating the antibody. Extrapolation of this linear line results in a Y-intercept that is characteristic of the degree of homology. As is shown in Figure 1, this intercept is not altered by the degree of purity of the competing antigen. The heterologous antigen (229E) results in very little competition relative to that of the uninfected cell control.

In Figure 2, this method is used to determine the relationship between viruses SK, A59, OC43, and 229E. Figure 2A demonstrates that when SK is bound to plastic, both viruses A59 and OC43 compete at a comparable level for the antibody directed against SK while virus 229E does not compete. In Figure 2B, OC43 is bound to the microELISA plates and anti-OC43 serum is the competed antibody. The results of this experiment demonstrate that SK appears to be more closely related to the OC43 antigen than does A59. This observation confirms the results of the neutralization test (Table I) in which this antisera also recognized isolates SK or SD more readily than the mouse virus A59.

Immunoprecipitation of coronavirus SK or SD S^{35} methionine labeled cytoplasmic extracts. Viral specific polypeptides immunoprecipitated from SK-infected and SD-infected 3T3 cells are identical as is shown in Figure 3. The viral specific polypeptides are defined as those precipitated by immune serum from infected cells, but not detected in preimmune sera immunoprecipitations of infected cells or immune sera immunoprecipitation of uninfected cells. Molecular weight estimates relative to VSV markers indicate that coronavirus polypeptides have molecular weights of 180,000 (180K), 90,000 (90K), 50,000 (50K), 24,000 (24K), and 22,000 (22K). An additional polypeptide of 42,000 (42K) is observed in variable amounts in either SK or SD infections. Similar polypeptides are also observed in SK-infected cytoplasmic extracts that are immunoprecipitated with either anti-A59, SD, or OC43 sera (Figure 4). The inverse experiment (Figure 5) confirms that these same polypeptides are immunoprecipitated from A59 infection by

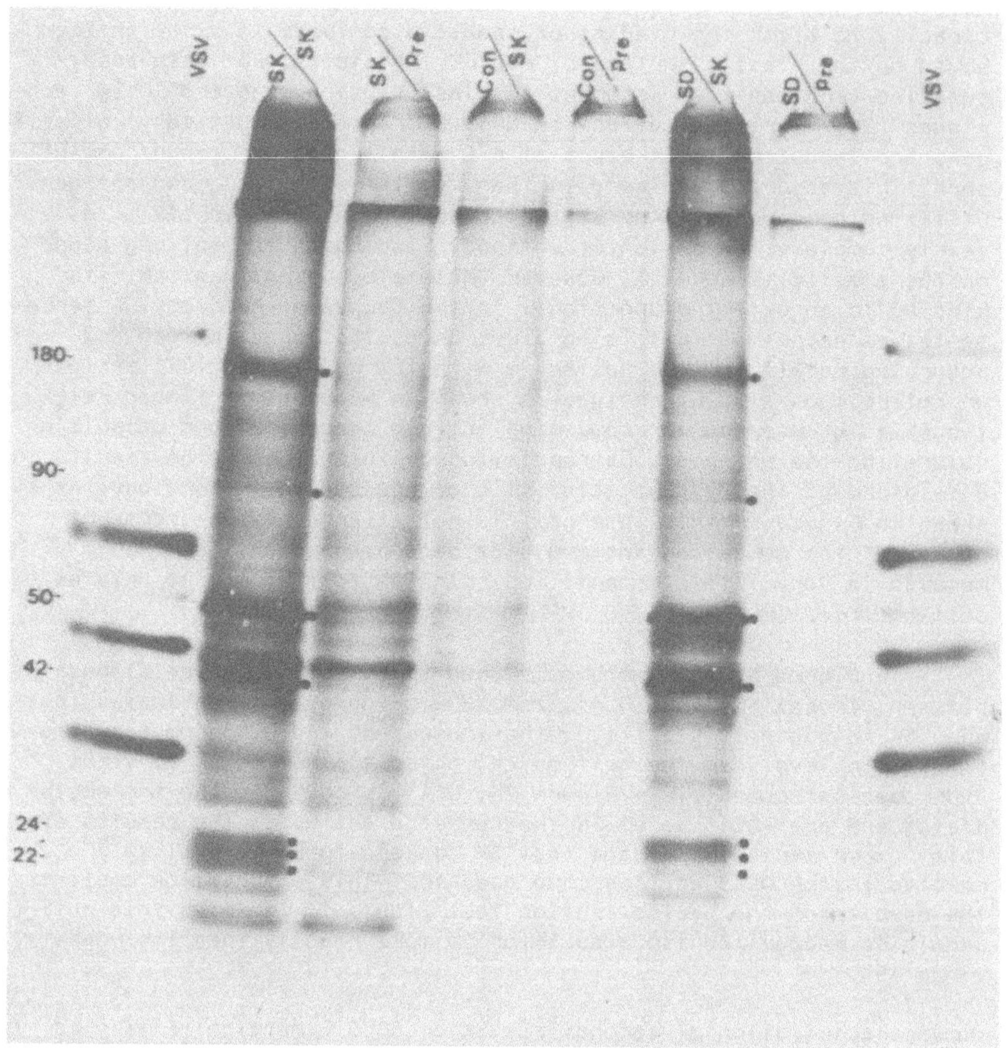

Figure 3: Polyacrylamide gel electrophoresis of S^{35} labeled polypeptides immunoprecipitated from SK or SD infected 17Cl-1 cytoplasmic extracts. Viral polypeptides are identified by black dots and estimated molecular weights given in kilodaltons. SK/SK = SK infected cell extract precipitated by anti-SK serum. SK/pre = SK infected cell extract precipitated with preimmune serum. Con/SK = uninfected cell extract precipitated with anti-SK serum. SD/pre = SD infected cell extract precipitated with preimmune serum. SD/SK = SD infected cell extract precipitated with anti-SK serum.

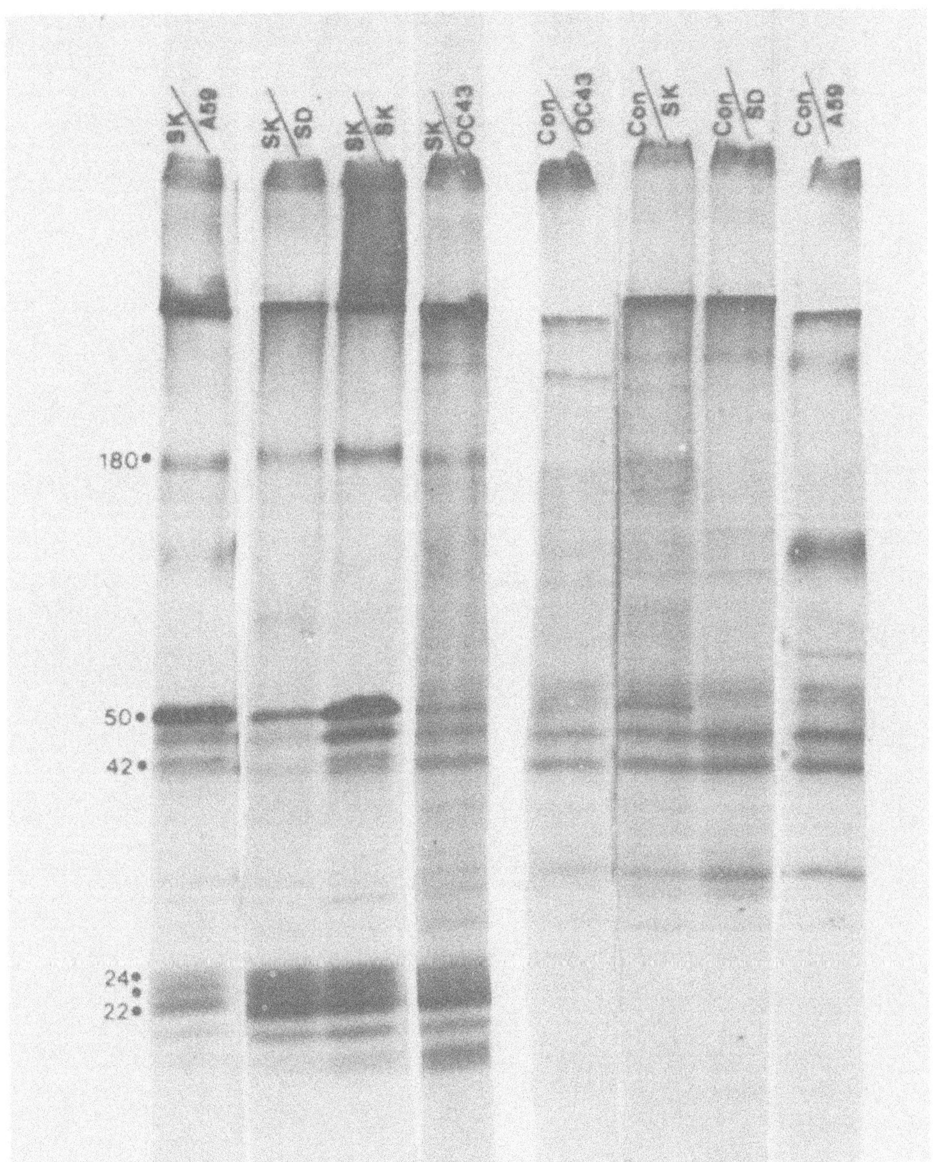

Figure 4: Polyacrylamide gel electrophoresis of S^{35} labeled polypeptides immunoprecipitated from SK infected 17Cl-1 cytoplasmic extracts utilizing homologous and heterologous antisera. SK/SK, SK/A59, SK/SD, SK/OC43 = polypeptides precipitated from SK infected cell extract by antisera directed against SK, A59, SD, and OC43. Con/SK, Con/A59, Con/SD, Con/OC43 = polypeptides precipitated from uninfected cell extract by antisera directed against SK, A59, SD, and OC43.

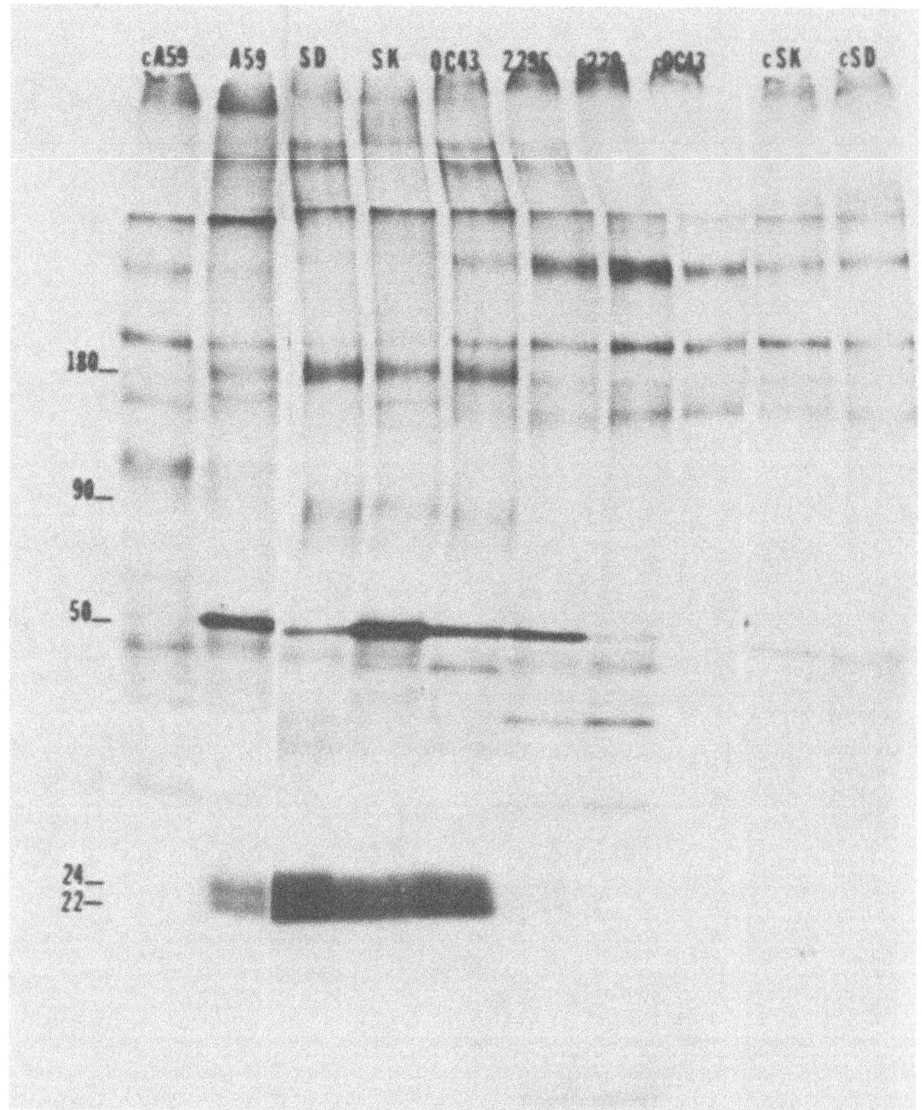

Figure 5: Polyacrylamide gel electrophoresis of S^{35} labeled polypeptides immunoprecipitated from A59 infected 17Cl-1 cytoplasmic extracts utilizing homologous and heterologous antisera. A59, SK, SD, OC43, 229E = polypeptides precipitated from A59 virus infected 3T3 cytoplasmic extract by antisera directed against A59, SK, SD, OC43, or 229E. cA59, cSK, cSD, cOC43 = polypeptides precipitated from uninfected 3T3 cytoplasmic extract by antisera directed against A59, SK, SD, 229E, or OC43.

antisera directed against A59, SD, SK, or OC43. Antiserum directed against human virus 229E recognizes only the 50K protein.

DISCUSSION

Antigenic cross-reactivity between human virus OC43 and various MHV strains has previously been reported by several investigators (2,7,16,17). For these studies cross-reactivity was demonstrated by fluorescent antibody, serum neutralization, or complement fixation tests. Our results suggest that coronaviruses SK and SD also belong in this antigenic group.

Utilizing cross-neutralization values and competitive enzyme linked immunoabsorbent assays, MS isolate SK is more closely related to human virus OC43 than is mouse virus A59. However, the more qualitative assay of immunoprecipitation suggests some degree of homology between OC43, A59, SD, and SK for all of the major component polypeptides. Since human and mouse coronaviruses share antigenic determinants, the identification of the species origin of unknown coronaviruses is not possible on the basis of antigenicity. In summary, we have shown that MS isolates SD and SK differ from human coronaviruses OC43 and 229E and mouse coronaviruses JHM and A59. However, coronaviruses A59, SD, SK, and OC43 all share antigenic determinants.

REFERENCES

1. Bonner, WM and Laskey, RA: A film detection method for tritium-labeled proteins and nucleic acids in polyacrylamide gels. Eur. J. Biochem. 46:83-88, 1974.

2. Bradburne, AF: Antigenic relationships amongst coronaviruses. Arch. ges Virusforsch. 31:352-364, 1970.

3. Burks, JS, DeVald, BL, Jankovsky, LD, and Gerdes, JC: Two coronaviruses isolated from central nervous system tissue of two multiple sclerosis patients. Science 209:933-934, 1980.

4. Cheever, FS and Mueller, JH: Epidemic diarrheal disease of suckling mice. I. Manifestations, epidemiology, and attempts to transmit the disease. Exp. Med. 85:405-416, 1947.

5. Gerdes, JC, Klein, I, DeVald, B., and Burks, JS: Multiple sclerosis virus isolates SK and SD are serologically related to murine coronaviruses A59 and JHM and human coronavirus OC43, but not to human coronavirus 229E. J. Virol. Submitted.

6. Heine, JW, Honess, RW, Cassai, E, and Roizman, B: The proteins specified by herpes simplex virus. XII. The virion polypeptides of type I strains. J. Virol. 14:640-651, 1974.

7. Hierholzer, JC, Broderson, JR, and Murphy, FA: New strain of mouse hepatitis virus as the cause of lethal enteritis in infant mice. Infect. Immun. 24:508–522, 1979.

8. Hirano, N, Fujiwara, K, Hino, S, and Matumoto, M: Replication and plaque formation of mouse hepatitis virus (MHV-2) in mouse cell line DBT culture. Arch. Gesamte Virusforsch 44:298–302, 1974.

9. Hierholzer, JC, Suggs, MT, and Hall, EC: Standardized viral hemagglutination and hemagglutination-inhibition tests. II. Description and statistical evaluation. Appl. Microbiol. 18:824–833, 1969.

10. Kaye, HS, Hierholzer, JC, and Dowdle, WR: Purification and further characterization of an "IBV-like" virus (coronavirus). Proc. Soc. Exp. Biol. Med. 135:457–463, 1970.

11. Kaye, HS and Dowdle, WR: Some characteristics of hemagglutination of certain strains of "IBV-like" virus. J. Infect. Dis. 120:576–581, 1969.

12. Kessler, SW: Rapid isolation of antigens from cells with staphylococcal protein A-antibody absorbent: parameters of the interaction of antigen-antibody complexes with protein A. J. Immunol. 115:1617–1624, 1975.

13. Laemmli, UK: Cleavage of structural proteins during the assembly of the head of bacteriophage T4. Nature (London) 227:680–685, 1970.

14. Lai, MMC and Stohlman, SA: RNA of mouse hepatitis virus. J. Virol. 26:236–242, 1978.

15. McIntosh, K, Becker, WB, and Chanock, RM: Growth in suckling mouse brain of "IBV-like" viruses from patients with upper respiratory tract disease. Proc. Natl. Acad. Sci. 58:2268–2273, 1967.

16. McIntosh, KA, Kapikian, AZ, Hardison, KA, Hartley, JW, and Chanock, RM: Antigenic relationships among the coronaviruses of man and between human and animal coronaviruses. J. Immunol. 102:1109–1118, 1969.

17. Pedersen, NC, Ward, J., and Mengeling, WL: Antigenic relationship of the Feline Infectious Peritonitis Virus to coronaviruses of other species. Arch. Virol. 58:45–53, 1978.

18. Rowe, WP, Hartley, JW, and Capps, WI: Mouse hepatitis virus infection as a highly contagious, prevalent, enteric infection of mice. Proc. Soc. Exp. Biol. Med. 112:161-165, 1963.

19. Sturman, LS, Holmes, KV, and Behnke, J: Isolation of coronavirus envelope glycoproteins and interaction with the viral nucleocapsid. J. Virol. 33:449-462, 1980.

20. Voller, A, Bidwell, D, and Bartlett, A: Microplate enzyme immunoassays for the immunodiagnosis of virus infections. In Manual of Clinical Immunology. N.R. Rose, H. Friedman, ed., ASM, pp. 506-512, 1976.

21. Wagner, RR, Prevec, L, Brown, F, Summers, DF, Sokol, F, and MacLeod, R: Classification of rhabdovirus proteins: a proposal. J. Virol. 10:1128-1230, 1972.

ACKNOWLEDGMENT

We thank Lyle Hileman, Irene Johnson, and Doubravka Kett for excellent technical assistance, and Karen Michelsen for typing the manuscript.

This research was supported by The Kroc Foundation and the Veterans Administration grant #1169-01.

THE RNA AND PROTEINS OF HUMAN CORONAVIRUSES

John C. Hierholzer, Maurice C. Kemp, and
Gregory A. Tannock*

Respiratory Virology Branch, Virology Division, Center
for Disease Control, Atlanta, Georgia, U.S.A. 30333; and
*G.A.T.: Division of Clinical Investigation, Faculty of
Medicine, University of Newcastle, New South Wales 2308,
Australia

Coronaviruses were classified as a distinct group of viruses in 1968[1] and are now recognized as the etiologic agents of an increasing number of diseases of man and animals[2-7]. At least four members of the group are human respiratory pathogens. Others have been suggested to be involved in neurologic and enteric disease processes in man, although none of these strains have yet been isolated in the true sense of the word.[8-18] Respiratory strain B814 was the first human coronavirus discovered, having been isolated in human embryonic tracheal organ culture by Tyrrell & Bynoe in 1960.[19] Strain 229E was recovered in secondary human fetal kidney cell cultures by Hamre & Procknow in 1962.[20] Strain OC-43 and many related strains were then found by organ culture techniques in 1966 by McIntosh et al.[21] Strain 692 was identified by immune electron microscopy in 1966 by Kapikian et al.[22]

None of these strains are readily adaptable to laboratory procedures. They replicate poorly if at all in conventional cell cultures; they tend to be highly labile under conditions of virus purification; and they do not produce soluble antigens which can be measured by routinely available serologic tests. For these reasons, detailed analyses of the protein and nucleic acid structure of the respiratory coronaviruses have not kept pace with similar studies on avian and mammalian coronaviruses.

Despite the difficulties, much has been learned about the structure of two of the human respiratory coronaviruses in the past 5 years. In this paper, we will review these data to bring the human coronaviruses into perspective with the biochemistry and biology of the other animal coronaviruses.

BIOLOGICAL ACTIVITY TESTS FOR STRAINS OC-43 AND 229E

The original strains OC-43 and 229E, as well as other isolates of these same "types," have been thoroughly checked for antigenic relatedness to animal coronaviruses by complement-fixation (CF) and immunodiffusion (ID) tests.[23,24] In addition to CF, human infections by both strains are readily detected by indirect fluorescent antibody (IFA) tests on shed respiratory cells and secretions[25] and on acute and convalescent serum specimens.[26] Antibody to both OC-43 and 229E can also be measured by single radial hemolysis (SRH) tests.[27,28]

Strain OC-43, adapted to suckling mouse brain and grown to high infectivity titer, was found to possess a hemagglutinin (HA) for human "O", vervet monkey, chicken, rat, and mouse cells.[29] This HA activity has been essential in virus purification studies as a readily quantifiable marker[30-32] and is useful in documenting human infection by hemagglutination-inhibition (HI) tests on patients' acute and convalescent serum specimens.[26-29,33,34] OC-43 has also been detected in cell cultures by hemadsorption (HAd) tests with rat or mouse cells.[34] A plaque-reduction neutralization test for OC-43 in MA-321 microcultures has been described which appears to be more sensitive than the HI test for measuring human serologic response to infection.[33] Finally, antibody response to OC-43 infection measured by solid-phase radioimmunoassay (RIA) was found to be comparable to that measured by CF, HI, or SRH tests.[35]

Strain 229E is readily identified by serum neutralization (SN) tests in various cell cultures.[23,26,36] In addition, sensitive indirect hemagglutination (IHA) and immune-adherence hemagglutination (IAHA) tests were developed to measure serum antibodies.[36,37] An indirect ELISA test was recently used for 229E but has not yet been applied to human serology.[38]

PROTEINS OF STRAIN OC-43

Utilizing its properties of hemagglutination and high-titered growth in suckling mouse brain, OC-43 was extensively purified by temperature-dependent adsorption to and elution from fresh human "O" erythrocytes and by batch $CaHPO_4$ chromatography.[31] The final purified virus suspension was concentrated by ultrafiltration with XM-300 Diaflo membranes (Amicon Corp.). The virus was purified to a 5000-fold decrease in total protein with a yield of 90% and a final HA titer of 1.3×10^5. The purity of the virus was confirmed by immunologic procedures, density gradient centrifugation, electron microscopy, and analytical procedures.[30] Electron microscopy at low and high magnifications showed very clean fields of particles exhibiting the pleomorphism typical of this virus. Analytical ultracentrifugation revealed a sharp peak at 15,000 rpm with as little as 1.0 mg protein in the sample; this peak had the same sedimentation rate as one of several broad peaks observed when crude virus (at 2-4 mg protein/.4 ml) was sedimented under identical conditions. Acrylamide gels loaded with untreated concentrated supernatant fluids obtained from centrifugation (23,800g, 2 hr) of purified virus suspensions revealed no protein bands.[30]

Mouse ascitic fluid and mouse antiserum prepared against crude virus and against purified virus gave predominantly single bands (of identity) with pure or crude virus in standard ID tests. However, tests with guinea pig and chicken anti-crude and anti-pure virus sera showed two precipitin bands of complete identity between pure and crude virus, and one additional band of identity between pure virus, crude virus, and normal mouse brain. These results suggest that the OC-43 virion contains at least one mouse-brain antigen. Additional evidence of host antigen in the intact virion was found by an identical line between anti-normal mouse-brain serum and the three concentrated antigens. Immunoelectrophoresis of these same antigen-antiserum combinations demonstrated three or four precipitin arcs with crude virus and two or three arcs with purified virus, and confirmed the presence of a mouse-brain protein associated with the purified virus.[30]

The virus was solubilized with SDS/mercaptoethanol/urea, and the resulting polypeptides were separated by PAGE. The staining patterns with Coomassie blue revealed a minimum of six bands, five of which might be considered major. One additional faint band was occasionally observed between the top two bands.[30]

The molecular weights of the viral proteins were determined by co- and companion electrophoresis with proteins of known molecular weight (Table 1). Gels were also stained for lipid and carbohydrate. The lipid content of the single lipoglycopolypeptide was more evident in gels in which the sample was not heated than in those in which it was heated at 100°C for 1 min. However, the classification of the polypeptides as glyco- or lipoglycoproteins must be considered as only tentative, since the chemical nature of these complexes cannot be precisely defined by differential staining techniques. The use of more sensitive procedures to confirm the nature of these proteins awaits the successful adaptation of OC-43 to high-titered growth in cell cultures.

The peplomers on the virion surface have previously been associated with HA activity and are thought to comprise the major antigens measured by both the HI and CF tests. Hence the envelope-associated antigens, unlike influenza virus, appear to consist of a single species. Absence of neuraminidase was confirmed using highly sensitive assay systems. Attempts to determine directly which polypeptides comprise the external antigen, by eluting bands from acrylamide gels in PBS, dialyzing, and titrating for direct and

Table 1. Polypeptides of Strains OC-43 and 229E

Virus	Polypeptide number[a]	Approx. MW (mean)	% comp. (mean)	Probable function/location	Reference
OC-43	VLGP-191	191,200	13	peplomer dimer	Hierholzer et al (1972)[30]
	VP-165	165,000	2	peplomer base	
	VGP-104	104,000	8	peplomer monomer	
	VGP-60	59,500	22	double-shelled envelope	
	VP-47	47,100	16	core (RNA-associated)	
	VP-30	30,500	25	double-shelled envelope	
	VGP-15	15,000	14	peplomer	
229E	VLGP-196	196,100	15	peplomer dimer	Hierholzer (1976)[40]
	VGP-165	165,000	3	peplomer base	
	VGP-106	105,500	8	peplomer monomer	
	VGP-66	65,500	21	double-shelled envelope	
	VP-47	47,300	16	core (RNA-associated)	
	VGP-31	31,400	20	double-shelled envelope	
	VGP-17	16,900	17	peplomer	
229E	VGP-160	160,000	ND	surface projections	Macnaughton (1980)[42]
	VGP-105	105,000	ND	surface projections	
	VP-50	50,000	ND	internal component	
	VGP-24	24,000	ND	?	
	VP-22	22,000	ND	?	

[a]Designated as V=viral, L=lipo, G=glyco, P=protein

indirect hemagglutination, were unsuccessful because residual SDS adversely affected the erythrocytes. Repeated attempts to determine the composition of the external antigen by selectively removing the entire peplomer from the virus envelope also were of limited value. So, membrane-associated components were identified indirectly by bromelin digestion in a reducing buffer with dithiothreitol. The effect of bromelin treatment on purified virus was monitored every 30 minutes under the electron microscope. The club-shaped projections were completely degraded after 2 hours of incubation at 37°C with 0.13% bromelin. The 2-hour test samples, along with the appropriate virus and enzyme controls, were repurified on 5-40% aqueous neutral potassium tartrate gradients at 75,000*g* for 8 hr. The untreated control virus banded in the 1.18 g/cm^3 region of the gradient and was associated with a sharp HA peak; by EM this band consisted of typical virions. The bromelin-treated virus banded in the 1.15 g/cm^3 region of the gradient; by EM this band contained fully enveloped virions which lacked surface projections. All biological activity was lost by the enzyme treatment (Table 2). Polypeptides of the repurified virion control and of the bromelin-treated virions were analyzed by SDS-PAGE. Two major polypeptides, both glycoproteins, and the minor VP-165 were absent in the bromelin-treated sample. However, exactly which proteins comprise the peplomers remains to be confirmed, because the molecular weight

Table 2. Properties of Bromelin-treated OC-43 Virus

Sample[a]	Buoy. dens. (g/cm^3)	Infectivity ($\log_{10}LD_{50}$/ 0.02 ml, SMB)	Antigen titer[b]		No. bands in PAGE	No. of preci. arcs in IE
			HA	CF		
1 Control virus	1.18	9.8	32,768	128	7	3
2 Bromelin-treated v.	1.15	0.7	<1	<2	4	1
3 Bromelin control	--	0.0	<1	<2	0	0

[a]Harvests from potassium tartrate gradients after equilibrium centrifugation at 75,000 *g* for 8 hr: No. 1 was purified virus incubated for 2 hr at 37°C with 0.1 M Tris-HCl buffer, pH 7.2, containing 0.001 M EDTA and 0.005 M DTT (final concentration), and collected from the 1.18-1.19 g/cm^3 region of the gradient; No. 2 was purified virus treated with 0.13% bromelin in the above buffer at the same conditions, and collected from 1.15-1.16 g/cm^3 region of the gradient; No. 3 was the equivalent amount of bromelin and buffered medium incubated with PBS and collected from a gradient in a manner identical to sample No. 2.

[b]Titers expressed as reciprocals of the endpoint dilution.

estimates of proteins by acrylamide gels are often highly inaccurate at both the high and the low ends of the standard curve. In fact, we suspect that the MW estimate of VGP-104 is probably high under the gel systems used, and that VGP-104 might really be the monomeric form of VLGP-191. This is currently being investigated by more precise methods.

Analytical ultracentrifugation of intact, purified virus (HA titer = 2.6×10^5) at 15, 16, and 18,000 rpm revealed a single distinct peak with a sedimentation coefficient ($s_{20,b}$) of $368 \pm 14 \times 10^{-13}$ sec. Corrections for physical/chemical parameters and for virus concentration gave a fully corrected sedimentation coefficient ($S^{\circ}_{20,w}$) of 390 ± 16 S. The apparent molecular weight was then calculated to be $112 \pm 5 \times 10^6$ daltons, so that the particle weight of one OC-43 virion is approximately $18 \pm 1 \times 10^{-17}$ g.[30]

Our data, therefore, indicate that the HA, CF, and infectious virus activities of OC-43 are associated with the peplomers, and that the intact virion has a density of 1.18 g/cm^3 and a sedimentation coefficient of approximately 390 S.[30] Other workers have reported somewhat different data. Pokorny et al. found the maximum CF activity of OC-43 in sucrose gradients to be in the ribosomal region of 1.14 g/cm^3, HA activity and intact virus to be in the microsomal fraction (1.16 g/cm^3), and incomplete or damaged particles to be in the mitochondrial fraction (1.19 g/cm^3).[32] Sheboldov et al. reported that the density of OC-43 virus in CsCl gradients was 1.24 g/cm^3 and of OC-43 ribonucleoprotein was 1.31 g/cm^3.[39] From sucrose gradient centrifugation data, they found the sedimentation coefficient of the virion to be 280 S and that of the RNP to be 180 S.[39] However, calculation of sedimentation coefficients by this procedure is very approximate, as none of the controls or physical correction factors can be applied.

PROTEINS OF STRAIN 229E

As a prerequisite for studying the polypeptide composition of 229E, it was necessary to closely define its growth parameters in cell culture.[40] Optimum growth was achieved using a medium consisting of Eagles MEM with twice the normal concentrations of amino acids and vitamins and 2% fetal calf serum. Growth characteristics for an MOI of 0.1 and 1.0 are shown in Fig. 1.

Peaks of infectious virus were obtained at 24 hr, with a rapid decline occurring after this time indicating that the virus is highly labile. The growth of infectious virus was paralleled by the extracellular incorporation of labeled amino acids into TCA-precipitable material. Slightly lower titers were obtained for multiplicities of 10.0 and much lower for MOI's of 0.01 and 0.05. When additional vitamins and amino acids were not used, the yield was decreased by 300-fold. Preliminary amino acid analyses on purified virus showed

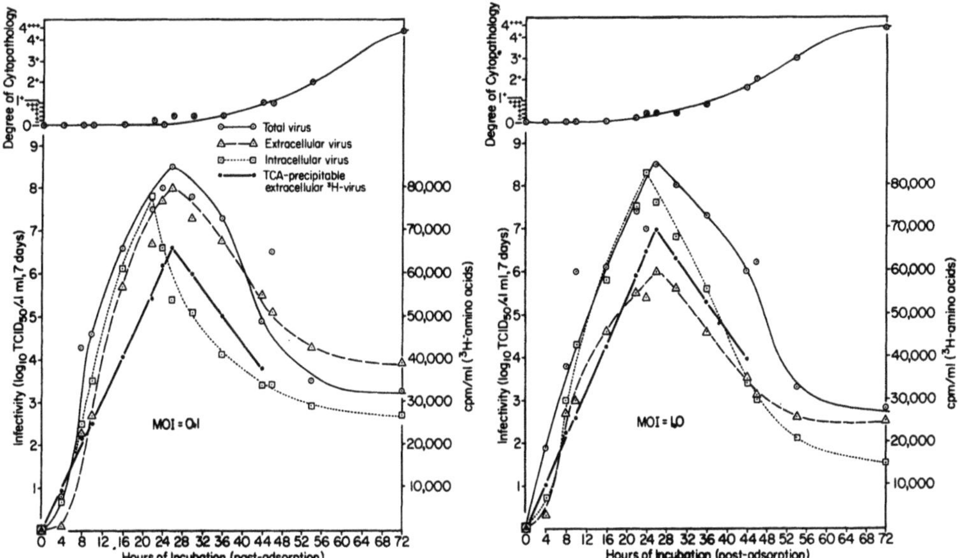

Fig. 1. Growth curves of 229E in HELF cells at MOI = 0.1 & 1. Peak titers of infectious intracellular virus at 22-24 hr were followed by peak titers of infectious extracellular and total virus and by peak levels of ^{3}H-labeled virus at 26 hr postadsorption, when CPE was minimal. Maximum CPE was coincident with rapid autolysis of the virus as it remained at 35°C. CPE was scaled from $\pm$ (5% of cells visibly affected) to +++ (20%) to 1^+ (25%) to 4^+ (100%) to 4^{+++} (all cells totally destroyed).

that 229E contains five amino acids in concentrations of >8 mol%: aspartic acid, glutamic acid, leucine, serine, and valine. Possibly it is the additional requirement for one or more of these amino acids which results in increased virus yield in fortified cultures.[40]

Similar infectious virus results were obtained by Macnaughton et al., who found highest infectivity titers of 229E in MRC fibroblasts 32 hr after infection.[41] In their study, discrete foci of virus were found by indirect immunofluorescence as early as 8 hr after infection, and numbers of foci were correlated with increasing infectivity titers.

Strain 229E is a relatively poor test antigen and a weak immunogen. The IHA and CF antigen titers are considerably lower than one would expect from nine logs of virus, and the IHA, CF, and SN titers (1:80, 1:128, 1:40, respectively) of antiserum to purified virions also are much lower than expected. Although Bradburne reported two precipitin lines in ID tests between 229E and human 229E-convalescent sera,[23] we consistently found only one line in both ID and IE tests with convalescent human sera and with rabbit antiserum versus 10-log preparations of crude or purified virus.[40]

Virus synthesized under optimum conditions of growth was purified for analysis of constituent proteins by PAGE. Two purification schemes were used: (1) the procedure described for OC-43 utilizing adsorption to and elution from human "O" erythrocytes, followed by dialysis and adsorption to calcium phosphate gel; the gel was sequentially washed with phosphate buffers of 0.001 to 0.2 M, pH 7.2, and the virus eluted with 0.3 M buffer;[30] and (2) precipitation of clarified extracts with PEG-6000 and centrifugation to equilibrium through shallow glycerol/tartrate gradients; the virus band was then recentrifuged through steep glycerol/tartrate equilibrium gradients for 16 hr or rate zonal gradients for 4.5 hr.[40]

Procedure (1) gave a mean 5800-fold reduction in total protein with a 67% yield. Procedure (2) gave a mean 5100-fold reduction in total protein with a 96% yield. Both schemes were approximately equal in their removal of host cell proteins, with the final products containing <0.02% of crude tissue culture proteins and <0.007% of crude culture radioactivity. The criteria of purity established for OC-43 were met for 229E as well.

Absorption spectra of different lots of purified 229E at weighed concentrations of 1 mg/ml or less revealed a mean maximum at 256 nm and a mean minimum at 241.2 nm. The mean O.D. 260/280 ratio was 1.53; the specific extinction coefficient, k, for a 1% solution and a 1-cm light path was $51.8_{O.D.260}$ and $34.0_{O.D.280}$; the extinction coefficient, $E^{1\%}_{1cm}$, had a mean value of 54.3 at 256 nm. All values were corrected for light scattering.

Gel electrophoresis was carried out in continuous phosphate gels as used for OC-43[30] and in discontinuous Tris-glycine gels.[40] Gels were stained for protein, phosphoprotein, glycoprotein, and lipoprotein and scanned as before.[30] Seven polypeptides were consistently found, six of which appeared to contain carbohydrate and one lipid (Table 1). None contained phosphate at a level exceeding 0.6% of the virion by weight.

Electropherograms of labeled virus harvested 26-30 hr after adsorption supported both the purity of the 229E preparations and the composition of the virus as determined by gels stained for protein and carbohydrate (Fig. 2). Again, seven polypeptides in proportions similar to those obtained in stained gels were observed, and only VP-47 was not glycosylated.[40] Our results are somewhat different from those of Macnaughton,[42] who found five major proteins, three of which were glycosylated and two of which were associated with the peplomers (Table 1).

Bromelin treatment of purified 229E removed VGP-106 and VGP-17 entirely and appeared to significantly reduce VGP-165 and VLGP-196. Further studies on the glycoproteins of 229E are in progress and are summarized in the last section of this review.

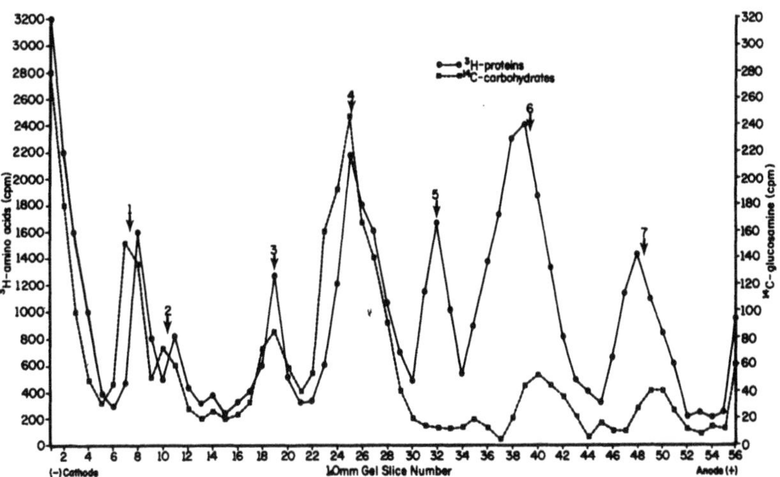

Fig. 2. Radioactive profile of purified 229E virus with ^{3}H-labeled proteins and ^{14}C-labeled carbohydrates. The viral proteins were electrophoresed in 3%/8% gels in the discontinuous Tris buffer system.

Sedimentation coefficients for 229E were measured between 15,000 and 19,000 rpm on Schlieren optics. Uncorrected coefficients averaged 359 x 10^{-13} sec. Values corrected for solvent density and viscosity, for partial specific volume of the virus, and for infinite dilution gave a sedimentation coefficient of $S^{\circ}_{20,w}$ = 381 S. Equilibrium runs with 229E were of limited value due to the rapid disintegration of the virus at 20°C.

RNA OF STRAIN OC-43

The RNA of strain OC-43 was examined by prelabeling 4-day-old suckling mice intracerebrally with approximately 320 µCi of ^{32}P orthophosphate, followed at 8 hr with $10^{4.22}$ LD_{50} of virus by the same route.[43,44] Brains were harvested at 40 hr and virus present was purified by freezing and thawing the suspension 4x, clarifying, and adsorbing to and eluting from human "O" cells. The final eluate was concentrated and centrifuged to equilibrium at 97,100*g* for 15 hr through a 25-65% sucrose gradient in NET buffer at 7°C. The lower coincident peak of radioactivity, hemagglutinin, and CF activity was then recentrifuged through a 15-65% sucrose velocity gradient for 1 hr at 43,200*g*. The upper peak of radioactivity and hemagglutinin was used as the starting material for RNA studies. RNA extraction was carried out by five different methods in an effort to find the method best suited for OC-43 RNA.

RNA was prepared from two samples of ^{32}P OC-43 virus by the warm phenol-SDS (WPS) method and from two other samples by the SDS-lysis (SL) method.[45,46] Profiles of OC-43 and marker RNAs from each gradient after centrifugation are shown in Fig. 3. When the WPS method was used and the RNAs were examined in 15-30% sucrose gradients (Fig. 3A), most RNA was distributed broadly in the 15-50S region of the gradient, with a smaller quantity of 4S RNA also present. Analysis in 5-20% gradients (Fig. 3B) suggested that the

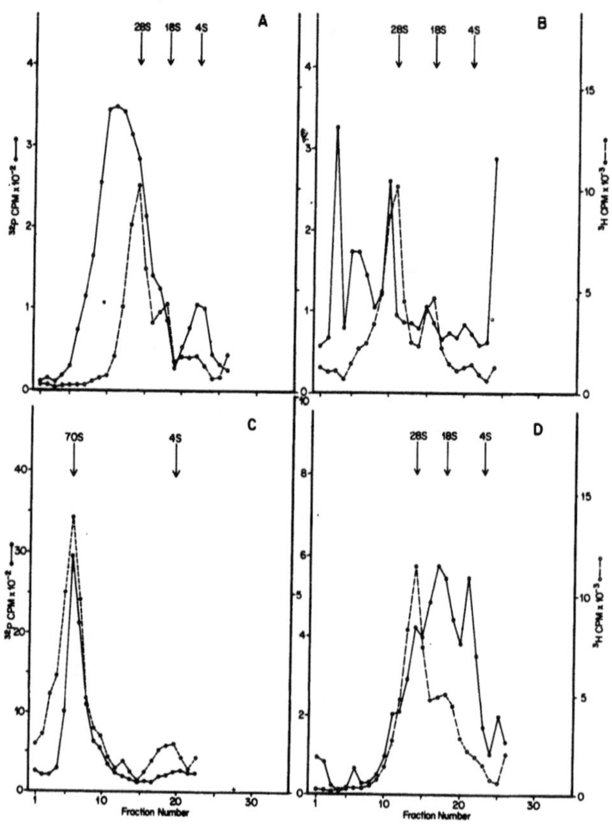

Fig. 3: Sucrose gradient analysis of OC-43 RNA prepared by extraction methods used for other coronaviruses. RNA was extracted from two samples of ^{32}P OC-43 virus by the WPS method (A & B). After extraction, carrier and ^{3}H-uridine ribosomal RNA were added and all RNAs were precipitated with ethanol. Each precipitate was dissolved in 0.5 ml NET and analyzed by ultracentrifugation in 4.4 ml 15-30% (A) or 5-20% (B) sucrose gradients. RNA from two further samples (C & D) was released by the SL method. Sample C was mixed with 0.1 ml of ^{3}H-uridine RSV RNA. Sample D was first mixed with 0.1 ml of ^{3}H-uridine ribosomal RNA and 100 μg carrier RNA, and all RNAs were precipitated with ethanol, resuspended in 0.5 ml NET, and analyzed by centrifuging through 15-30% sucrose gradients. The profiles of acid-insoluble radioactivity, fractionated onto paper strips, are hown for OC-43 (—●—) and ribosomal or RSV (--O--) RNA.

RNA was distributed throughout the gradient, and no resolution between the smaller 4S and larger heterogeneous RNA classes was possible. When the SL method was used to release viral RNA (Fig. 3C), a single large homogeneous RNA was obtained with a sedimentation coefficient identical to the major (70S) component of Rous Sarcoma Virus (RSV) RNA. The OC-43 RNA is best described as a 70S RNA on the basis of repeated sucrose gradients cocentrifuged with various RNA markers. When RNA was released by the SL method, precipitated with ethanol, and reconstituted in NET (Fig. 3D), a smaller and more heterogeneous range of RNA species was obtained, suggesting a breakdown of the large RNA noted in Fig. 3C.[43]

In view of differences in the RNA profile for OC-43 noted in Fig. 3, RNA profiles were obtained by the SDS-pronase (SP), phenol-chloroform (PC), and perchlorate-chloroform-isoamyl alcohol (PCIA) extraction methods.[43,47,48] By the SP method, a more homogeneous major RNA component with a sedimentation coefficient of 45-50S and a minor 4S component were apparent (Fig. 4A). Extraction by the PC method (Fig. 4B) revealed a heterogeneity in the RNA fragments comprising the major class similar to that noted with the WPS method (Fig. 3A); a minor 4S component also was present. Complete RNA degradation occurred after extraction by the PCIA method, indicating its unsuitability for OC-43 RNA extraction (Fig. 4C). Degradation is probably caused by an interaction between outer virion components oxidized by perchlorate treatment and virion RNA, similar to that described for periodate treatment of myxoviruses. The PC

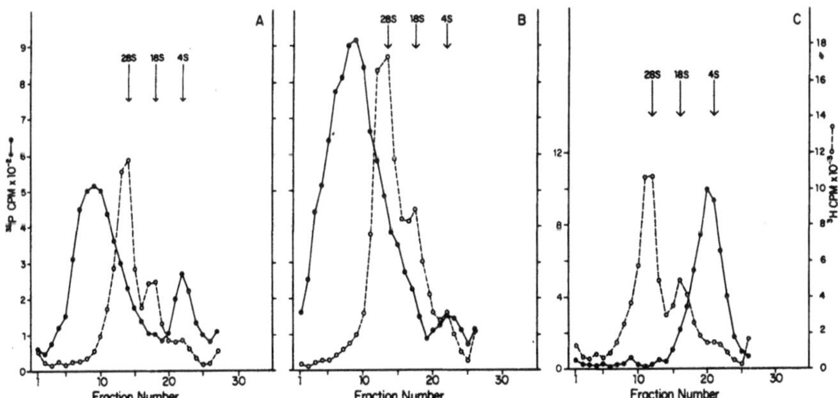

Fig. 4: RNA profiles for OC-43 virus obtained by other extraction procedures. ^{32}P OC-43 RNA was extracted by the (A) SP, (B) PC, and (C) PCIA procedures. Each extract was combined with 0.1 ml ^{3}H-uridine ribosomal and 100 µg of carrier RNA and precipitated with ethanol. The precipitates were resuspended in 0.5 ml NET and analyzed in 15-30% sucrose gradients. The distributions of acid-insoluble radioactivity are shown for OC-43 (—●—) and ribosomal (--O--) RNAs.

method was used for all subsequent extractions involving phenol because of the greater RNA yields obtained and the observation that phenol-chloroform mixtures conserved polyadenosine sequences in RNA.[43]

The profile obtained for OC-43 RNA by sucrose-gradient centrifugation was compared with one obtained by PAGE. The RNA typically migrated as a homogeneous complex with an electrophoretic mobility similar to that of 45S ribosomal precursor RNA. Acrylamide gels electrophoresed at 23°C revealed considerable breakdown of the complex; this thermolability of OC-43 RNA was confirmed in later experiments. The electrophoretic profiles of OC-43 RNA, after preparation by the PC and SP methods, were then determined at 5°C. Clearly, the PC method resulted in considerable breakdown of the large complex into a range of RNA fragments with electrophoretic mobilities between 45S and 18S (Fig. 5A). A minor 4S component was also present; it was similar to that found for IBV RNA after extraction by the WPS method.[45] RNA prepared by the gentler SP method was more homogeneous (Fig. 5B), but some degradation, evidenced by apparent trailing of the major peak, and a minor 4S component can still be seen. The latter appears to be released from the major 70S complex by the WPS, PC, and SP methods.

A semilogarithmic plot of molecular weight versus electrophoretic mobility of the data from replicate experiments gave a mean apparent molecular weight of 6.1×10^6 for the undegraded RNA complex. OC-43 RNA, when prepared by the SL method, has an identical electrophoretic mobility to 70S RSV RNA.[43] Because of the complexity of RSV RNA, however, it was not used as a molecular weight marker.

Garwes et al. reported that RNA complexes from the porcine coronaviruses TGEV and HEV were degraded if extracted by SDS lysis at temperatures above 60°,[46] as has been noted for the RNAs of Retroviridae. To confirm this with OC-43 RNA, preparations of OC-43 virus were treated with 1% SDS by the SL method at 23°, 37°, and 60° C. The distributions of acid-insoluble radioactivity for each gradient suggest that some breakdown of the 70S complex into smaller 4S fragments occurred at 37°C and a more generalized breakdown to a range of intermediate species occurred at 60°C. Because little dissociation of the HEV and TGEV RNAs occurred at temperatures less than 60°C,[46] the OC-43 RNA complex seems even more labile than that of the porcine coronaviruses. Additionally, the 4S RNA component obtained by the two phenol extraction methods or the SP method appears to be derived from the larger 70S complex.

Heterogeneity in the major RNA component of OC-43 after phenol extraction (Figs. 3,4,5) may have been caused by (1) mechanical disruption by phenol of noncovalent bonds linking the OC-43 RNA fragments which form the 70S complex or (2) specific release or

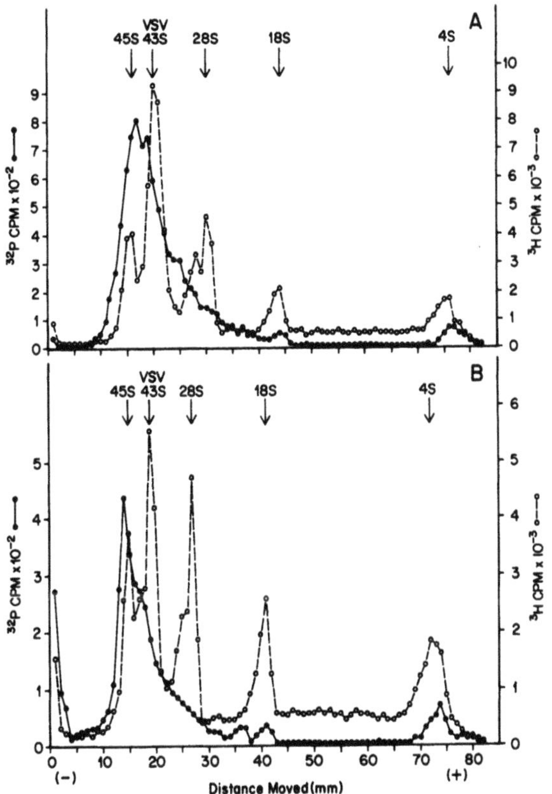

Fig. 5: PAGE of ^{32}P OC-43 RNA extracted by (A) the PC and (B) the SP methods. ^{3}H-uridine ribosomal and ^{3}H-uridine VSV RNA and 50 μg of carrier RNA were added to each, and all RNAs were precipitated with ethanol. The precipitates were dissolved in 100 μl NET; sucrose and bromphenol blue were added to final concentrations of 10% and 0.01%, respectively; and 60 μl aliquots were electrophoresed. The distributions of radioactivity for OC-43 (—●—) and ribosomal and VSV (--O--) RNAs are shown.

activation of virion ribonucleases in the extraction procedure. To examine these possibilities, we coextracted RNAs from mixtures of ^{32}P OC-43 virus and ^{3}H-uridine TMV or ^{3}H-uridine RSV by the PC method. TMV RNA contains a single piece of RNA with a sedimentation coefficient of 31S. The major 70S RNA of RSV is comprised of smaller fragments of variable size and linked by noncovalent bonds; a number of minor RNA components are also present. RNAs in each mixture, after preparation, were precipitated with ethanol in the presence of carrier RNA and analyzed in sucrose gradients. The profiles of acid-insoluble radioactivity for each gradient showed the same heterogeneity for the major class of OC-43 RNA fragments already noted by the phenol extraction method (Figs. 3,4) and again confirm the presence of a minor 4S component. Both TMV RNA and 70S RSV RNA remained undegraded after extraction, suggesting that the heterogeneity of the major RNA class is caused not by the activation of ribonucleases but by disruption of noncovalent linkages between RNA fragments which are much weaker than similar linkages within the 70S RSV RNA. Sedimentation coefficients for the major RNAs released by phenol (15-55S) were less than the homogeneous 70S peak obtained by the SL method (Fig. 3C).

Further evidence that OC-43 70S RNA is a complex of fragments held together by weak, noncovalent bonds was obtained by (1) isolation of 70S OC-43 RNA by SDS-lysis and centrifugation, followed by PC extraction in the presence of TMV RNA, and (2) isolation of RNA by the SL method and centrifugation in DMSO gradients. OC-43 70S RNA was lysed with SDS and centrifuged to isolate the RNA complex. The profile for total (acid-soluble and -insoluble) radioactivity from aliquots of each gradient fraction revealed a sharp peak of ^{32}P radioactivity in the 70S region (the RNA complex) and a much larger peak of low density material at the top of the gradient. Similarly located but much smaller peaks for acid-insoluble, ribonuclease-resistant radioactivity are seen in Fig. 3C. It, therefore, seems likely that SDS-lysis separates RNA from large amounts of acid-soluble components, some acid-insoluble phospholipids, and perhaps other components in the outer virion coat.

PC extraction in the presence of ^{3}H-uridine TMV RNA followed by ethanol precipitation and analysis in sucrose gradients revealed completely degraded OC-43 70S RNA but intact TMV RNA. This confirms earlier evidence that the 70S complex is held together by weak noncovalent bonds which are destroyed by phenol extraction (Figs. 3,4) or gentle heating. The breakdown of isolated 70S RNA by the PC extraction method is more complete than by similar extraction of purified virions. It does not appear to be due to ribonuclease activity because TMV RNA within the same mixture remains intact.

Since DMSO has been used as a critical test for noncovalent linkages in RSV 70S RNA, we investigated its effect on 70S OC-43 RNA prepared by SDS-lysis. The profile for total radioactivity showed a complete breakdown of the 70S RNA complex to smaller fragments which sediment slightly faster than structural phospholipids at the top of the gradient.

In summary, human coronavirus RNA was characterized using OC-43 virus propagated in suckling mouse brain in the presence of ^{32}P orthophosphate. When isolated from purified virions by SDS-lysis, a single RNA species is obtained which has a sedimentation coefficient of 70S, a molecular weight of 6.1×10^6, and is heat-labile. Phenol extraction isolates a range of RNAs with sedimentation coefficients of 15 to 55S, and some 4S RNA is present as a minor component.[43] We then proceeded to examine OC-43 RNA for the presence of genomic polyadenylic acid (poly (A)) sequences by affinity column chromatography and for the presence of a virion transcriptase with systems optimal for the transcriptases of myxoviruses and paramyxoviruses.[44]

^{32}P-OC-43 RNA was extracted from purified virions by the PC method, precipitated with ethanol in the presence of carrier RNA, and dissolved in NET. Mixtures consisting of OC-43 and a) ^{3}H-uridine poliovirus RNA, b) ^{3}H-uridine VSV RNA, or c) ^{3}H-uridine RSV RNA were applied to poly (U)-Sepharose 4B columns and the filtrates were collected. Nonadherent RNA was removed with washes, and poly (A)-containing RNAs were eluted with a formamide-NET buffer. For each mixture, a significant proportion of OC-43 RNA was removed with the elution buffer, indicating that poly (A) sequences were present. In the controls, significant amounts of poliovirus and RSV RNA (each containing poly (A)) in mixtures (a) and (c) were also eluted, but very little VSV RNA (containing no poly (A)) remained after the washing steps.

The size of the poly (A) residues in OC-43 RNA was determined by sucrose density centrifugation after ribonuclease digestion and passage through a poly (U)-Sepharose 4B column (Fig. 6). The profiles for acid-insoluble radioactivity showed that the poly (A) was present as a single peak with a sedimentation coefficient of 2S located near the top of the gradient. The peak was well resolved from what appeared to be some incompletely digested RNA fragments too large to contain poly (A) alone. The molecular weight of the 2S poly (A) was calculated to be 6645, which corresponds to a stretch of approximately 19 adenylate residues.

Similar profiles were obtained in two further experiments. When pancreatic ribonuclease was omitted from the RNA-enzyme mixture, a larger peak with a sedimentation coefficient of 4S was obtained, indicating that small amounts of nucleotides other than A were present. The polyadenylate 2S fragment represents approximately 0.3% of the total RNA before digestion. The latter figure is a minimal value, however, because larger, incompletely digested, poly (A)-containing fragments were also found (see Fig. 6), which could be due to regions of base pairing within the RNA genome. These may or may not be related to the 2S fragment.

Transcriptase experiments were carried out with systems optimal for influenza and for Newcastle Disease Virus (NDV), along with appropriate controls. For the influenza-type system, transcriptase activity was also measured in mixtures in which i) 2-mercaptoethanol was added, ii) manganous chloride was omitted, and iii) magnesium chloride was omitted. The incorporation obtained for each set of conditions is shown in Fig. 7. For influenza (Fig. 7A), maximum incorporation of 77 pmol UMP/mg virus protein

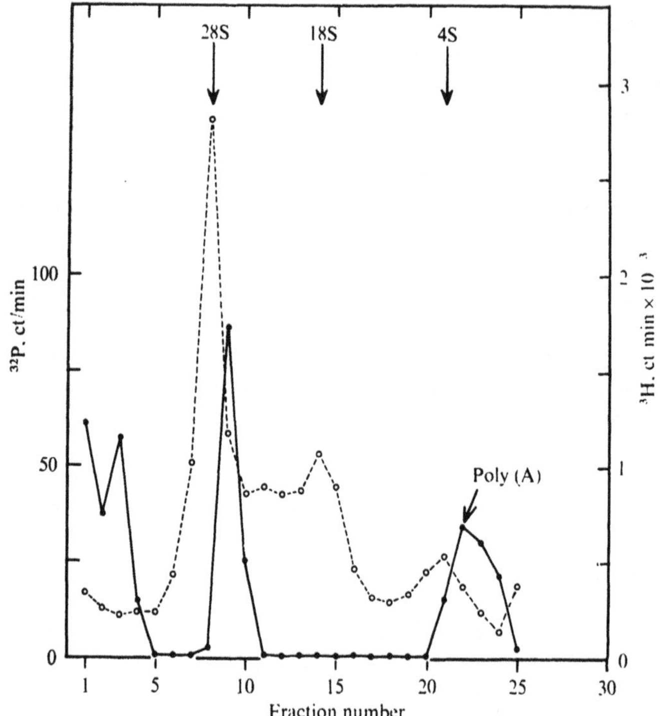

Fig. 6: Sizing of poly (A) sequences in OC-43 RNA. One ml of ^{32}P-OC-43 RNA prepared by PC extraction in NET (0.1 M NaCl, 0.01 M EDTA, 0.01 M Tris, pH 7.4) was incubated with 50 units of ribonuclease T_1 and 10 μg of pancreatic ribonuclease for 60 min at 34°C. The mixture was extracted three times by the PC method and precipitated with ethanol in the presence of carrier RNA. The precipitate was taken up with NET and passed through a poly (U)-Sepharose 4B column. The eluates were further precipitated with ethanol in the presence of carrier and ^{3}H-uridine ribosomal RNA and analyzed in a sucrose-density gradient. The distributions of acid-insoluble, ^{32}P-OC-43 poly (A) (—●—) and ^{3}H-ribosomal RNAs (--O--) are shown.

was obtained after 60 min at 37°C in the standard reaction mixture and in mixtures i and ii. When magnesium chloride was omitted (iii), no incorporation occurred above background. In the same system for OC-43 (Fig. 7B), no incorporation above background occurred under any conditions. With NDV in an NDV-type system (Fig. 7C), incorporation occurred to a maximum of 7 pmol UMP/mg virus protein after 1 hr at 32°C, but no incorporation above background was noted for OC-43 (Fig. 7D). An OC-43 RNA transcriptase was therefore not detected with systems optimal for the transcriptases of morphologically-similar viruses.[44]

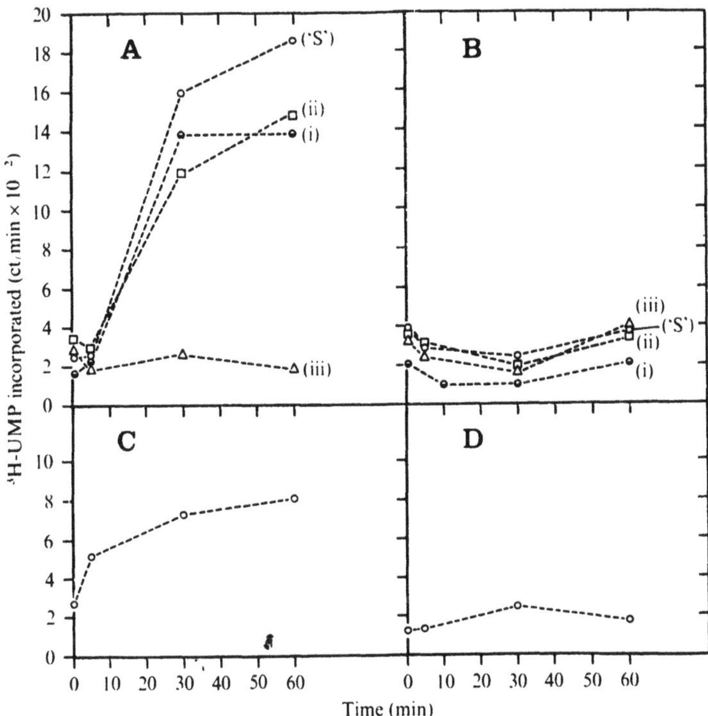

Fig. 7: Tests for the presence of OC-43 virion transcriptase. Transcriptase activity, according to the extent of acid-insoluble ^{3}H-UMP incorporation, was measured for (A) influenza and (B) OC-43, with an influenza-type system, and for NDV (C) and OC-43 (D), with an NDV-type system. For the influenza-type system, besides the standard reaction mixture ('S')additional mixtures were prepared in which (i) 2 µl of 10% 2-mercaptoethanol was added, and (ii) manganous chloride and (iii) magnesium chloride was omitted. The influenza-type system was incubated at 37°C and the NDV-type system at 34°C.

Thus, poly (A) is present in 15-55S OC-43 RNA obtained by PC extraction but absent from the minor 4S RNA, suggesting different functions for each RNA class. A segment of about 19 AMP residues was obtained by T_1 and pancreatic ribonuclease digestion. The function of OC-43 4S RNA in PC extracts is unknown. It may be that the same 4S RNA which is freed from the 70S complex by heating functions as a specific t-RNA, as is the case with retrovirus RNA. Evidence as to whether the poly (A) in OC-43 RNA is internal or is located at the 3' terminus is still incomplete.

RNA OF STRAIN 229E

Studies described above showed that the genome of OC-43 has a molecular weight of approximately 6.1 x 10^6. During ongoing studies of 229E RNA, we attempted to determine the molecular weight of the 229E genome in similar fashion. Virion RNA was labeled with ^{32}Pi and extracted by the phenol-chloroform method. The labeled RNA was then electrophoresed on acid-urea agarose gels with molecular weight markers, and the separated RNA species were visualized by autoradiography.[49] The results showed that the 229E genome has a molecular weight of approximately 6.5 x 10^6. In addition, three other RNA species ranging in size from 16-26S were resolved. Preliminary data indicate that these RNA species are not breakdown fragments of the 70S genomic RNA, but may in fact represent defective interfering RNA molecules.

The estimated size of the 229E genome may be low, since the genome of IBV has been estimated to have a molecular weight of 6.9 x 10^6 by gel electrophoresis and 8.1 x 10^6 by complexity measurements.[50] The size estimate of the 229E genome obtained in our laboratory is somewhat higher than the value of 5.8 x 10^6 reported by Macnaughton & Madge.[51]

In our studies, no replication occurred in the presence of actinomycin-D, even at concentrations of 0.5 µg/ml.[40] However, this and all higher concentrations were toxic for human embryonic lung fibroblasts and, therefore, the inability of the virus to replicate does not necessarily indicate a concomittant requirement for nuclear function. Kennedy & Johnson-Lussenburg found inhibition of replication of 229E with actinomycin D levels as low as 0.1 µg/ml, but this inhibition did not apparently involve viral RNA synthesis.[52] The fact that 229E has a single-stranded RNA[40] and has been shown in ongoing studies to have polyadenylate residues in its genome suggests that its RNA acts as a primary messenger which would obviate the need for a virion transcriptase. Further studies are needed to resolve this question.

BIOSYNTHESIS AND ASSEMBLY OF HUMAN CORONAVIRUSES

Little information has been obtained on the biosynthesis and assembly of OC-43 and 229E. Morphologically, both viruses form by budding into the cisternae of the endoplasmic reticulum between membranes.[53-56] In the earliest stages of development, altered segments of cisternal or reticulum membrane bulging from the cytoplasm into the vesicular lumen were observed in 229E-infected cells.[53] The membrane that seemed destined to become part of the envelope of the virion appeared to be a bilayer. Thus the budding mechanism is not unlike that described for other enveloped viruses that mature at the plasma membrane of infected cells. The morphogenesis of OC-43 seems to be similar to that of 229E, but discrete steps in the budding process were not observed.[54]

Although direct evidence has not been presented, the dense crescent-shaped structure which forms at the cisternal membrane of 229E-infected cells is probably comprised of a ribonucleoprotein complex (RNP). Such a complex has been isolated from purified virions and shown to consist of a tightly coiled helical or linear nucleocapsid.[57-59] A number of workers agree that the density of the RNP complex is 1.27 g/cm^3, but the reported diameter of the RNP complex ranges from 9-16 nm in width.[57-59] A preliminary analysis of the RNP complex proteins showed that a 45,000-dalton protein was associated with the viral RNA.[57]

The synthesis and assembly of the viral membrane components of a number of enveloped viruses have been studied. First, viral glycoproteins appear to be synthesized on membrane-bound polyribosomes, and glycosylation occurs in association with cytoplasmic membranes. Secondly, glycoproteins appear to migrate from rough endoplasmic reticulum to smooth or Golgi-complex membranes with further modification of viral glycoprotein oligosaccharides. Thirdly, the glycoproteins are inserted into the plasma membrane of virus-infected cells and assembled into virions.[60-62] This pathway has been clearly demonstrated for well characterized members of the myxo- and rhabdovirus groups. But coronaviruses, as described above, do not bud from the plasma membrane of infected cells. Instead, the virions bud into the vesicular lumen and egress from the cell by lysis of the cell or by rupture of virion-containing vesicles at the plasma membrane.[54,56] In fact, the presence of human coronavirus glycoproteins on the surface of the cellular plasma membrane has not yet been demonstrated. Thus, we sought to determine if coronavirus glycoproteins contain glycosyl sidechains similar to those of Sindbis,[63-65] influenza,[66-68] and rhabdovirus virions.[69,70]

To answer this question, coronavirus 229E glycoproteins labeled with ^{3}H-glucosamine were purified and the protein constituents were solubilized and separated by SDS-PAGE as previously described.[71,72] After electrophoresis, the glycoproteins were visualized by fluorography[72] and gel segments corresponding to VLGP-196 (or simply "gp190") were excised and prepared for glycopeptide analysis.[71,72] The gp190 glycopeptides of 229E were co-chromatographed on a Bio-Gel P6 column with ^{14}C-glucosamine-labeled glycopeptides of influenza A/WSN virus.[66] The elution profile of the gp190 oligosaccharide moieties is shown in Fig. 8. The major size class of glycopeptides found corresponded in size to the 2900-dalton influenza glycopeptides.

The 2900-dalton influenza glycopeptides are designated type I and contain glucosamine, mannose, galactose, and fucose.[66]

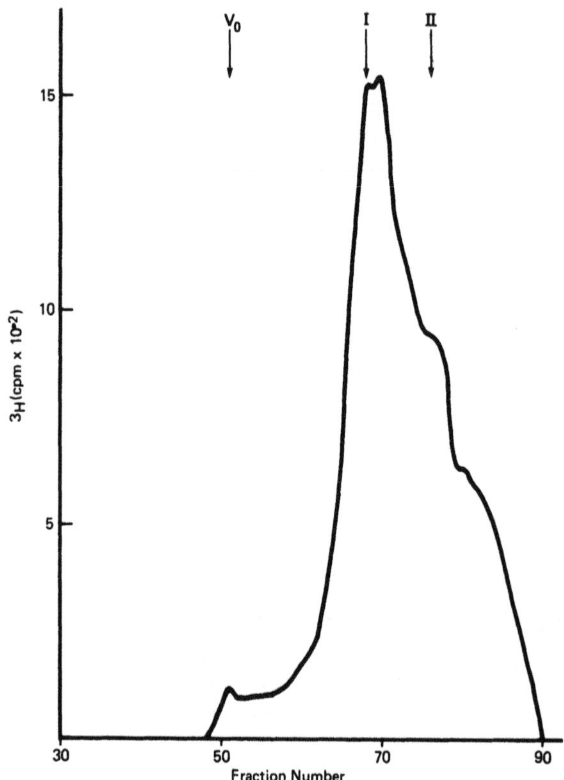

Fig. 8: Analysis of ^{3}H-glucosamine-labeled gp190 glycopeptides of 229E by Bio-Gel P6 gel filtration. ^{14}C-glucosamine-labeled glycopeptides of influenza A/WSN grown in MDBK cells were co-chromatographed as internal molecular weight markers. The elution positions of the type I glycopeptides (MW = 2900) and smaller type II glycopeptides (MW = 2200) are indicated by solid arrows; V_o = the void volume.

Thus, the major glycopeptide constituent of gp190 appears to contain glycopeptides similar to those of viruses which bud from the plasma membrane.[63-72] Therefore, even though coronaviruses are assembled at sites within the endoplasmic reticulum, the mechanism of synthesis and glycosylation of strain 229E glycoproteins does not appear to differ from that of other well-studied, enveloped viruses.

REFERENCES

1. D. A. J. Tyrrell, J. D. Almeida, D. M. Berry, C. H. Cunningham, D. Hamre, M. S. Hofstad, L. Mallucci, and K. McIntosh, Coronaviruses, Nature 220:650 (1968).
2. A. F. Bradburne and D. A. J. Tyrrell, Coronaviruses of man, Progr. Med. Virol. 13:373 (1971).
3. J. C. Hierholzer, J. R. Broderson, and F. A. Murphy, New strain of mouse hepatitis virus as the cause of lethal enteritis in infant mice, Inf. Imm. 24:508 (1979).
4. K. McIntosh, Coronaviruses: A comparative review, Current Topics in Microbiol. Immunol. 63:85 (1974).
5. A. S. Monto, Coronaviruses, Yale J. Biol. Med. 47:234 (1974).
6. J. A. Robb and C. W. Bond, Coronaviridae, Comprehensive Virology 14:193 (1979).
7. D. A. J. Tyrrell, D. J. Alexander, J. D. Almeida, C. H. Cunningham, B. C. Easterday, D. J. Garwes, J. C. Hierholzer, A. Kapikian, M. R. Macnaughton, and K. McIntosh, Coronaviridae: Second report, Intervirology 10:321 (1978).
8. H. W. Ackermann, G. Cherchel, J. P. Valet, J. Matte, S. Moorjani, and R. Higgins. Experiences sur la nature de particules trouvées dans der cas d'hepatite virale: type coronavirus, antigène Australia et particules de Dane, Can. J. Microbiol. 20:193 (1974).
9. K. Apostolov, P. Spasić, and N. Bojanić, Evidence of a viral etiology in endemic (Balkan) nephropathy, Lancet 2:1271 (1975).
10. J. S. Burks, B. L. DeVald, L. D. Jankovsky, and J. C. Gerdes, Two coronaviruses isolated from central nervous system tissue of two multiple sclerosis patients, Science 209:933 (1980).
11. E. O. Caul and S. K. R. Clarke, Coronavirus propagated from patient with non-bacterial gastroenteritis, Lancet 2:953 (1975).
12. E. O. Caul and S. I. Egglestone, Further studies on human enteric coronaviruses. Arch. Virol. 54:107 (1977).
13. E. O. Caul, W. K. Paver, and S. K. R. Clarke, Coronavirus particles in faeces from patients with gastroenteritis, Lancet 1:1192 (1975).
14. L. Georgescu, P. Diosi, I. Butiu, L. Plavosin, and G. Herzog, Porcine coronavirus antibodies in endemic (Balkan) nephropathy, Lancet 1:163 (1978).
15. A. W. Holmes, F. Deinhardt, W. Harris, F. Ball, and G. Cline, Coronaviruses and viral hepatitis, J. Clin. Invest. 49:45a (1970).
16. M. Mathan and V. I. Mathan, Coronaviruses and tropical sprue in southern India, in: Fourth Int. Cong. for Virol., The Hague, Behring Inst., Frankfurt Germany (1978).
17. R. D. Schnagl, I. H. Holmes, and E. M. Mackay-Scollay, Coronavirus-like particles in aboriginals and nonaboriginals in western Australia, Med. J. Australia 1:307 (1978).

18. A. J. Zuckerman, P. E. Taylor, and J. D. Almeida, Presence of particles other than the Australia-SH antigen in a case of chronic active hepatitis with cirrhosis, Brit. Med. J. 1:262 (1970).
19. D. A. J. Tyrrell and M. L. Bynoe, Cultivation of a novel type of common-cold virus in organ cultures, Brit. Med. J. 1:1467 (1965).
20. D. Hamre and J. J. Procknow, A new virus isolated from the human respiratory tract, Proc. Soc. Exp. Biol. Med. 121:190 (1966).
21. K. McIntosh, J. H. Dees, W. B. Becker, A. Z. Kapikian, and R. M. Chanock, Recovery in tracheal organ cultures of novel viruses from patients with respiratory disease, Proc. Nat. Acad. Sci. 57:933 (1967).
22. A. Z. Kapikian, H. D. James, S. J. Kelly, and A. L. Vaughn, Detection of coronavirus strain 692 by immune electron microscopy, Inf. Imm. 7:111 (1973).
23. A. F. Bradburne, Antigenic relationships amongst coronaviruses, Arch. Gesamte Virusforsch. 31:352 (1970).
24. K. McIntosh, A. Z. Kapikian, K. A. Hardison, J. W. Hartley, and R. M. Chanock, Antigenic relationships among the coronaviruses of man and between human and animal coronaviruses, J. Immun. 102:1109 (1969).
25. K. McIntosh, J. McQuillin, S. E. Reed, and P. S. Gardner, Diagnosis of human coronavirus infection by immunofluorescence: Method and application to respiratory disease in hospitalized children, J. Med. Virol. 2:341 (1978).
26. A. S. Monto and L. M. Rhodes, Detection of coronavirus infection of man by immunofluorescence, Proc. Soc. Exp. Biol. Med. 155:143 (1977).
27. J. C. Hierholzer and G. A. Tannock, Quantitation of antibody to non-hemagglutinating viruses by single radial hemolysis: Serological test for human coronaviruses, J. Clin. Microbiol. 5:613 (1977).
28. H. Riski, T. Hovi, P. Väänänen, and K. Penttinen, Antibodies to human coronavirus OC 43 measured by radial haemolysis in gel, Scand. J. Inf. Dis. 9:75 (1977).
29. H. S. Kaye and W. R. Dowdle, Some characteristics of hemagglutination of certain strains of "IBV-like" virus, J. Inf. Dis. 120:576 (1969).
30. J. C. Hierholzer, E. L. Palmer, S. G. Whitfield, H. S. Kaye, and W. R. Dowdle, Protein composition of coronavirus OC 43, Virology 48:516 (1972).
31. H. S. Kaye, J. C. Hierholzer, and W. R. Dowdle, Purification and further characterization of an "IBV-like" virus (coronavirus), Proc. Soc. Exp. Biol. Med. 135:457 (1970).
32. J. Pokorny, M. Bruckova, and M. Ryc, Biophysical properties of coronavirus strain OC-43, Acta Virol. 19:137 (1975).
33. G. Gerna, E. Cattaneo, P. M. Cereda, M. G. Revelo, and G. Achilli, Human coronavirus OC-43 serum inhibitor and neutralizing antibody by a new plaque-reduction assay, Proc. Soc. Exp. Biol. Med. 163:360 (1980).

34. A. Z. Kapikian, H. D. James, S. J. Kelly, L. M. King, A. L. Vaughn, and R. M. Chanock, Hemadsorption by coronavirus strain OC-43, Proc. Soc. Exp. Biol. Med. 139:179 (1972).
35. T. Hovi, H. Kainulainen, B. Ziola, and A. Salmi, OC 43 strain-related coronavirus antibodies in different age groups, J. Med. Virol. 3:313 (1979).
36. G. Gerna, G. Achilli, E. Cattaneo, and P. Cereda, Determination of coronavirus 229E antibody by an immune-adherence hemagglutination method, J. Med. Virol. 2:215 (1978).
37. H. S. Kaye, S. B. Ong, and W. R. Dowdle, Detection of coronavirus 229E antibody by indirect hemagglutination, Appl. Microbiol. 24:703 (1972).
38. C. A. Kraaijeveld, M. H. Madge, and M. R. Macnaughton, Enzyme-linked immunosorbent assay for coronaviruses HCV 229E and MHV 3, J. Gen. Virol. 49:83 (1980).
39. A. V. Sheboldov, L. Y. Zakstelskaya, and V. M. Zhdanov, Sedimentation and density characteristics of coronavirus, Vopr. Virusol. 1:59 (1973).
40. J. C. Hierholzer, Purification and biophysical properties of human coronavirus 229E, Virology 75:155 (1976).
41. M. R. Macnaughton, B. J. Thomas, H. A. Davies, and S. Patterson, Infectivity of human strain 229E, J.Clin.Micr. 12:462 (1980).
42. M. R. Macnaughton, The polypeptides of human and mouse coronaviruses, Arch. Virol. 63:75 (1980).
43. G. A. Tannock, and J. C. Hierholzer, The RNA of human coronavirus OC-43, Virology 78:500 (1977).
44. G. A. Tannock, and J. C. Hierholzer, Presence of genomic polyadenylate and absence of detectable virion transcriptase in human coronavirus OC-43, J. Gen. Virol. 39:29 (1978).
45. G. A. Tannock, The nucleic acid of infectious bronchitis virus, Arch. Gesamte Virusforsch. 43:259 (1973).
46. D. J. Garwes, D. H. Pocock, and T. M. Wijaszka, Identification of heat-dissociable RNA complexes in two porcine coronaviruses, Nature 257:508 (1975).
47. M. W. Pons, Influenza virus messenger ribonucleoprotein, Virology 67:209 (1975).
48. M. Adesnik, and J. E. Darnell, Biogenesis and characterization of histone messenger RNA in HeLa cells, J. Mol. Biol. 67:397 (1972).
49. B. P. Holloway, and J. F. Obijeski, Rabies virus-induced RNA synthesis in BHK-21 cells, J. Gen. Virol. 49:181 (1980).
50. D. F. Stern, and S. I. T. Kennedy, Coronavirus multiplication strategy. I. Identification and characterization of virus-specified RNA, J. Virol. 34:665 (1980).
51. M. R. Macnaughton, and M. H. Madge, The genome of human coronavirus strain 229E, J. Gen. Virol. 39:497 (1978).
52. D. A. Kennedy, and C. M. Johnson-Lussenburg, Inhibition of coronavirus 229E replication by actinomycin D, J. Virol. 29:401 (1978).
53. W. B. Becker, K. McIntosh, J. H. Dees, and R. M. Chanock,

Morphogenesis of avian infectious bronchitis virus and a related human virus (strain 229E), J. Virol. 1:1019 (1967).
54. R. A. Bucknall, A. R. Kalica, and R. M. Chanock, Intracellular development and mechanism of hemadsorption of a human coronavirus, OC43, Proc. Soc. Exp. Biol. Med. 139:811 (1972).
55. H. A. Davies, and M. R. Macnaughton, Comparison of the morphology of three coronaviruses, Archives of Virology 59:25 (1979).
56. L. S. Oshiro, J. H. Schieble, and E. H. Lennette, Electron microscopic studies of coronavirus, J. Gen. Virol. 12:161 (1971).
57. E. O. Caul, C. R. Ashley, M. Ferguson, and S. I. Egglestone, Preliminary studies on the isolation of coronavirus 229E nucleocapsids, FEMS Microbiol. Letters 5:101 (1979).
58. D. A. Kennedy, and C. M. Johnson-Lussenburg, Isolation and morphology of the internal component of human coronavirus strain 229E, Intervirology 6:197 (1976).
59. M. R. Macnaughton, H. A. Davies, and M. V. Nermut, Ribonucleoprotein-like structures from coronavirus particles, J. Gen. Virol. 39:545 (1978).
60. J. Lenard, and R. W. Compans, The membrane structure of lipid-containing viruses, Biochem. Biophys. Acta 344:51 (1974).
61. R. W. Compans, and M. C. Kemp, Membrane glycoproteins of enveloped viruses, in: "Current Topics in Membranes and Transport" (R. L. Juliano and A. Rothstein, eds.), Vol. 11, Academic Press, New York, (1978).
62. R. W. Compans, and H. -D. Klenk, Viral membranes, in: "Comprehensive Virology," (H. Fraenkel-Conrat and R. R. Wagner, eds.), Vol. 13, Plenum Press, New York (1979).
63. B. W. Burge, and J. H. Strauss, Glycopeptides of the membrane glycoprotein of Sindbis virus, J. Mol. Biol. 47:449 (1970).
64. B. Sefton, and K. Keegstra, Glycoproteins of Sindbis virus: Preliminary characterization of the oligosaccharides, J. Virol. 14:522 (1974).
65. K. Keegstra, B. Sefton, and D. Burke, Sindbis virus glycoproteins: Effect of the host cell on the oligosaccharides, J. Virol. 16:613 (1975).
66. K. Nakamura, and R. W. Compans, Glycopeptide components of influenza viral glycoproteins, Virology 86:432 (1978).
67. K. Nakamura, and R. W. Compans, Biosynthesis of the oligosaccharides of influenza viral glycoproteins, Virology 93:31 (1979).
68. R. T. Schwarz, M. F. G. Schmidt, U. Anwer, and H. -D. Klenk, Carbohydrates of influenza virus. I. Glycopeptides derived from viral glycoproteins after labeling with radioactive sugars, J. Virol. 23:217 (1977).
69. S. A. Moyer, J. M. Tsang, P. H. Atkinson and D. F. Summers, Oligosaccharide moieties of the glycoprotein of vesicular stomatitis virus, J. Virol. 18:167 (1976).

70. J. R. Etchison, J. S. Robertson, and D. F. Summers, Partial structural analysis of the oligosaccharide moieties of the vesicular stomatitis glycoprotein by sequential chemical and enzymatic degradation, Virology 78:375 (1977).
71. M. C. Kemp, S. Basak, and R. W. Compans, Glycopeptides of murine leukemia viruses. I. Comparison of two ecotropic viruses. J. Virol. 31:1 (1979).
72. M. C. Kemp, N. G. Famulari, P. V. O'Donnell, and R. W. Compans, Glycopeptides of murine leukemia viruses. II. Comparison of xenotropic and dual-tropic viruses, J. Virol. 34:154 (1980).

GENOME STRUCTURE OF MOUSE HEPATITIS VIRUS: COMPARATIVE ANALYSIS BY OLIGONUCLEOTIDE MAPPING

Michael M.C. Lai and Stephen A. Stohlman

University of Southern California School of Medicine

2025 Zonal Avenue, Los Angeles, CA 90033

ABSTRACT

Several natural variants of mouse hepatitis viruses have been compared by the T_1-oligonucleotide fingerprinting technique. In general, they have diverged quite extensively. However, MHV-3, a hepatotropic strain, and A59, a nonpathogenic strain, were found to be extremely related. Yet, each of them contains 2-4 specific oligonucleotides. One of the MHV-3-specific oligonucleotides was mapped in 30S poly(A)-containing RNA or 6-7 Kb from the 3-end and the other near the 5'-end of the genome. These two genetic regions might be associated with viral pathogenicity. In addition, two JHM plaque variants, DL producing large plaques and DS producing small plaques, were also compared. They share almost all T_1-oligonucleotides, but each contains one unique spot. The DL-specific oligonucleotide was mapped in 21S poly(A)-containing RNA or at about 4 kb from the 3'-end. Finally, the MHV genome was found to contain the "cap" structure, confirming that it is a positive-stranded RNA.

INTRODUCTION

Mouse hepatitis viruses (MHV) are members of the coronavirus group which includes viruses infecting a variety of animals (Mc-Intosh, 1973). MHV infections occur primarily as natural, latent infections of mice (Gledhill and Niven, 1955) and have been isolated from many laboratory strains of mice (Calisher and Row, 1966). Experimentally, they induce a variety of pathological findings in animals: while most MHV strains cause fulminating hepatitis, a few strains are able to induce acute and chronic neurological diseases (Herndon et al, 1975; Virelizier et al, 1975). For instance, the JHM strain induces demyelinating encephalomyelitis (Weiner, 1973) and MHV-3 strain induces chronic choriodoependymitis and meningitis in some strains of mice (Virelizier et al, 1975). Still another strain, A59, has very low pathogenicity (Robb and Bond, 1978). The diversity in the disease potential of MHV offers a system for the study of mechanism of viral pathogenesis.

The genome of MHV has been shown to consist of a single piece of single-stranded 60S RNA (Lai and Stohlman, 1978; Wage et al, 1978). At least one third of the genomic RNA contains polyadenylated sequences and is infectious. Therefore, the MHV genome appears to be positive-stranded, although the presence of negative-stranded RNA in the MHV virion has not been ruled out. To study the genetic basis of viral pathogenicity, we have first characterized the RNA genome of various MHV strains by oligonucleotide mapping. We have identified some gene sequences which might be associated with pathogenicity of the different diseases caused by MHV. This approach thus proves to be useful for the study of molecular basis of viral pathogenicity.

MATERIALS AND METHODS

Viruses: MHV-1, MHV-3, and MHV-S were originally isolated from mice dying of acute hepatitis (Gledhill and Andrews, 1951; Dick, Niven, and Gledhill, 1956; and Rowe et al, 1963) and were obtained from Dr. Michael Collins, Microbiological Associates, Bethesda, Maryland. MHV-2 and MHV-A_{59} were also isolated from animals with acute hepatitis (Nelson, 1952; Manaker et al, 1961) and were obtained from K. Fujiwara, Tokyo, Japan and L. Sturman, Albany, N.Y. respectively. MHV-JHM was originally isolated from a mouse with hindleg paralysis and demyelination (Cheever et al, 1949; Bailey et al, 1949). The origin of plaque variant, designated DL, has been previously described (Lai and Stohlman, 1978). The DS variant was obtained from the 8th suckling mouse brain passage (Weiner, 1972) and cloned to homogeneity by 8 passages of single plaques using DBT cells and was used at the 6th subsequent *in vitro* passage in DBT cells for this study.

Oligonucleotide Mapping: Growth and purification of virus and extraction of RNA were carried out as previously described (Lai and Stohlman, 1978). The ^{32}P-labeled RNA was exhaustively digested with RNase T_1 and analyzed by two-dimensional polyacrylamide gel electrophoresis according to a modification of the pro-

Fig. 1 Oligonucleotide fingerprints of the genomic RNA of different MHV strains: The spots indicated by triangles are the oligonucleotides shared with the MHV-3 specific spots. The spots indicated by arrows are the oligonucleotides shared with the A59 specific oligonucleotides (see Fig. 3 for comparison).

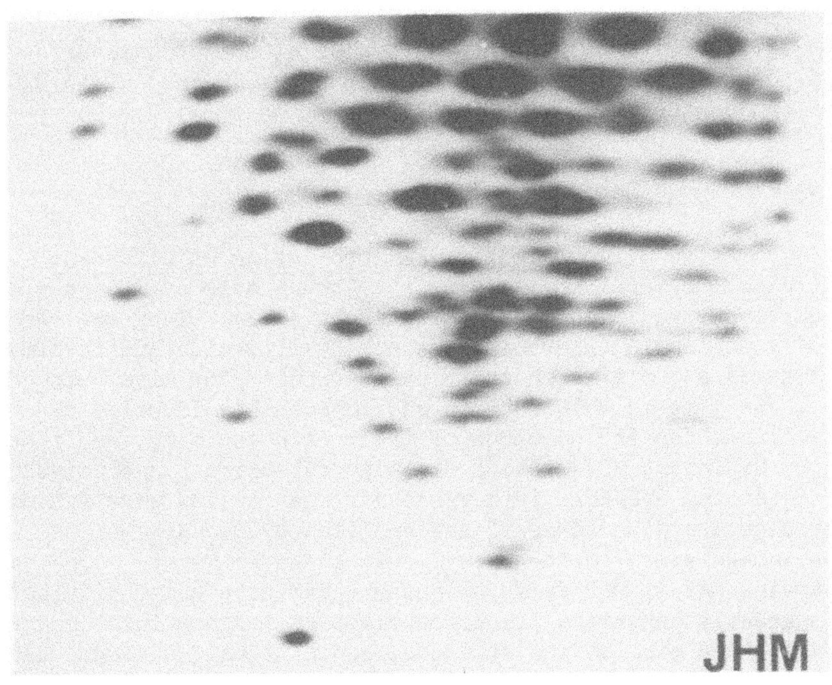
JHM

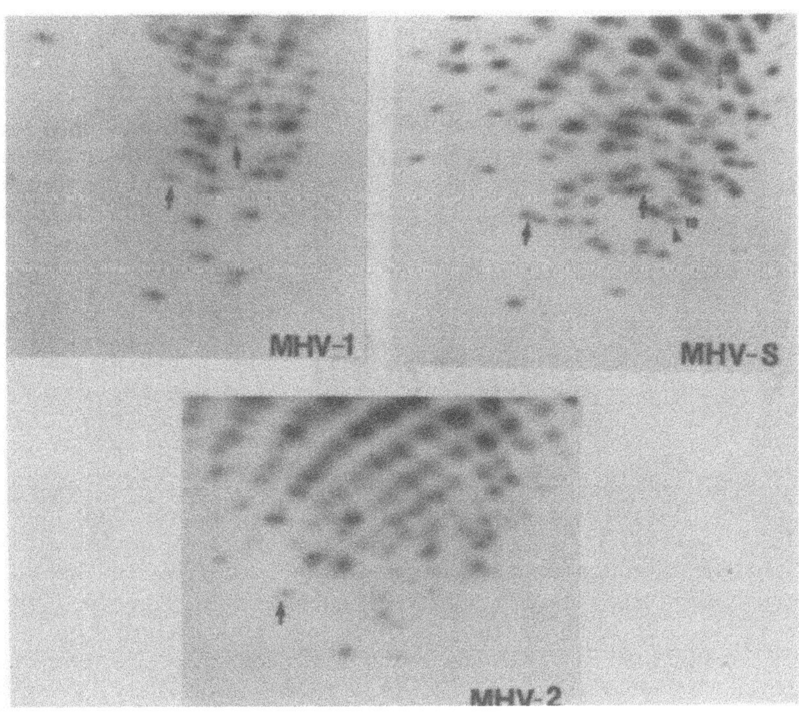
MHV-1
MHV-S

cedure by deWachter and Fiers (1972). The first dimension was performed on 8% polyacrylamide gel slabs (30 x 10 x 0.15 cm.) at pH 3.3, 700 $\bar{v}$ for 4 hours. The second dimension was performed on 22% polyacrylamide gel slabs (40 x 35 x 0.075 cm.) at pH 8.0, 650 $\bar{v}$ for 16 hours.

RESULTS

Comparative Oligonucleotide Fingerprinting of Different MHV Strains: Several MHV strains have been isolated independently from different mouse colonies (McIntosch, 1973). They are serologically separable (Hierholzer et al, 1979; Childs and Stohlman, unpublished) and differ in their pathogenicity for mice. To study their genetic relationship and to possibly identify the genetic basis for the spectrum of their pathogenicity, we first compared different MHV strains by oligonucleotide fingerprinting. The ^{32}P-labeled 60S RNAs from various virus strains were exhaustively digested with RNase T_1 and analyzed by two-dimensional polycrylamide gel electrophoresis. As shown in Figure 1, pathogenic MHV strains MHV-1, MHV-2, MHV-S and MHV-JHM have quite distinct and apparently unrelated T_1-oligonucleotide fingerprints, suggesting that all these strains isolated independently have diverged very extensively. In an attempt to understand the genetic basis for pathogenicity, we have compared these strains with a nonpathogenic strain MHV-A59. The fingerprints of the RNA mixtures of MHV-A59 and the other viruses (pictures not shown) were compared with the fingerprints of each individual viral RNA. As shown in Figure 2, these viruses share various degrees of homology with MHV-A59. If we assume that the large T_1-oligonucleotides are representative of the viral genome, the degree of sequence relatedness of different virus strains to MHV-A59 varies from 29% to 59%, except for MHV-3 (Figure 3), which has 97% sequence homology to A59 (Table 1). We therefore further studied MHV-3 and MHV-A59 extensively.

MHV-3 and MHV-A59 share about 95 out of 98 T_1-oligonucleotides which can be identified (Figure 3). But MHV-3 contains two spots, a and b, which are not present in MHV-A59, and MHV-A59 contains 4 spots, #13, #28, #19 and #9 which are MHV-A59 specific (the numbers of each spot are shown in Figure 5). Since these two strains are closely related antigenically (Childs and Stohlman, unpublished) and have similar protein profiles (Stohlman and Lai, 1979) but differ in their pathogenicity, some or all of these unique oligonucleotides might be derived from the genetic sequences which are associated with the pathogenic properties of the virus. If this is indeed the case, then all of the MHV strains having similar pathogenicity might contain the identical or related oligonucleotides. To test this possibility, we examined all MHV strains for the presence of these MHV-A59- or MHV-3-specific

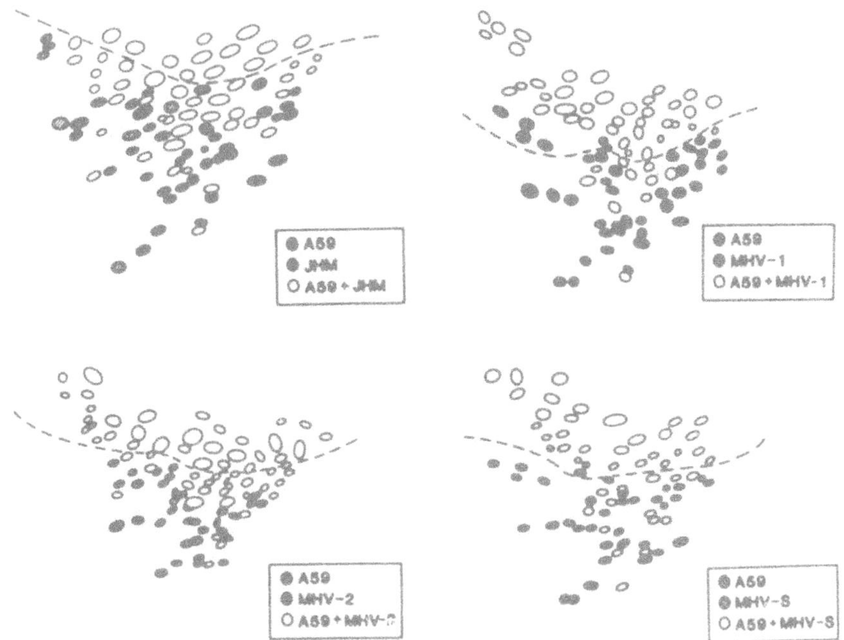

Fig. 2 Schematic drawing of the fingerprints of the RNA mixtures of A59 and other MHV strains: Equal amounts of ^{32}P-labeled RNAs from A59 and other MHV strains were mixed, digested with Rnase T_1 and analyzed by two-dimensional polyacrylamide gel electrophoresis. The origin of each spot was determined by comparing these fingerprints with the fingerprints of individual RNAs.

Table 1

Sequence relationship between MHV-A59 and other MHV strains

	The number of oligonucleotide spots shared with A59[a]	
MHV-1	8/28	(28%)
MHV-2	24/43	(55%)
MHV-3	95/98	(97%)
MHV-S	14/28	(50%)
JHM	32/54	(59%)

[a]) only the large T_1-oligonucleotides below the dashed lines in each fingerprints in Figure 2 were considered

oligonucleotides. Examination of Figure 1-3 reveals that one of the MHV-3 specific spots, a, is present in all 4 hepatotropic strains, but not in MHV-A59 or MHV-JHM, both of which cause minimal hepatitis (Table 2). The other spot, b, is present in MHV-1, MHV-3, and MHV-S, but not in MHV-2, A59 or JHM (Table 2). Therefore, these spots, particularly, spot a, appear to be widely preserved in and unique to most of the hepatotropic strains. On the other hand, among the 4 MHV-A59-specific oligonucleotides, #19 is present also in MHV-S, a hepatotropic strain of reduced virulence. #9 was occasionally seen in MHV-3; therefore, it is probably not a real MHV-A59 specific oligonucleotide. Thus, only #13 and #28 are unique to the nonpathogenic MHV-A59.

Mapping of MHV-3- or A59-specific oligonucleotides on the RNA genome: Since MHV-3 causes hepatitis in most strains of

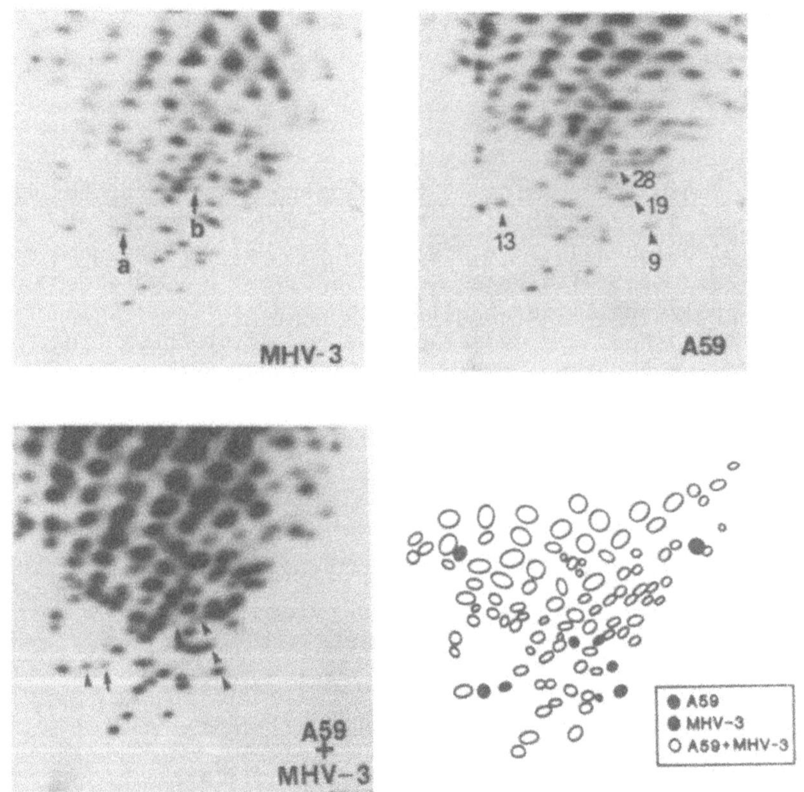

Fig. 3 Oligonucleotide fingerprints of MHV-3, A59 and their schematic drawing: The spots indicated by triangles and arrows are MHV-3 and A59 specific oligonucleotides, respectively.

Table 2

Distribution of MHV-3 and A59-specific oligonucleotides in different MHV strains*

	a	b	13	28	19	9
MHV-3	+	+	-	-	-	±
MHV-1	+	+	-	-	-	-
MHV-2	+	-	-	-	-	-
MHV-S	+	+	-	-	+	-
A59	-	-	+	+	+	+
JHM	-	-	-	-	-	-

* The data were obtained from Figure 1-3

mice and MHV-A59 has very low pathogenicity (Robb and Bond, 1978), the oligonucleotide spots unique to either virus could come from a region of the RNA genome which is associated with viral pathogenicity. It is, therefore, of interest to understand the localization of these specific spots on the RNA genome. To map these oligonucleotides, the ^{32}P-labeled 60S RNA was briefly degraded and passed through oligo(dT) cellulose column (Aviv and Leder, 1973). The poly(A)-containing RNA fractions were selected and separated by sucrose gradient sedimentation. The RNAs of different size fractions were then analyzed individually by oligonucleotide fingerprinting. Such an analysis of MHV-A59 is shown in Figure 4. From the oligonucleotides present in different size fractions of poly(A)-containing RNA, a map of oligonucleotide spots on the genome was obtained (Figure 5). It is seen that among the four probably MHV-A59-specific oligonucleotides, #28 is located near the extreme 5'-end of the genome; #13 is located in 30S poly(A)-containing RNA, or at about 6-7 kb from the 3'-end, and the other two spots, #19 and #9 are located in the 5'-half of the genome. Therefore, these 4 spots appear not to be contiguous on the genome.

Similar studies have been performed with MHV-3 RNA, and the oligonucleotide map is also presented in Figure 5 for comparison with MHV-A59. Since MHV-3 and MHV-A59 share most of the oligonucleotide spots, the oligonucleotides of MHV-3 were given numbers as corresponding to the spots identified in MHV-A59, except for the two MHV-3 specific spots. All of the shared oligonucleotides in MHV-3 were localized at exactly the same map positions as the corresponding spots in MHV-A59, confirming the genetic homology between the two viruses (The MHV-3 oligonucleotides which are identical to those of MHV-A59 are not represented in Figure 5).

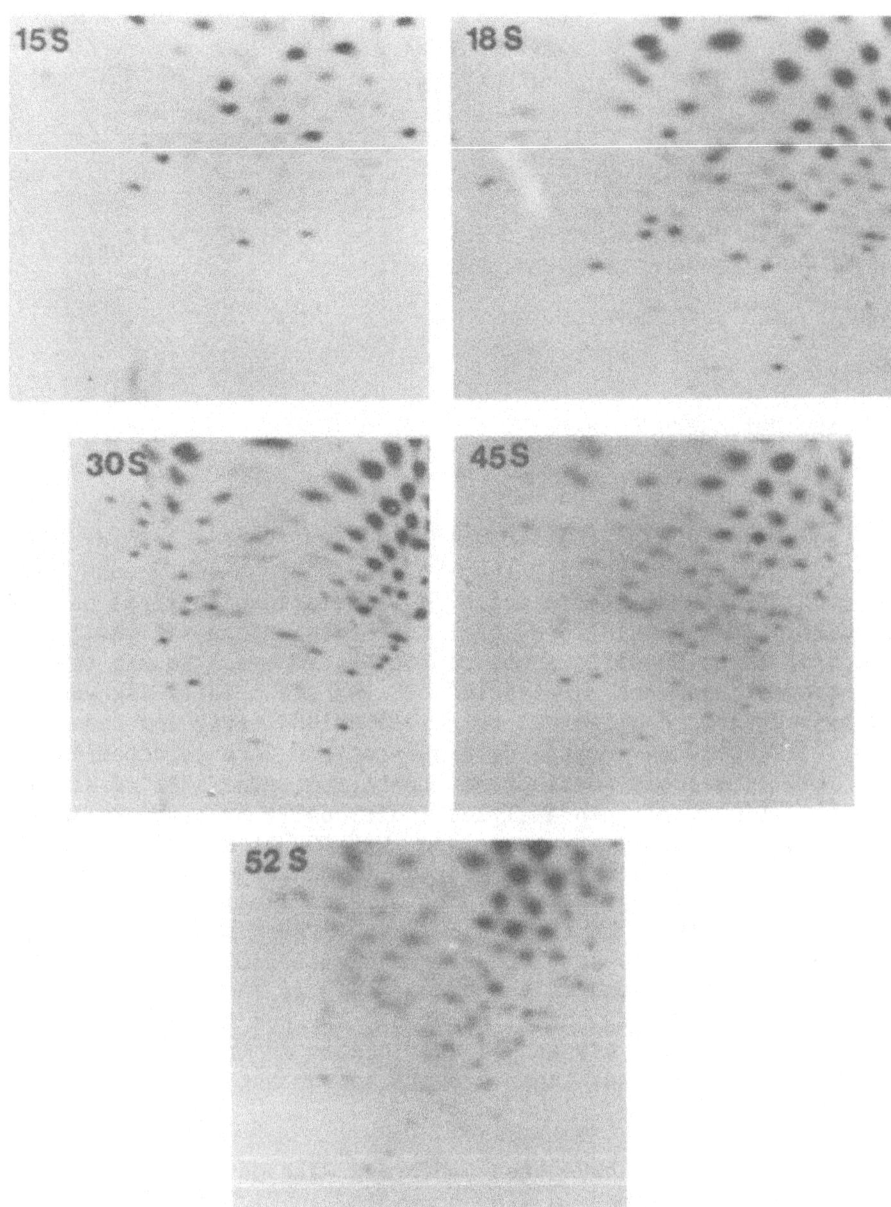

Fig. 4 Oligonucleotide fingerprints of the different size fractions of poly(A)-containing RNA of A59: The ^{32}P-poly(A)-containing A59 RNA was selected by oligo dT column, separated by sucrose gradient sedimentation and each size fraction was fingerprinted individually.

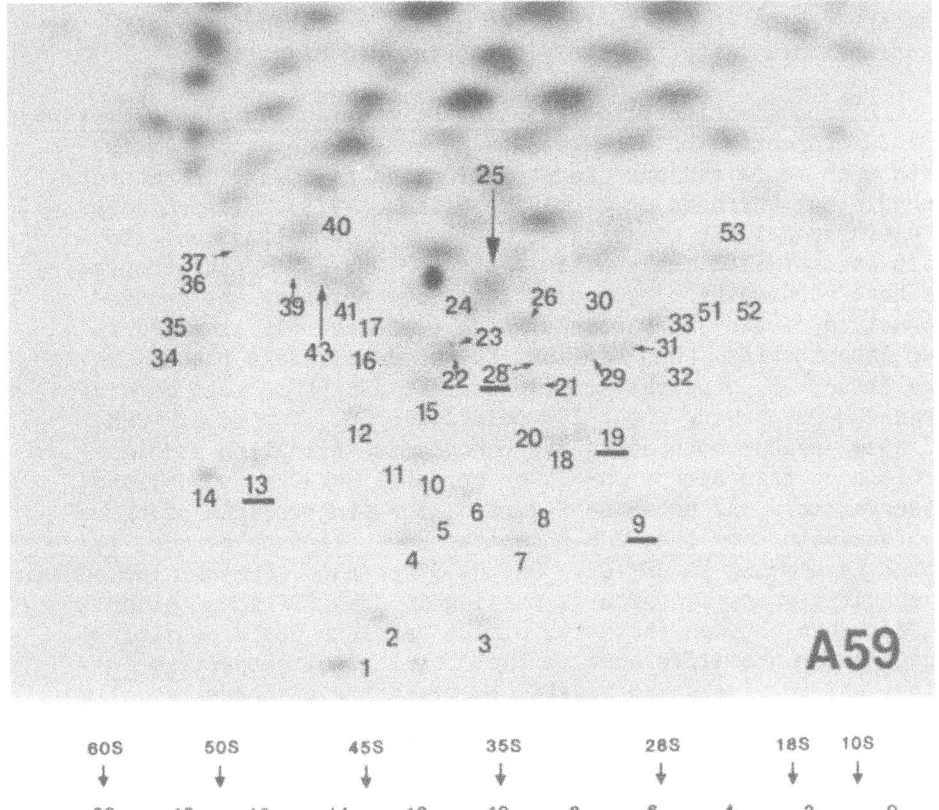

Fig. 5 Maps of the oligonucleotides on the RNA genome of A59 and MHV-3: The numbers of oligonucleotides were arbitrarily assigned. The numbers circled are A59-specific spots. The position of each oligonucleotide on the genome was estimated from the sedimentation values of different RNA size fractions. The map positions of all of the MHV-3 spots are identical to those of A59. Only the MHV-3-specific spots, a and b, are shown on the map.

As shown in Figure 5,one of the MHV-3 specific spots, a, was mapped at exactly the same location as the MHV-A59-specific spot #13, while the other MHV-3 specific spot, b, was mapped at the 5'-end, the same location as the MHV-A59-specific spot, #28. This suggests that a and #13, and b and #28 are probably related in their sequences, and represent the corresponding genetic regions in A59. It also suggests that these two regions, the 5'-end and the region at 6-7 kb from the 3'-end are associated with viral pathogenicity, possibly virus-induced hepatitis.

Oligonucleotide fingerprinting of the two JHM plaque variants: MHV-JHM infection of mice results in acute encephalomyelitis with both acute and chronic demyelination following intracerebral inoculation (Herndon et al, 1975; Weiner, 1973). It provides a useful model for studying virus-induced demyelination. To gain insight into the genetic basis for MHV-JHM's neurotropism, we have studied by oligonucleotide fingerprinting the genome structure of two JHM variants which were recently isolated in our laboratories. One variant, DL, produces large plaques while the other, DS, produces small plaques. JHM-DL is much more virulent than JHM-DS, having about 200-fold lower LD_{50} for mice. JHM-DS also induces both acute and chronic demyelination at higher efficiency than either JHM-DL or parental MHV-JHM (unpublished observation). As shown in Figure 6, the fingerprints of these two variants show that JHM-DS contains an oligonucleotide, x, which is missing in JHM-DL. On the other hand, JHM-DL also contains a specific spot, Z, which is missing in JHM-DS. These minor differences between these two plaque variants could possibly account for the difference in their biological properties *in vitro* and *in vivo*. The genetic localization of these two oligonucleotides is being investigated. Preliminary data showed that the JHM-DL specific spot, Z, was mapped in 21S poly(A)-containing RNA, or at 4 kb from the 3'-end (data not shown). The JHM-DS specific spot, x, was probably localized in 35S poly(A)-containing RNA or 9-10 kb from the 3'-end. Which of these two genetic regions is responsible for plaque size or demyelination is being studied.

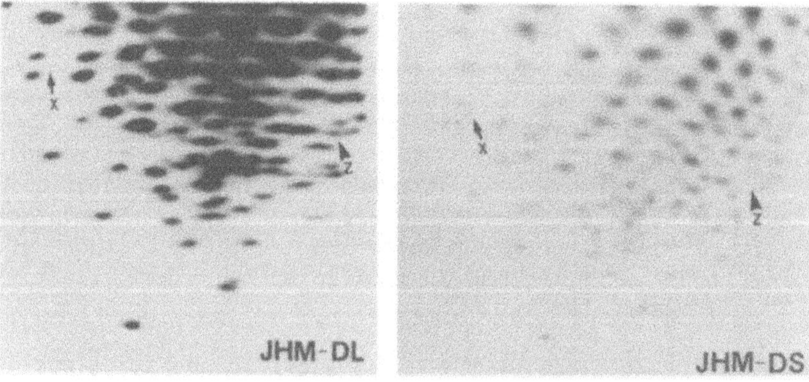

Fig. 6 Oligonucleotide fingerprints of JHM-DS and JHM-DL: The spots indicated by arrows are JHM-DS and JHM-DL specific spots.

The MHV RNA contains 5'-"cap" structure: Since the 60S RNA of MHV is a positive-stranded RNA, we wanted to know whether it contained a "cap" structure at its 5'-end (Shatkin, 1974; Furuich and Miura, 1975). The ^{32}P-labeled 60S MHV RNA was digested with a mixture of Rnase A, T1 and T2 and then electrophoresed on DEAE-cellulose paper at pH 3.5. Under this condition, the entire sequences of the RNA are digested into mono- or di- nucleotides except the "cap" structure, which has a characteristic electrophoretic mobility (Shatkin, 1974; Wang et al, 1977). As shown in Figure 7, the MHV RNA contains a "cap" structure which has similar electrophoretic mobility to that of the cap structure in Rous sarcoma virus (Wang et al, 1977; Keith and Fraenkel-Conrat, 1975), providing further evidence that MHV genome is a positive-stranded RNA.

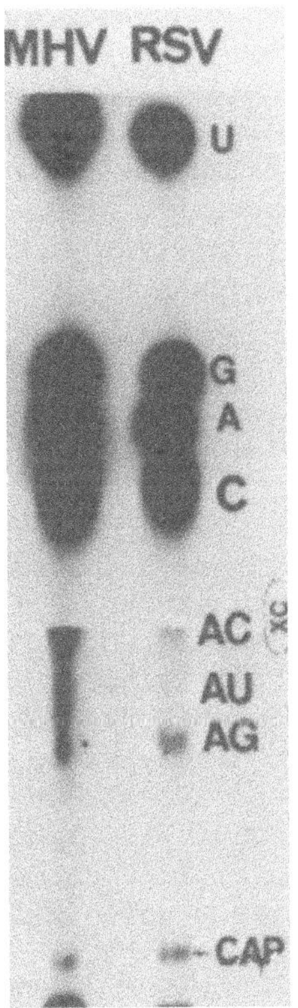

Fig. 7 Electrophoretic separation of RNA digests of A59: The ^{32}P-A59 RNA was digested with RNase A, T_1, and T_2 and then separated by electrophoresis on DEAE cellulose paper at pH 3.5 at 1500 v for 3 hours. The position of the "cap" structure was indicated on the electrophoregram. The lower part of the electrophoregram was exposed with an intensifying screen.

DISCUSSION

The studies presented in this communication represent our first attempts to understand the molecular basis of the pathogenesis of the diseases produced by MHV. Two major groups of diseases are caused by these viruses: hepatitis and demyelinating neurological disorders (McIntosch, 1973; Weiner, 1973; Herndon et al, 1974). Our oligonucleotide fingerprinting studies on a hepatotropic strain, MHV-3, and a nonpathogenic strain, MHV-A59, suggest that the genetic sequences associated with hepatitis might be localized at the region around 6-7 kb from the 3'-end, and possibly also at the 5'-end region. The latter location was inferred from the location of one of the MHV-3 specific oligonucleotides, b. However, this spot is not present in all of the hepatotropic strains and may be correlated with other diseases caused by MHV-3 (Virelizier et al, 1975). Therefore, the biological significance of the 5'-end sequences is questionable at the moment. In contrast, the region at 6-7 kb from the 3'-end contains the other MHV-3-specific oligonucleotide, a, which is present in all of the hepatotropic strains. If mouse hepatitis virus has the same mRNA structure as avian coronavirus, Infectious Bronchitis Virus, i.e. various virus-specific mRNAs have nested structure (Stern and Kennedy, 1980), it will suggest that the genetic sequences associated with viral pathogenicity will be present in the mRNA species with molecular weight of about $2.0\text{-}2.5 \times 10^6$, or 30S, and probably also the mRNA of the genome size. The translation products of such mRNA will be candidate proteins responsible for the difference in the biological and pathogenic properties of MHV-3 and MHV-A59.

The interpretation of our data is complicated by the fact that MHV-3 and A59 are natural variants of MHV. Therefore, it could not be ruled out that these two strains might differ in more respects than pathogenicity alone. Thus, the difference detected in their genome sequences does not necessarily reflect the pathogenicity. However, since pathogenicity is the only major difference between these two strains, it is likely that at least one of these two genetic locations might be associated with either hepatitis or other diseases caused by MHV-3 (Virelizier et al, 1975). More definitive studies will have to be performed with laboratory-derived virus mutants.

Studies on the neurotropic properties of MHV-JHM plaque variants had just begun. The small difference in their oligonucleotide fingerprints suggests that the difference between them is very minor, possibly involving only minor base substitutions. Since these two variants vary both in plaque size *in vitro* and in pathogenicity *in vivo* it is possible that they differ in more than one genetic location. Preliminary data mapped the two unique oligonucleotides at two different locations. The biological functions of these genetic regions is being investigated.

ACKNOWLEDGEMENTS

This investigation received partial financial support from Public Health Service grants NS 112967, CA 16113 from the National Institutes of Health and grant PCM-7904567 from the National Science Foundation.

REFERENCES

Bailey, O.T., Pappenheimer, A.M., Cheever, F.S., and J.B. Daniels. 1949. A murine virus (JHM) causing disseminated encephalomyelitis with extensive destruction of myelin. II. Pathology. J. Exp. Med. 90:195-212.

Calisher, C.H. and W.P. Rowe. 1966. Mouse hepatitis, Reo-3 and Theiler viruses. Nat. Cancer Inst. Monogr. 20:67-75.

Cheever, L.S., Daniels, J.B., Pappenheimer, A.M., Bailey, O.T. 1949. A murine virus (JHM) causing disseminated encephalomyelitis with extensive destruction of myelin. I. Isolation and biological properties of the virus. J. Exp. Med. 90: 181-194.

De Wachter, R. and W. Fiers. 1972. Preparative two dimensional polyacrylamide gel electrophoresis of ^{32}P-labeled RNA. Anal. Biochem. 49:184-197.

Dick, G.W., Niven, J. and A. Gledhill. 1956. A virus related to that causing hepatitis in mice (MHV). Brit. J. Exp. Path. 38:90-96.

Furuich, Y. and K. Miura. 1975. A blocked structure at the 5' terminus of mRNA from cytoplasmic polyhedrosis virus. Nature 253:374-375.

Gledhill, A. and O.C. Andrews. 1951. A hepatitis virus of mice. Brit. J. Exp. Path. 32:559-568.

Gledhill, A.W. and J.S.F. Niven. 1955. Latent virus as exemplified by mouse hepatitis virus (MHV). Vet. Rev. Annot. 1:82-90.

Herndon, R.M., Griffin, D.E., McCormick, U., and Weiner, L.P. 1975. Mouse hepatitis virus-induced recurrent demyelination. Arch. Neurol. 32:32-35.

Hierholzer, J.C., Broderson, J.R. and F. Murphy. 1979. New strain of mouse hepatitis virus as the cause of lethal enteritis in infant mice. Inf. Immun. 24:508-522.

Keith, J. and H. Fraenkel-Conrat. 1975. Identification of the 5'-end of Rous sarcoma virus RNA. Proc. Natl. Acad. Sci. USA 72:3347-3358.

Lai, M.M.C. and Stohlman, S.A. 1978. The RNA of mouse hepatitis virus. J. Virol. 26:236-242.

Manaker, R.A., Piczak, C., Miller, A. and M. Stanton. 1961. A hepatitis virus complicating studies with mouse leukemia. J. Natl. Canc. Inst. 27:29-51.

McIntosh, K. 1973. Coronaviruses: A comparative review. Curr. Top. Microbiol. Immunol. 63:85-129.

Nelson, J.B. 1952. Acute hepatitis associated with mouse leukemia. I. Pathologic features and transmission of the disease. J. Exp. Med. 196:293-300.

Robb, J.A. and C.W. Bond. 1979. Pathogenic murine coronaviruses. I. Characterization of the biological behavior in vitro and virus-specific intracellular RNA of strongly neurotropic JHMV and weakly neurotropic A59V viruses. Virology 94:352-370.

Rowe, W., Hartley, J. and W. Capps. 1963. Mouse hepatitis virus infection as a highly contagious, prevalent enteric infection of mice. Proc. Soc. Exp. Biol. Med. 112:161-165.

Shatkin, A.J. 1974. Methylated messenger RNA synthesis in vitro by purified reovious. Proc. Natl. Acad. Sci. USA 71:3204-3207.

Stern, D.F. and S.I.T. Kennedy. 1980. Coronavirus multiplication strategy. I. Identification and characterization of virus-specific RNA. J. Virol. 34:665-674.

Stohlman, S.A. and M.M.C. Lai. 1979. Phosphoproteins of murine coronaviruses. J. Virol. 32:672-675.

Virelizier, J.L., Dayan, A.D. and Allison, A.C. 1975. Neuropathological effects of persistent infection of mice by mouse hepatitis virus (MHV-3). Infection and Immunity 12:1127-1140.

Wang, L.H., P.H. Duesberg, T. Robins, et al. 1977. The terminal oligonucleotides of avian tumor virus RNAs are genetically linked. Virology 82:472-492.

Wege, H., A. Muller, and V. ter Meulen. 1978. Genomic RNA of the murine coronavirus of JHM. J. Gen. Virol. 41:217-228.

Weiner, L.P.: Pathogenesis of demyelination induced by a mouse hepatitis virus (JHM virus). Arch. Neurol. 28:298-303.

THE STRUCTURE OF THE CANINE CORONAVIRUS

David J. Garwes

Agricultural Research Council
Institute for Research on Animal Diseases
Compton, Nr. Newbury, Berks., U.K.

During a survey of canine sera in 1970, Norman and his associates detected antibodies to porcine transmissible gastroenteritis (TGEV). Since many of the dogs had never been in contact with pigs it was unlikely that this reflected infection with the porcine virus, suggesting the existence of a canine virus that was serologically related to TGEV. Further evidence to support this was provided by the study by Cartwright and Lucas (1972) of an outbreak of gastroenteritis in a kennel of 40 dogs in which rising antibody titres to TGEV were found. Although neither of these studies could find evidence of transmission of TGEV from pigs to dogs, this possibility could not be discounted since Haelterman (1962) had clearly demonstrated that dogs and foxes could be infected with the porcine virus. Dogs that were experimentally infected with TGEV showed no clinical signs but the virus could be reisolated from faeces and TGEV-neutralizing antibodies were produced in the serum.

The picture became clearer, however, when Binn and his associates (1975) reported their isolation of a canine enteric coronavirus, designated 1-71, from American military dogs suffering from diarrhoea. This virus was readily cultivated in puppies, in which it caused severe gastroenteritis, but would not infect piglets. It was antigenically related to TGEV but lacked the ability to infect porcine cells.

Our interest in the canine coronavirus (CCV) grew out of our studies on TGEV. For the past few years there has been very little TGEV in the U.K. although the pigs would seem to be fully susceptible. Since it is in the national interest to keep the number of TGEV outbreaks down to the minimum we became interested in the role of the dog and the cat (Reynolds and Garwes, 1979) as potential carriers of the virus. In both of these instances, the epizootiology is confused by the presence of TGEV-related coronaviruses in the carrier, i.e. canine coronavirus and feline infectious peritonitis virus (Reynolds et al., 1977). We have studied the serological relationships of these viruses (Reynolds et al., 1980) and compared the structures of CCV and TGEV (Garwes and Reynolds, 1980). This paper summarizes our findings for the structural polypeptides of these two coronaviruses.

We used the 1-71 isolate of CCV for this study, grown in secondary dog kidney cells. To ensure that we were not working with a mixed population of virus we developed a plaque assay procedure and used this to clone the virus three times. Several clones were selected at each plaquing step and were subsequently tested to determine whether any obvious differences in their structural polypeptides could be detected but they were indistinguishable from each other and from the parent stock by this method.

Like many other coronaviruses, the growth of CCV in primary and secondary cell cultures does not result in very high titres. Yields of 10^6-10^7 $TCID_{50}$/ml were achieved but we did not consider that these were adequate to carry out chemical studies on the virus and we therefore resorted to the use of radiolabelled precursors, incorporated into the growth medium.

The virus was purified by the procedure that we had established for TGEV; removal of cell debris by low speed centrifugation, concentration of the virus by ammonium sulphate precipitation followed by 2 rounds of centrifugation in sucrose gradients (Garwes and Pocock, 1975). Following dissociation of the purified virus by sodium dodecyl sulphate and β-mercaptoethanol, the polypeptides were separated by electrophoresis on 5% acrylamide gels crosslinked with ethylene diacrylate using a phosphate buffer system.

The electropherograms shown in Fig. 1 were obtained from virus that had been grown in the presence of ^{3}H-leucine (a), ^{35}S-methionine (b) and ^{3}H-glucosamine hydrochloride (c). It can be seen that there are 4 major polypeptides of which 3 are glycosylated. The presence of minor components cannot be excluded but the small peaks and humps between the first and second major polypeptides tended to be inconsistent from preparation to preparation. By comparison with the rates of migration of proteins of known molecular weights, the sizes of the 4 major polypeptides of CCV were estimated from 18 determinations using 13 different batches of virus and this is summarised in Table 1. The molecular weights of gp 204, gp 32 and gp 22 are only approximate as the carbohydrate present on these glycopolypeptides will affect their migration rates.

We had previously shown that the high molecular weight glycopolypeptide of TGEV was associated with the peplomers that

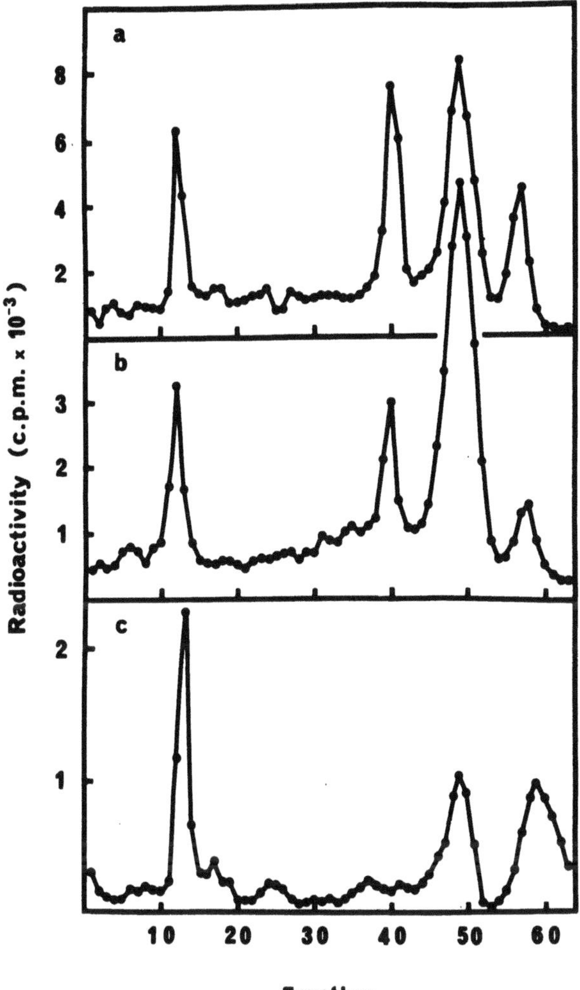

Fig. 1. Polyacrylamide gel electropherograms of CCV polypeptides labelled with (a) ^{3}H-leucine, (b) ^{35}S-methionine and (c) ^{3}H-glucosamine. Migration was from the left.

Table 1. The Structural Polypeptides of Canine Coronavirus

Polypeptide Designation	Molecular Weight	Standard Deviation	Glycosylation
gp 204	203,800	6,400	+
p 50	49,800	900	-
gp 32	31,800	1,100	+
gp 22	21,600	1,500	+

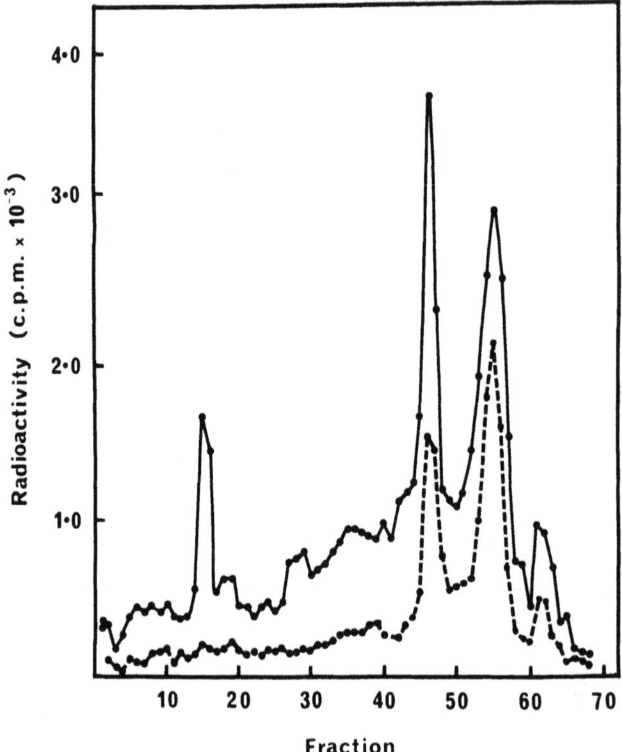

Fig. 2. Polyacrylamide gel electropherograms of CCV polypeptides. Control, ●—● : NP40-treated, ●--●. Migration was from the left.

protrude from the surface of the virion and that these could be removed from the virus following solubilisation of the lipid envelope with detergent (Garwes et al., 1976). A similar procedure was attempted with CCV; purified virus was treated with 1% Nonidet P40 at room temperature for 15 minutes and then centrifuged through a sucrose gradient. The RNA-containing subviral particles were recovered from the gradient and compared with virus that had been treated with water and then centrifuged as a control. The resultant electropherograms of these 2 preparations are shown in

Fig. 2. The polypeptide profile of the detergent-treated virus resembles that of the control in most respects but it is obvious that gp 204 is lacking from the subviral particle. This is only circumstantial evidence for the role of gp 204 in the structure of the CCV peplomer, however, as electron microscopy of the subviral particles revealed structures that, although lacking the characteristic coronavirus projections, were so morphologically altered that there is no certainty that peplomers would be seen even if they were present (Fig. 3).

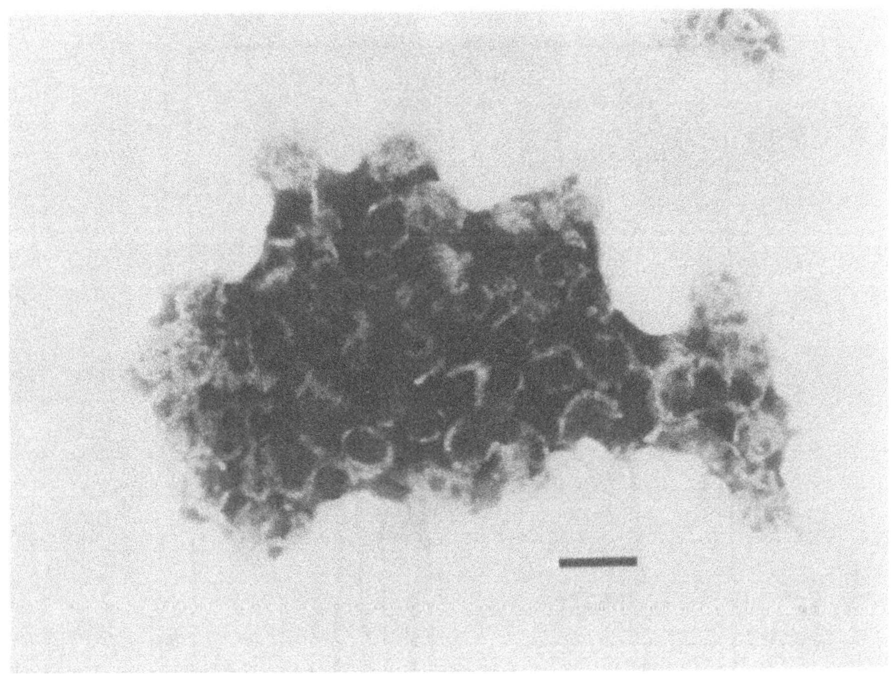

Fig. 3. Electron micrograph of CCV subviral particles. 2% sodium phosphotungstate, pH 7.2. The bar represents 100 nm.

The apparent molecular weights of the CCV polypeptides were strikingly similar to those found for TGEV (Garwes and Pocock, 1975). For an accurate comparison to be made between the two viruses, differences that might be caused by host-induced glycosylation patterns or by variation between polyacrylamide gels would need to be avoided. To this end, TGEV was grown in secondary dog kidney cells under identical conditions to those used for CCV. The titre of virus achieved was similar to that for CCV but TGEV produced much greater cytopathic changes in the cells, resulting in cell rounding and detachment within 18h after infection. We were unable to show any replication of CCV in secondary pig thyroid cells, the culture system employed by us for TGEV (D. Reynolds, personal communication).

In order to analyse TGEV and CCV in the same polyacrylamide gel, we used ^{3}H-leucine and ^{35}S-methionine for double label experiments. When purified preparations of CCV that had been grown in ^{3}H-leucine and ^{35}S-methionine were pooled and subjected to gel electrophoresis,

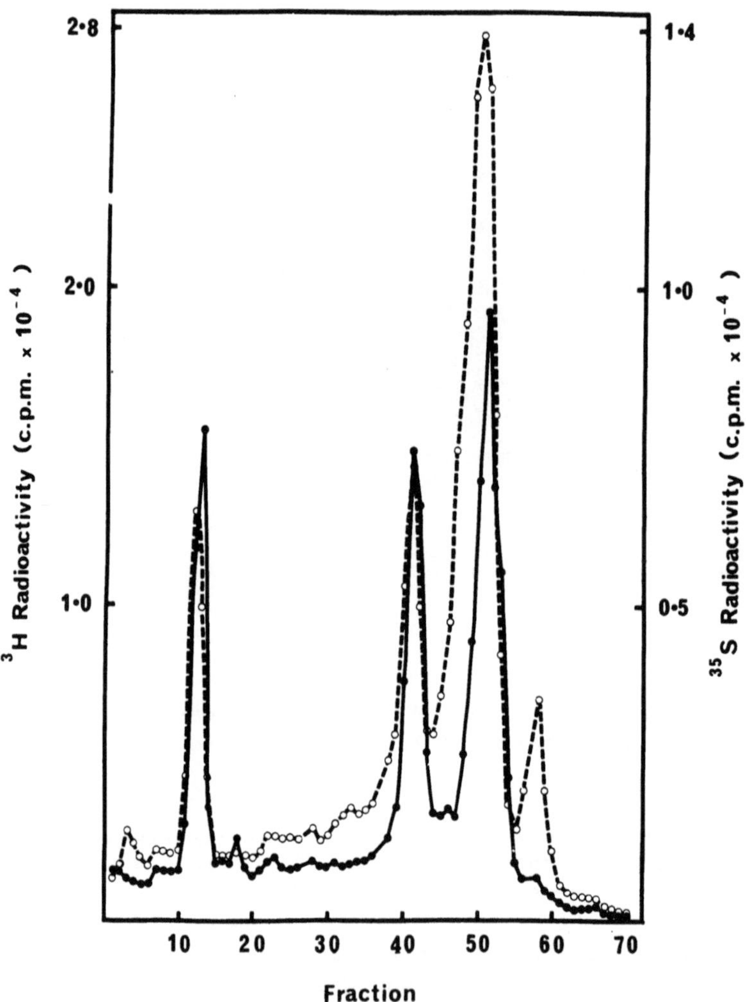

Fig. 4. Polyacrylamide gel electropherogram of the structural polypeptides of ^{35}S-methionine-CCV (O) and ^{3}H-leucine-TGEV (●). Migration was from the left.

the resulting peaks coincided exactly, showing that the substitution of one label for another had no noticeable effect on the migration rates of the polypeptides. There was a marked difference in the relative proportions of ^{3}H-leucine and ^{35}S-methionine in gp 32, comparable with Sturman's observation of a relative richness of methionine in the membrane glycopolypeptide of the murine coronavirus A59 (Sturman, 1977).

Co-electrophoresis of CCV and TGEV that had been grown in different labels showed several differences. An example of ^{3}H-leucine-TGEV and ^{35}S-methionine-CCV is illustrated in Fig. 4 but a similar profile was obtained with ^{35}S-methionine-TGEV and ^{3}H-leucine-CCV (except for the height of the gp 32 peak of CCV, as just mentioned). Whereas p50 of both CCV and TGEV exactly coincided, gp 204 and gp 32 of CCV were slightly, but reproducibly, larger than their equivalents in TGEV. More noticeable, however, was the absence of a major polypeptide of 22,000 daltons in TGEV. We cannot rule out the possibility that TGEV may have a gp 22 (or equivalent) as a minor constituent but it is clearly not present in the quantities seen in CCV. It was possible that CCV gp 22 was a cleavage product of one of the other major viral polypeptides but this seems unlikely if one examines the candidates: gp 204 is removed by detergent but gp 22 is not; p50 is not glycosylated whereas gp 22 is; gp 32 is rich in methionine but gp 22 does not appear to be. It appears that CCV may have 2 membrane glycopolypeptides, a feature shown by several other coronaviruses (Garwes, 1980) including, as previously suggested (Garwes and Pocock, 1975), TGEV.

In conclusion, then, we can say that CCV and TGEV are related in their polypeptide structure as well as antigenically. Considering the lack of similarity between TGEV and other coronaviruses, including the other porcine member haemagglutinating encephalomyelitis virus, the close relationship between CCV and TGEV strongly suggests that they were derived either one from the other or both from a common parent during the evolution of the Coronaviridae. One might speculate that a mutation of CCV, resulting in a decrease in the size of gp 204 and gp 32 and in the loss of gp 22, allowed the modified CCV to grow in porcine cells yielding TGEV. Further, the new virus TGEV could grow in its old host (dog) as well as its new (pig) whereas the CCV stock could not grow in pig cells. This is, however, pure speculation but it is possible that more information on the evolution of this antigenic subgroup of coronaviruses will become available when the structure of the third member of the group, feline infectious peritonitis virus, is elucidated.

I gratefully acknowledge the close collaboration of Mrs. D. Reynolds in this study, the able technical assistance of

Miss Fiona Stewart-Smith and the generous gift of primary dog kidney cells by Dr. A. Whitaker, Wellcome Research Laboratories, Beckenham, U.K.

References

Binn, L.N., Lazar, E.C., Keenan, K.P., Huxsoll, D.L., Marchwicki, R.H. and Strano, A.J., 1975, Recovery and characterization of a coronavirus from military dogs with diarrhoea, Proc. 78th Meeting U.S. Anim. Hlth. Assoc., 359.

Cartwright, S.F. and Lucas, M.H., 1972, Vomiting and diarrhoea in dogs, Vet. Rec., 91:571.

Garwes, D.J., 1980, Structure and physicochemical properties of coronaviruses, in: "Viral Enteritis in Humans and Animals", I.N.S.E.R.M., Grignon, France.

Garwes, D.J. and Pocock, D.H., 1975, The polypeptide structure of transmissible gastroenteritis virus, J. gen. Virol., 29:25.

Garwes, D.J., Pocock, D.H. and Pike, B.V., 1976, Isolation of subviral components from transmissible gastroenteritis virus, J. gen. Virol., 32:283.

Garwes, D.J. and Reynolds, D.J., 1980, The polypeptide structure of canine coronavirus and its relationship to porcine transmissible gastroenteritis virus, J. gen. Virol., in the press.

Haelterman, E.O., 1962, Epidemiological studies of transmissible gastroenteritis of swine, Proc. 66th Ann. Meeting U.S. Livestock Sanit. Assoc., 305.

Norman, J.O., McClurkin, A.W. and Stark, S.L., 1970, Transmissible gastroenteritis (TGE) of swine : Canine serum antibodies against an associated virus, Can. J. Comp. Med., 34:115.

Reynolds, D.J. and Garwes, D.J., 1979, Virus isolation and serum antibody responses after infection of cats with transmissible gastroenteritis virus, Arch. Virol., 60:161.

Reynolds, D.J., Garwes, D.J. and Gaskell, C.J., 1977, Detection of transmissible gastroenteritis virus neutralising antibody in cats, Arch. Virol., 55:77.

Reynolds, D.J., Garwes, D.J. and Lucey, S., 1980, Differentiation of canine coronavirus and porcine transmissible gastroenteritis virus with canine, porcine and feline sera, Vet. Microbiol., in the press.

Sturman, L.S., 1977, Characterization of a coronavirus. 1. Structural proteins : Effects of preparative conditions on the migration of protein in polyacrylamide gels, Virology, 77:637.

CHARACTERISATION OF VIRAL RNA IN CELLS INFECTED WITH THE MURINE CORONAVIRUS JHM

Helmut Wege, Stuart Siddell, Margarete Sturm and Volker ter Meulen

Institute for Virology and Immunobiology, University of Würzburg, Federal Republic of Germany

SUMMARY

The murine coronavirus JHM induces in Sac(-) cells seven major and two minor RNA species. These RNAs are polyadenylated and single stranded. Their sizes were estimated by electrophoresis in agarose gels containing methylmercury hydroxide. The mol. wts. for the major species are 6.67×10^6 for RNA of genome size, 3.42×10^6 for RNA 2, 2.76×10^6 for RNA 3, 1.35×10^6 for RNA 4, 1.19×10^6 for RNA 5, 0.93×10^6 for RNA 6 and 0.62×10^6 for RNA 7. The minor species have a size of 4.7×10^6 (RNA a) and 1.5×10^6 (RNA b). No essential difference in the number and proportion of each RNA species was found between total cytoplasmic RNA, polyadenylated cytoplasmic RNA and RNA extracted from pelleted polysomes, nor was any difference found during the infection cycle. The major RNA species are likely to be subgenomic mRNAs.

INTRODUCTION

Mouse hepatitis viruses deserve special attention because of their potential for experimental studies of acute and chronic diseases. These agents induce a variety of diseases in small rodents (Robb et al. 1979). In tissue culture systems, both lytic and persistent infections are readily established (Lucas et al., 1978; Stohlman et al., 1979). The strain JHM is particularly interesting because of its ability to cause chronic disorders of the central nervous system in mice and rats (Weiner et al., 1973; Nagashima et al., 1979). However, little is known on the replication of this virus in lytic and persistent infections, a prerequisite for studies of the pathogenesis of these diseases.

The essential features of the JHM virus structure are now established. The genome of JHM virus consists of a single stranded polyadenylated RNA which is infectious and has a mol. wt. (in millions) of at least 5.6 (Lai and Stohlman, 1978; Wege et al., 1978). Purified virus consists of six major proteins with a mol. wt. between 23.000 and 170.000. Four of the proteins are glycosylated (Wege et al., 1979). In the infected cell, several virus specific polypeptides are synthesized and their possible relationship to the structural proteins have been investigated (Siddell et al., 1981; Bond et al., 1979). The cell free translation of RNA extracted from JHM infected cells provides strong evidence for the existence of several subgenomic mRNAs (Siddell et al., 1980). As a basis for the final characterisation of the mRNAs of JHM virus and their translation products we describe here the number and size of JHM virus specific RNA synthesized in infected cells.

MATERIAL AND METHODS

Details of virus growth, maintenance of cells, radioactive labelling, virus purification and extraction of RNA are described in previous communications (Wege et al. 1978 and 1979, Siddell et al., 1980).

Virus and cells. The JHM virus was originally obtained from L. Weiner, Johns Hopkins University, as a suckling mouse brain suspension. It was adapted to Sac (-) cells, a permanent murine Moloney sarcoma cell line (Weiland et al., 1978) and cloned by plaque passages.

Electrophoresis of RNA. RNA was elctrophoresed in 0.9 % agarose gels after denaturation with glyoxal-DMSO

(McMaster and Carmichael 1977). Alternatively, 0,9 % agarose gels containing 5 mM methylmercury hydroxide (Bailey & Davidson, 1976) were used. For fluorography, gels were soaked in Enhance (NEN-Chemicals), transferred into water, dried and exposed at - 70° C to Kodak XR5 film. RNA species were recovered from composite agarose polyacrylamide urea gels (Floyd et al., 1974) by excision, homogenisation and reextraction with phenol SDS. The extracted RNAs were poly A selected on poly U sepharose columns.

RESULTS

Kinetics of viral growth and RNA synthesis.

Suspension cultures of Sac (-) cells were infected with a m.o.i. of 4 p.f.u. per cell and pulsed at various

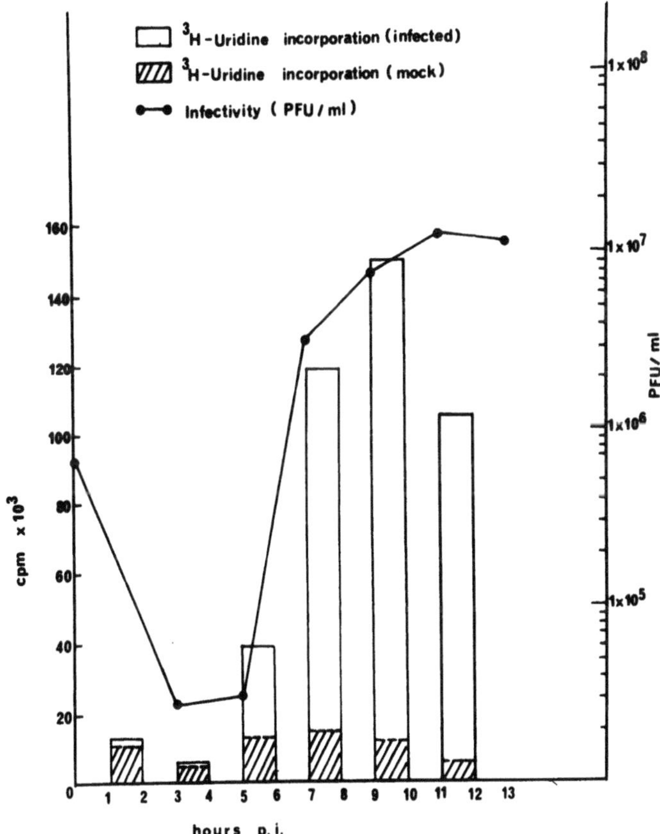

Fig.1: Rate of RNA synthesis and release of infectious virus from JHM infected Sac (-) cells (m.o.i. 4 p.f.u/cell).

times for 1 h. Actinomycin D (1 µg/ml) was added before labelling with 3 H-uridine. At this concentration actinomycin D does not inhibit the growth of infectious virus. The rate of virus specific RNA synthesis was measured by determination of trichloracetic acid precipitable radioactivity from cytoplasmic lysates.

As Fig. 1 shows, an increase of virus specific RNA synthesis was first detected at about 4 h p.i. and the rate of RNA synthesis reached a peak at 9 h p.i.. Infectious virus was released into the culture medium in parallel to the production of RNA.

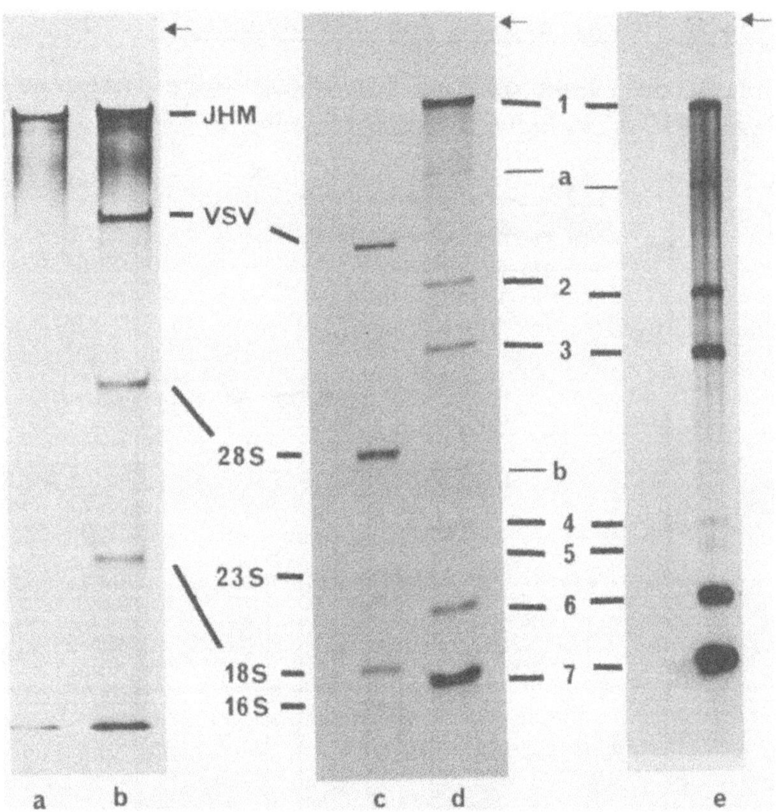

Fig. 2 Fluorograms of JHM-RNAs separated by electrophoresis in 0.9 % agarose gels. Denaturation of RNA samples either with glyoxal (slot a, b, c and d) or methylmercury hydroxide (slot e). a) and b) JHM virion RNA, c) marker-RNAs. Ribosomal RNA of E. coli and L-cells, VSV virion RNA, d) total cytoplasmic RNA denatured with glyoxal DMSO, e) total cytoplasmic RNA denatured with methylmercury hydroxide.

Virion RNA and total viral cytoplasmic RNA

Virion RNA labelled with 3 H uridine was extracted from purified virus and electrophoresed after glyoxal-DMSO treatment. The majority of the virion RNA migrated as a single homogeneous band considerably slower then the genome RNA of vesicular stomatitis virus (Fig. 2 a and b). Virion RNA comigrates with a cytoplasmic RNA species of the same size and the mol. wt. (in millions) of both species was determined to be 6.67. This value is bigger than estimated previously under non denaturing conditions.

For the preparation of cytoplasmic RNA, cells were labelled with 3 H uridine in the presence of actinomycin D for 4 - 6 1/2 h p.i. under single cycle growth conditions. The total cytoplasmic RNA was extracted by phenol SDS. Electrophoresis of total cytoplasmic RNA reproducibly revealed seven major and two minor species (Fig. 2 d). The major RNA species are numbered in order of decreasing size starting with the RNA of genome size as No. 1. The minor species designated with the letter "a" was detected at the same intensity in all preparations of cytoplasmic RNA, whereas the minor species "b" varied to some extend from batch to batch and was not always visible.

An essentially identical RNA pattern was obtained after denaturation of total cytoplasmic RNA with methylmercury hydroxide (Fig. 2 e). This more rigorous chaotropic agent was used for the determination of the mol. wts. of the individual RNA species (Fig. 3 a). The mol. wts. were obtained by coelectrophoresis and mixing of cytoplasmic RNA with radioactively labelled marker RNAs consisting of E.coli 16 S and 23 S RNA, ribosomal 18 S and 28 S L-cell RNA and vesicular stomatitis virion RNA. The standard deviations for each RNA species were obtained by measurements in at least four independent gels and are listed in Fig. 3 b. The values of the mol. wts. determined after glyoxal-DMSO treatment differ only slightly from this figures.

The cytoplasmic RNA pulse labelled early (4 h p.i.) and late(9 h p.i.) during a single growth cycle were analysed. The same number and quantity of RNA species were found. By chromatography on poly U sepharose 50 - 60 % of the cytoplasmic RNA was found to be polyadenylated. Electrophoresis of polyadenylated RNA reveals the same pattern as shown for total cytoplasmic RNA (Fig. 4 b)

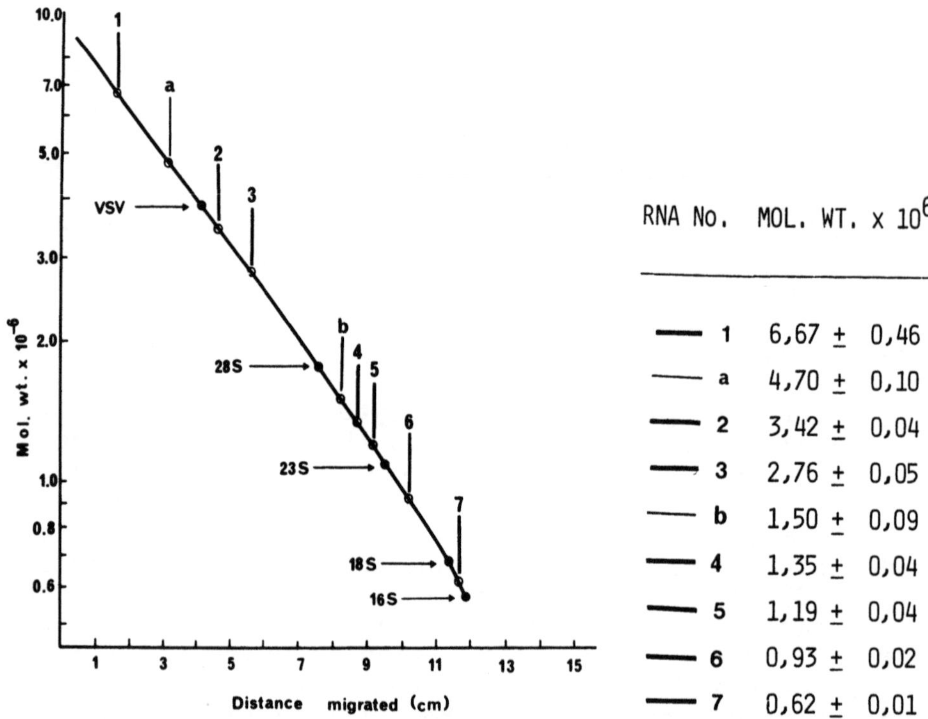

RNA No.	MOL. WT. x 10^6
1	6,67 ± 0,46
a	4,70 ± 0,10
2	3,42 ± 0,04
3	2,76 ± 0,05
b	1,50 ± 0,09
4	1,35 ± 0,04
5	1,19 ± 0,04
6	0,93 ± 0,02
7	0,62 ± 0,01

Fig. 3 a) Calibration curve for determination of mol. wts. obtained by electrophoresis of RNAs in 0.9 % agarose-methylmercury hydroxide gels. The following marker RNAs were used: Vesicular stomatitis virus genome (mol. wt. in millions 3.8, Repik and Bishop, 1971), ribosomal 18 S and 28 S RNA from L-cells (mol. wts. in millions 0.68 and 1.74, Loening, 1968) E. coli 16 S and 23 S RNA (mol. wt. in millions 0.55 and 1.07, Stanley & Bock, 1965). The positions of the individual intracellular RNAs relative to the marker RNAs are indicated by vertical bars.
b) Table of mol. wt. of JHM-RNAs.

The RNA species numbered 1 - 7 are single stranded as judged by their sensitivity to digestion with pancreatic RNAse. For this purpose, 32 P labelled cytoplasmic polyadenylated RNA was separated by electrophoresis in polyacrylamide urea gels, cut out after localisation by autoradiography from the gel and reextracted by phenol SDS. The individual RNAs were digested with pancreatic RNAse and ribosomal RNA extracted from the same gels was used as a control. Therefore, these RNA species are most probably polyadenylated single stranded subgenomic mRNAs.

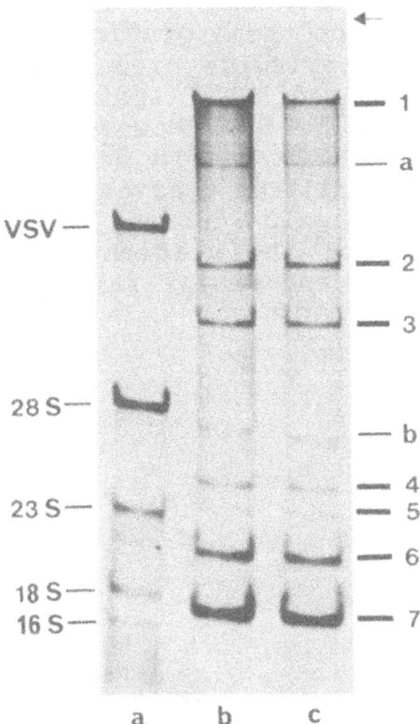

Fig. 4 Fluorogram of JHM-RNA electrophoresed after denaturation with glyoxal-DMSO in 0.9 % agarose slot a) same marker RNAs as in Fig. 2c, slot b) polyA selected cytoplasmic JHM RNA slot c) JHM RNA extracted from polysomes.

Additional support for this conclusion is the association of these RNA species with the polysomes of infected cells. Cytoplasmic extracts obtained by lysis with NP40 were centrifuged into 15 - 40 % sucrose gradients and fractionated. The fractions which sedimented faster than the monosomal 80 S peak were pooled and pelleted through a discontinuous gradient consisting of 2 M and 0.5 M sucrose. Electrophoresis of the RNA extracted from this preparation by phenol SDS revealed no essential difference in comparison to polyadenylated cytoplasmic RNA (Fig. 4 b and c). This polysomal pellet could still contain RNA incorporated into nucleocapsids, which might sediment through 2.0 M sucrose. Therefore, a polysomal pellet was resuspended and analysed on a 15 - 40 % sucrose gradient. As shown in Fig. 5a, the polysomal profile recorded at 260 nm is still conserved. The profile of radioactively labelled RNA showed a typical bimodal distribution. Analysis of RNA from individual fractions of this polysome gradient by electrophoresis in agarose polyacrylamide urea gels revealed, that most of the genome sized RNA 1 sediments in the region heavier than 200S (Fig. 5b). However, pretreatment of polysomal pellets by EDTA before density gradient centrifugation released all RNA species from the polysomes. Therefore, if nucleocapsids containing RNA 1 are existing in this region of the gradient, these structures might be very fragile and easily falling apart.

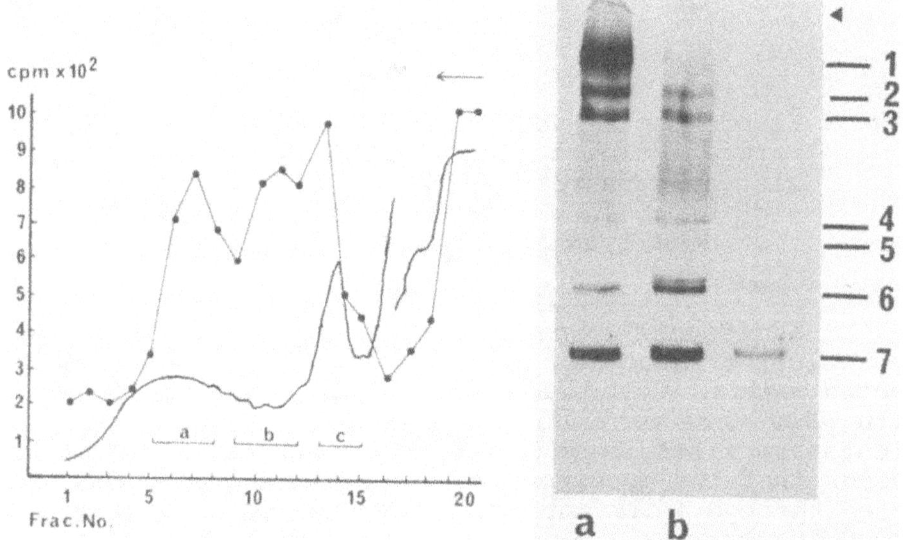

Fig. 5: Sedimentation of polysomes in 15 - 40 % sucrose gradients. a) Distribution of radioactivity (o--o) and optical density at 260 nm (---).b) Electrophoresis in agarose-polyacrylamide urea gels. slot a), b), RNA from the gradient as indicated by bars in Fig. 5a.

CONCLUSION

JHM virus infection of Sac(-) cells leads to the induction of RNA of genome size and six major polyadenylated single stranded subgenomic RNAs. Previous experiments have shown that the smallest RNA codes for a viral protein with a mol. wt. of 60,000 and the next smaller RNA for a viral protein with a mol. wt. of 23,000 (Siddell et al., 1980). Identical results were obtained by translation of RNA 7 (mol. wt. in millions 0.62) and RNA 6 (mol. wt. in millions 0.93) recovered from agarose polyacrylamide urea gels. These results and the translation of other RNA species (Siddell et al., this volume) support the conclusion that coronavirus proteins are synthesized by a set of several independent subgenomic RNAs, which are functionally monocistronic.

ACKNOWLEDGEMENTS

We thank Mrs. Hanna Wege for excellent technical assistance and Mrs. Christa Sieber for typing the manuscript. This work was supported by the Deutsche Forschungsgemeinschaft and the Österreichische Gesellschaft zur Bekämpfung der Muskelerkrankungen

REFERENCES

Bailey, J.M. and Davidson, N. (1976). Methylmercury as a reversible denaturing agent for agarose gel electrophoresis. Analytical Biochemistry 70, 75 - 85.

Bond, C.W., Leibowitz, J.L. and Robb, J.A. (1979). Pathogenic murine coronaviruses. II. Characterization of virus-specific proteins of murine coronavirus JHMV and A59V. Virology 94, 371-384.

Floyd, R.W., Stone, M.P. and Joklik, W.K. (1974). Separation of single-stranded ribonucleic acids by acrylamide-agarose-urea gel electrophoresis. Analytical Biochemistry 59, 599-609.

Lai, M.M.C. and Stohlman, S.A. (1978). RNA of Mouse hepatitis virus.
Journal of Virology 26, 236-242.

Loening, U.E. (1968). Molecular weights of ribosomal RNA in relation to evolution.
Journal of Molecular Biology 38, 355-365.

Lucas, A., Coulter, M., Anderson, R., Dales, S. and Flintoff, W. (1978). In vivo and in vitro models of demyelinating diseases. II. Persistence and host regulated thermosensitivity in cells of neuronal derivation.
Virology 88, 325 - 337.

McMaster, G.K. and Carmichael, G.G. (1977). Analysis of single and double-stranded nucleic acids on polyacrylamide and agarose gels by using glyoxal and acridine orange.
Proceedings of the National Academy of Science, U.S.A. 74,4835-4838.

Nagashima, K., Wege, H., Meyermann, R. and ter Meulen, V. (1979). Demyelinating encephalomyelitis induced by a long-term corona virus infection in rats. Acta Neuropathologica 45, 205 - 213.

Repik, P. and Bishop, D.H.L. Determination of the molecular weight of animal RNA viral genomes by nuclease digestion. I. Vesicular stomatitis virus and its defective T particle.
Journal of Virology 12, 969-983.

Robb, J.A. and Bond, C.W. (1979). Coronaviridae. In: H. Fraenkel-Conrat and R.R. Wagner (ed.), Comprehensive Virology 14, 193-247. Plenum Press, New York.

Stohlman, S.A., Sakaguchi, A.Y. and Weiner, L.P. (1979) Characterisation of the cold-sensitive murine hepatitis virus mutants rescued from latently infected cells by cell fusion.
Virology 98, 448-445.

Siddell, S., Wege, H., Barthel, A. and ter Meulen, V. (1981). Coronavirus JHM: Intracellular protein synthesis.
Journal of General Virology, in press.

Siddell, S., Wege, H., Barthel A. and ter Meulen, V. (1980). Coronavirus JHM: Cell-free synthesis of structural protein p60.
Journal of Virology 33, No. 1, 10-17.

Stanley, W.M. and Bock, R.M. (1965). Isolation and physical properties of the ribosomal ribonucleic acid of E. coli.
Biochemistry 7, 1302-1311.

Wege, H., Wege, Hanna, Nagashima, K. and ter Meulen, V. (1979). Structural polypeptides of the murine coronavirus JHM.
Journal of General Virology 42, 37-47.

Wege, H., Müller, A. and ter Meulen, V. (1978). Genomic RNA of the murine coronavirus JHM.
Journal of General Virology, 41, 217-227.

Weiland, E.M., Mussgay F. and Weiland, F. (1978). Nonproducer malignant tumor cells with rescuable sarcoma virus genome isolated from a recurrent Moloney sarcoma.
Journal of Experimental Medicine 148, 408-423.

Weiner, L.P. (1973). Pathogenesis of demyelination induced by a mouse hepatitis virus (JHM virus).
Archives of Neurology, 28, 293-303.

RELATEDNESS OF VIRION AND INTRACELLULAR PROTEINS OF THE MURINE CORONAVIRUSES JHM AND A59

Clifford W. Bond, Kevin Anderson, Susan Goss, and Lisa Sardinia

Department of Microbiology
Montana State University
Bozeman, MT. 59717

INTRODUCTION

Coronaviruses are a group of RNA viruses with positive polarity that cause a wide variety of diseases in many species including man. The structural proteins of coronaviruses have been studied extensively (reviewed in Robb and Bond, 1979). However, little attention has been focused on the intracellular proteins (Bond et al. 1979, Anderson et al. 1979, Siddel et al. 1980).

We have described 9 intracellular and viral-specific proteins of the murine coronaviruses JHM and A59 (Bond et al. 1979). Four of these 9 viral-specific proteins were identified as structural proteins.

In this communication, we compare the virion and intracellular viral-specific proteins of JHM and A59 viruses and describe post-translational events observed in murine coronaviral-specific protein synthesis.

MATERIALS AND METHODS

Cells

The source and growth of the murine cell lines 17CL-1 and DBT have been described previously (Sturman and Takemoto, 1972; Hirano et al. 1974; Bond et al. 1979).

Virus

The source and growth of the A59 and JHM virus stocks have been described previously (Bond et al. 1979). Cells were infected in suspension, and virus was adsorbed at 37° for 30 min at a cell density of 10^7 cells/ml. Adsorbed cells were centrifuged, resuspended in prewarmed (37°) Dulbecco's Modified Eagle's Medium with 2% fetal bovine serum (DME2) at a density of 2×10^6 cells/ml, plated into plastic culture dishes at a density of 3×10^5 cells/cm^2, and reincubated at 37°.

Preparation of Intracellular Proteins

Cells were infected by JHM or A59 virus at a multiplicity of infection (MOI) of 0.3 plaque forming units (PFU)/cell, and incubated at 37°. At the labeling time indicated in the experiment, the cell layers were washed twice with methionine-free DME2, and pulse-labeled with ^{35}S-methionine (100 µCi/ml) in methionine-free DME2 for the time period indicated. At the end of the pulse-period, the cell layers were washed twice with serum-free complete medium (DME0), and chased with DME2 or lysed *in situ*. Cells were lysed *in situ* at 0° with buffer B10 [10 mM Tris-HCl (pH 7.4), 5 mM $MgCl_2$, 0.5% (vol/vol) NP40, 0.1% (wt/vol) sodium dodecyl sulfate (SDS), 1% (vol/vol) Aprotinin, 50 µg/ml ribonuclease, 50 µg/ml deoxyribonuclease] and the cytoplasmic lysates were stored at -20°.

Immunoprecipitation

Cytoplasmic lysates were immunoprecipitated as follows. A cytoplasmic lysate representing 1.25×10^6 cells (50 µl) was diluted 10 fold with buffer B11 [50 mM Tris-HCl (pH 7.4), 150 mM NaCl, 5 mM EDTA, 0.02% (wt/vol) sodium azide, 0.05% (vol/vol) NP40, 1% (vol/vol) Aprotinin, 0.1% (wt/vol) bovine serum albumin]. Twenty µl of antisera (either mouse-anti-JHM virus or mouse-anti-A59 virus) were added to the suspension, incubated for one hr at 0°, and the immune complexes were precipitated with 50 µl of 10% (vol/vol) fixed *Staphylococcus aureus* (Cowan) by incubation for one hr at 0°. Antiviral antisera were prepared as previously described (Robb and Bond, 1979), and fixed *S. aureus* (Cowan) were prepared as described by Kessler (1975). The pellets were washed 3 times with buffer B11, and resuspended in 20 µl of 20 mM DTT, 1% (wt/vol) SDS. The proteins were eluted and reduced by incubation at room temperature for 15 min followed by heating at 60° for 5 min. The *S. aureus* (Cowan) were removed by centrifugation and the supernatant fraction was alkylated with N-ethylmaleimide at 0° for one hr as described by Crawford and O'Farrell (1979).

Preparation of Virion Proteins

Cells were infected by JHM virus or A59 virus at an MOI of 0.1 PFU/cell as described above and incubated at 33°. At 10 hrs PI, the infected cells were washed twice with methionine/5 DME2, and labeled with ^{35}S-methionine (50 µCi/ml) in methionine/5 DME2. The cell culture fluid was harvested at 70% cell lysis (24-30 hrs PI) and centrifuged at 2000 x g for 20 min. The supernatant fraction was layered onto a step gradient consisting of layers of 10%, 17%, and 40% (wt/wt) potassium tartrate in PNE buffer [30 mM PIPES (pH 6.5), 100 mM NaCl, 1 mM EDTA], and centrifuged at 153,400 x g for 90 min at 4°. The fraction containing infectious virus was diluted with PNE buffer, layered onto a linear gradient consisting of 10 to 40% (wt/wt) potassium tartrate in PNE buffer, and centrifuged to equilibrium at 208,800 x g for 5 hrs at 4°. Fractions were pooled on the basis of radioactivity, and Aprotinin was added to 1% (vol/vol). The suspension was dialyzed against 0.01 M NH_4HCO_3, lyophilized, and the resulting powder was resuspended in buffer B10. The suspension was adjusted to 20 mM DTT, 1% (wt/vol) SDS, and heated to 45° for 5 min. The proteins were alkylated with N-ethylmaleimide for one hr at 0° as described by Crawford and O'Farrell (1979).

Polyacrylamide Slab Gel Electrophoresis

Reduced and alkylated proteins were electrophoresed on 6%, 8%, or 10% polyacrylamide slab gels as described by Laemmli and Favre (1973) with the following exception. The resolving gel was supplemented with 0.5% (wt/vol) linear polyacrylamide. Volumes representing approximately equivalent cell numbers were loaded in each lane of the slab gel.

RESULTS

Cells (17CL-1) were infected with A59 virus or mock infected and labeled with ^{35}S-methionine for 30 min, 60 min, 120 min or 180 min beginning at 8 hrs PI (Figure 1). This time point was chosen because it was a time of maximum protein synthesis, and was during the time of logarithmic production of infectious virus at 37°. The density of the major viral-specific protein bands (150K, 60K, 57K, 54K, and 23K) was a function of the length of the labeling time. The 22K protein was not detectable until the length of the labeling period was 120 min. The 22K protein was readily detectable in a 180 min labeling period. An identical experiment was done with JHM virus, and similar data was obtained (data not shown). These data suggest that the 22K protein may be the result of posttranslational modification of a precursor protein. To test this hypothesis, the following experiment was done.

Cells (17CL-1) infected with A59 virus or mock infected were pulse-labeled with ^{35}S-methionine for 30 min, and chased for 0 min, 20 min, 40 min, 60 min, 80 min, and 100 min. Immunoprecipitates were electrophoresed on either 10% (Figure 2) or 6% (Figure 3) polyacrylamide slab gels. The results clearly indicate that the 23K protein band lost density, and the 22K protein band gained density during the chase (Figure 2). The density of the 150K band decreased during the chase (Figure 3). However, there was no concomitant increase of a corresponding protein during the chase. There was no significant evidence of posttranslational cleavage of precursor proteins in any other region of the gels. An identical experiment was done with JHM virus and similar data were obtained. Identical experiments were done using DBT cells infected by JHM virus or A59 virus, and similar results were obtained.

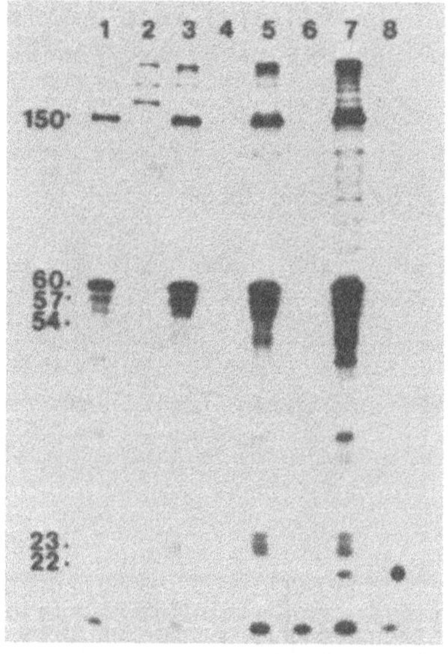

Fig. 1. The spectrum of viral-specific proteins synthesized by 17CL-1 cells infected by A59 virus or mock infected as a function of the length of the labeling period. Cells were infected with A59 virus (lanes 1, 3, 5, 7) or mock infected (lanes 2, 4, 6, 8), labeled with ^{35}S-methionine for 30 min (lanes 1, 2), 60 min (lanes 3, 4), 120 min (lanes 5, 6) or 180 min (lanes 7, 8), and immunoprecipitated. The immunoprecipitates were reduced and alkylated, and electrophoresed on an 8% polyacrylamide slab gel as described in Materials and Methods.

Structural proteins of purified JHM and A59 virions were compared with the intracellular proteins described in the previous experiments. The results are shown in Figure 4. The 63K intracellular protein of JHM virus and the 60K protein of A59 virus comigrate with the respective structural proteins of purified virions. The 150K and 22K proteins are not evident in the virion lanes of Figure 4. However, both were faintly evident in the original autoradiograms suggesting that these proteins are precursors to the slower migrating species. The 23K intracellular protein of JHM virus migrated slightly differently in comparison with the structural proteins of JHM virions. The 23K intracellular protein of A59 virus migrated slightly faster than the structural proteins of A59 virions. These data suggest that the 23K protein is not directly assembled into the virion without modification.

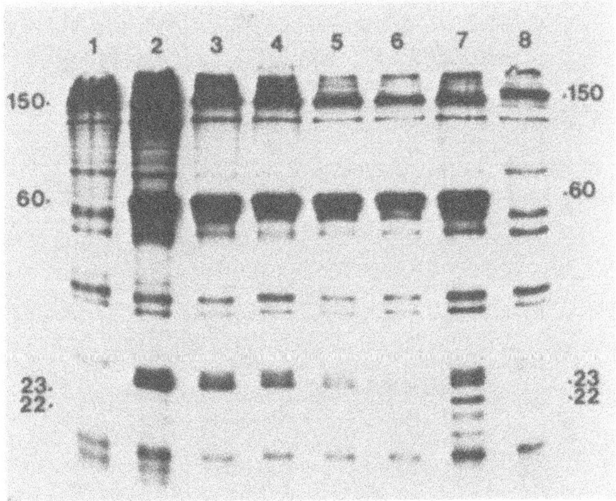

Fig. 2. Pulse-chase of viral-specific proteins synthesized by 17CL-1 cells infected by A59 virus or mock-infected. Cells infected by A59 virus (lanes 2-7) or mock infected (lanes 1, 8) were pulse-labeled with ^{35}S-methionine for 30 min, chased for 0 min (lanes 1, 2), 20 min (lane 3), 40 min (lane 4), 60 min (lane 5), 80 min (lane 6) or 100 min (lanes 7, 8), and immunoprecipitated. The immunoprecipitates were reduced and alkylated, and electrophoresed on a 10% polyacrylamide slab gel as described in Materials and Methods.

DISCUSSION

The data presented above demonstrate that the 23K intracellular protein of JHM and A59 viruses is processed to a 22K protein which is assembled into the virion. The 23K intracellular protein does not appear to be assembled directly into the virions of JHM and A59 without processing to the 22K species because it migrates differently than the structural proteins of these viruses. The 61K and 56K intracellular proteins of JHM virus, and the 57K and 54K intracellular proteins of A59 virus are not represented in the respective virions. Anderson et al. (1979) suggested that these proteins are the result of posttranslational modification of the 63K protein (JHM) or the 60K protein (A59). The data shown in Figures 2 and 3 do not support this contention.

The 150K intracellular protein bands of JHM and A59 viruses decrease in density during the chase (Figure 3). We have previously shown that this protein is glycosylated by glucosamine and mannose (Bond et al. 1979). This protein is incorporated into the virion

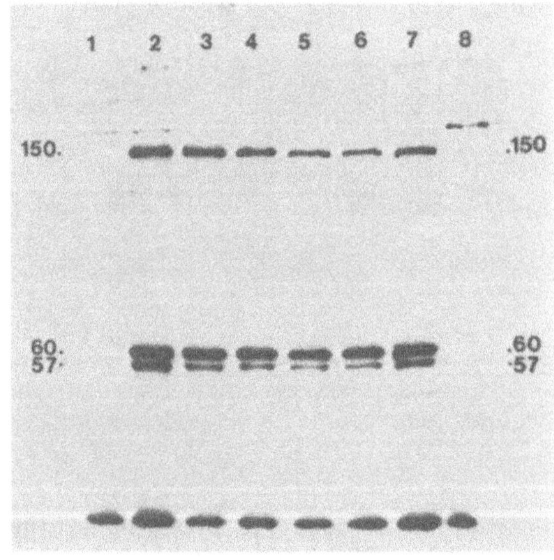

Fig. 3. Pulse-chase of viral-specific proteins synthesized by 17CL-1 cells infected by A59 virus or mock infected. The reduced and alkylated immunoprecipitates described in the legend to Figure 2 were electrophoresed in the corresponding lanes of a 6% polyacrylamide slab gel as described in Materials and Methods.

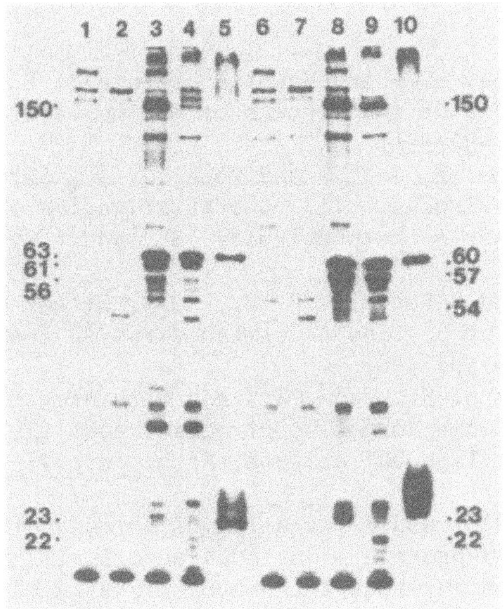

Fig. 4. Comparison of the intracellular and virion proteins of JHM virus and A59 virus. Cells were infected by JHM virus (lanes 3, 4), A59 virus (lanes 8, 9) or mock infected (lanes 1, 2, 6, 7), pulse-labeled with ^{35}S-methionine for 30 min, chased for 0 min (lanes 1, 3, 6, 8) or chased for 100 min (lanes 2, 4, 7, 9), and immunoprecipitated. Virion proteins of JHM (lane 5), and A59 (lane 10) were prepared as described in Materials and Methods. The immunoprecipitates and virion proteins were reduced and alkylated, and electrophoresed on an 8% polyacrylamide slab gel as described in Materials and Methods.

directly (Figure 4), and is probably then glycosylated to the slower migrating species found in the virion.

The pulse-chase experiments were done using DBT cells as well as 17CL-1 cells. Similar results were obtained. These results indicate that the posttranslational modifications are viral-specific, and not cellular artifacts. Aprotinin, a protease inhibitor, was utilized throughout the processing steps to eliminate protease activity that would result in cleavage artifacts.

Further work including tryptic peptide mapping of the structural and intracellular viral-specific proteins is in progress to further define the relatedness of the intracellular and virion proteins of the murine coronaviruses JHM and A59.

REFERENCES

Anderson, R., Cheley, S., and Haworth-Hatherell, E., 1979, Comparison of polypeptides of two strains of murine hepatitis virus, Virology, 97:492-494.

Bond, C. W., Leibowitz, J. L., and Robb, J. A., 1979, Pathogenic murine coronaviruses. II. Characterization of virus-specific proteins of murine coronaviruses JHMV and A59V, Virology, 94: 371-384.

Crawford, L. V. and O'Farrell, P. Z., 1979, Effect of alkylation on the physical properties of simian virus 40 T-antigen species, J. Virol., 29:587-596.

Hirano, N., Fujiwara, K., Hine, S., and Matumoto, M., 1974, Replication and plaque formation of mouse hepatitis virus (MHV-2) in mouse cell line DBT culture, Arch. ges. Virusforsch., 44: 298-302.

Kessler, S. W., 1975, Rapid isolation of antigens from cells with a Staphylococcal protein A-antibody adsorbent: Parameters of the interaction of antibody-antigen complexes with protein A. J. Immunol., 115:1617-1624.

Laemmli, U. K. and Favre, M., 1973, Maturation of the head of bacteriophage T4: I. DNA packaging events, J. Mol. Biol., 80:575-599.

Robb, J. A. and Bond, C. W., 1979a, Coronaviridae, in "Comprehensive Virology", vol. 14, H. Fraenkel-Conrat and R. R. Wagner, eds., pp. 193-247, Plenum Publishing Corp., New York.

Robb, J. A. and Bond, C. W., 1979b, Pathogenic murine coronaviruses. I. Characterization of biological behavior in vitro and virus specific intracellular RNA of strongly neurotropic JHMV and weakly neurotropic A59V viruses, Virology, 94:352-370.

Siddell, S. G., Wege, H., Barthel, A., and Ter Meulen, V., 1980, Coronavirus JHM: Cell-free synthesis of structural protein p60, J. Virol., 33:10-17.

Sturman, L. S. and Takemoto, K., 1972, Enhanced growth of a murine coronavirus in transformed mouse cells, Infection and Immunity, 6:501-507.

ASSEMBLY OF MOUSE HEPATITIS VIRUS STRAIN JHM

Andrew Massalski, Marion Coulter-Mackie and Samuel Dales

Cytobiology Group, Department of Microbiology and
Immunology, University of Western Ontario
London, Ontario N6A 5C1 Canada

INTRODUCTION

Coronaviruses have been characterized as a separate group (26), predominantly based on the morphology of their unique, massive peplomers and single stranded $^{+}$RNA genome (22). Electron microscopic studies on different members of this group revealed that assembly occurs in the cytoplasm, where progeny are formed by a budding process from membranes of either the endoplasmic reticulum and/or cytoplasmic vacuoles (9). The budding process has been described in some detail in the case of avian infectious bronchitis virus, the human agent, 229E (2), and other isolates (3, 7, 10, 16, 18, 23, 24, 25, 29, 30). Despite the preponderance of data favouring budding as the assembly mechanism some reservations have been made about the significance of this process (11, 27). The present electron microscopic study was undertaken to ascertain at high resolution the nature of coronavirus assembly, with particular attention to the incompletely characterized nucleocapsid.

MATERIAL AND METHODS

Cells and Viruses

Mouse 17Cl-1 cells of the passage are derivative of 3T3 BALB/c cells and were kindly provided by Dr. L.S. Sturman (Division of Laboratories and Research, N.Y. State Department of Health, Albany, N.Y.). They are routinely maintained in Eagle's minimal essential medium (MEM) supplemented with 10% heat-inactivated fetal bovine serum (Microbiological Associates), sodium bicarbonate (2 g/l), penicillin (100 u/ml) and streptomycin (100 mg/l) in a humidified atmosphere with 5% CO_2. The JHM strain of murine coronavirus was obtained from the American Type Culture Collection (Rockville, Maryland).

Growth and JHM Infection of Cells for EM

Cells were grown to monolayer in 30 mm plastic tissue culture dishes and infected with JHM at a multiplicity of 0.004 - 0.2 pfu/cell. After 1 hour adsorption at 32.5°, cultures were washed with phosphate buffered saline, overlaid with 2 ml MEM, and incubated at 32.5° for 24 or 48 hr prior to sampling. A range of multiplicities was employed in order to obtain samples representing various stages of infection at 24 and 48 hr, the two times chosen for sampling.

Electron Microscopy

Cell monolayers in which syncytia formation was evident were fixed in situ by flooding with 2% Glutaraldehyde in 0.05 M Phosphate buffer at pH 7.2 and postfixed with 1% OsO_4 according to our previous method (8). Following washing and dehydration in ethanol series, the cells were infiltrated with 1:1 mixture of absolute ethanol and Epon 812. The monolayers were finally covered with approximately 2-3 mm thick layer of Epon 812 and polymerized at 60°C for 24 hr. Small fragments of the hardened disks were cut out and mounted in orientations which permitted the monolayer to be sectioned both horizontally and vertically. Unsupported 200 mesh grids were used to collect sections, which were subsequently double-stained for 4 min with 5% Uranyl acetate in 50% Ethanol, followed by 3 mins with lead citrate solution (21). The specimens were examined in a Philips EM300 at an accelerating voltage of 60 or 80 KV.

RESULTS AND DISCUSSION

In order to facilitate sampling for examination of virus development by transmission electron microscopy, monolayers of Cl 17-1 cells were infected with JHM virus at multiplicities sufficiently low to initiate slow, progressive syncytiogenesis, described previously (14). The syncytia scattered throughout the monolayers are evident initially within 24 hr postinfection and become quite extensive by 48 hr. In order to preserve as faithfully as possible the structural relationship between sites of virus development and related cellular organelles as they may occur in the living state, fixation and embedding of attached cells were carried out in situ. This procedure facilitated a precise localization and selection of areas in the monolayer where syncytiogenesis was evident by light microscopy.

Examination of horizontally sectioned syncytia revealed presence of numerous vacuoles ranging in diameter from 150-160 nm

(Fig. 1). Absence of ribosomes on the cytoplasmic face of the vacuole membranes implies that these structures are derived from smooth endoplasmic reticulum (SER). Their random distribution, as ascertained by both vertical and horizontal sections implies that they occur throughout the cytoplasm. Occurrence of circular rather than flattened profiles of the sectioned vacuoles indicates that the SER becomes distended following infection. Virus assembly is confined to these vacuoles (Figs. 1 and 2), and has not been observed at either the plasma membrane or any other cellular surface. This is in agreement with other studies of the coronaviruses (22), but at variance with sites of assembly of enveloped viruses from the myxo-, paramyxo- and rhabdovirus groups (5, 20, 4, 12, 28).

An interpretation of the dynamic events during JHM virus assembly in the polykaryocytes was based upon a series of images ordered into a developmental sequence (Figs. 3-10). The most rudimentary stage was identified by presence of a short segment of dense material subjacent to the vacuolar membrane (Figs. 3-5). An associated unit membrane was clearly evident on the external surface (Figs. 3-5), and is presumed to represent the viral envelope covered by the peplomers (Figs. 9 and 10). Elongated structures, which in some images appeared to be tubular in nature, were organized on the cytoplasmic side of the modified vacuolar surface (Figs. 2-6). In the more advanced stages of budding the virus envelopes surrounded the elongated, internal component to a varying degree (Figs. 2 and 7-10). In favourable orientations the tubular nature of the internal component could be discerned (Figs. 7-8). These structures are highly reminiscent of the nucleoprotein helix of influenza virus (1). The external diameter of the coronavirus tubules is on the average 9.5 nm, ranging from 8.5 to 10.5 nm. These dimensions correspond to measurements made on the extruded coronavirus helical component evident by negative staining (13, 19), and a dense internal thread present within thinly sectioned infectious avian bronchitis virus (1). An internal component of a greater diameter has been recorded in one study (15). Our measurements also correspond to the diameter of the influenza virus nucleoprotein, measuring either 6-9 nm in sectioned virions (1) or 10-15 nm in whole mount preparations (5, 20). By contrast the diameter of the helical nucleocapsid of the paramyxoviruses, 15-19 nm in diameter is about double the width of the coronavirus tubular structure (4, 6, 12, 17). According to another recent interpretation the coronavirus nucleocapsid structure is described as a circular, dense, inner component, about 60 nm wide (10). Our new evidence, coupled with information obtained on disrupted negatively stained 229E virions (13, 15), and another representative of the group (19), indicates that the architecture of the coronaviruses simulates that of the myxo- and paramyxoviruses, although the coronaviruses unlike the other two groups, possess a single stranded RNA genome of the + sense. From this observation it may be

Figs. 1-10 Sections of infected Cl 17-1 cells sampled 48 hr after inoculation and perserved in situ to demonstrate assembly and distribution of virus progeny.

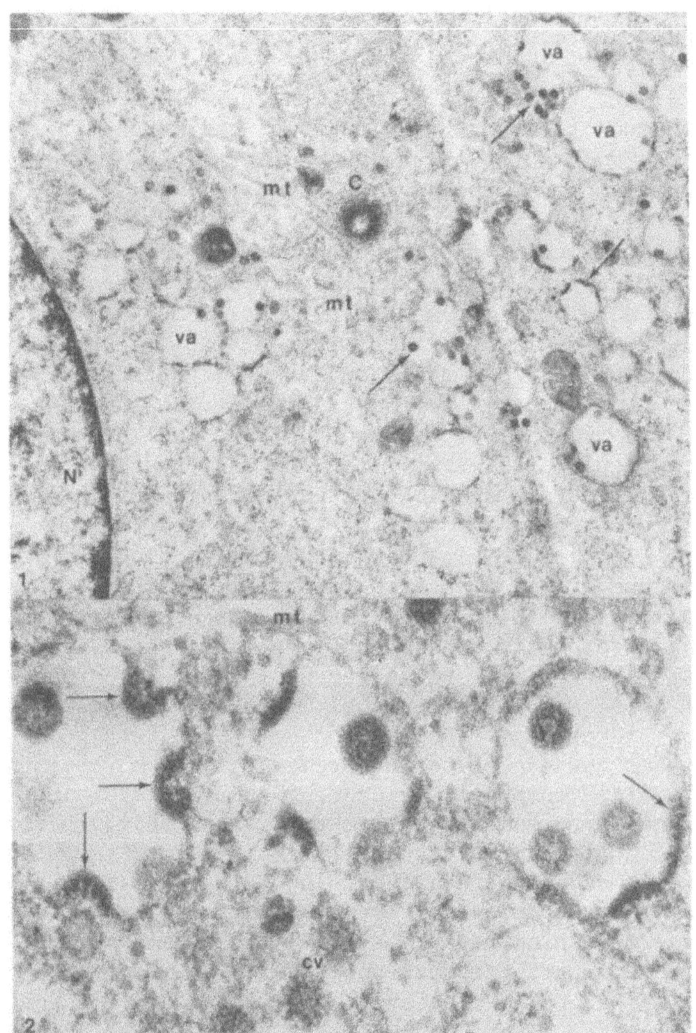

Fig. 1 Illustrates at lower magnification presence of cytoplasmic vacuoles (va) containing budding or free virus particles (arrows). C: centriole; mt: microtubules; N: nucleus. X 31,000.

Fig. 2 An example at higher resolution reveals stages of virus assembly at the membranes of vacuoles (arrows). mt: microtubule; cv: coated vesicle. X 138,000.

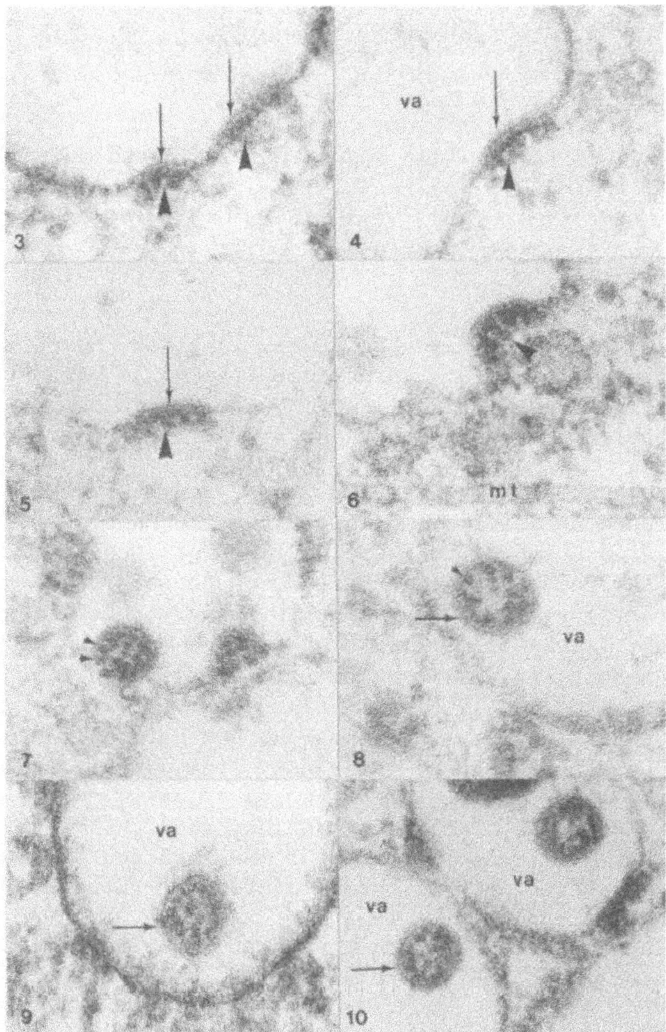

Figs. 3-10 Selected areas at high resolution demonstrating virus budding at membranes of vacuoles. The series represents reconstruction of the presumed assembly sequence. The virus envelope, either in continuity with the vacuole membrane (Figs. 3-7), or enclosing virions (Figs. 8-10), is indicated by arrows. The nucleocapsids indicated by arrowheads are evident as tubular structure in either the longitudinal aspect (Figs. 6 and 8), or in cross section (Fig. 7), during the formative stages (Figs. 3-7) and in completed virions (Fig. 8). mt: microtubule; va: vacuole. Fig. 8 X 240,000; all others X 200,000.

concluded that polarity of the RNA genome and helical conformation of the nucleoprotein are not necessarily interrelated.

ACKNOWLEDGEMENTS

Supported by the Medical Research Council and Multiple Sclerosis Society of Canada.

REFERENCES

1. K. Apostolov, T.H. Flewett, and A.P. Kendal, Morphology of Influenza A,B,C and Infectious Bronchitis Virus (IBV) Virions and their Replication, in: "The Biology of large RNA viruses", R.D. Barry and B.W.J. Mahy, ed., Academic Press, London-New York (1970).
2. W.B. Becker, K. McIntosh, J.H. Dees, and R.M. Chanock, Morphogenesis of avian infectious bronchitis virus and a related human virus (strain 229E), J. Virol. 1:1019 (1967).
3. D. Chasey, and D.J. Alexander, Morphogenesis of avian infectious bronchitis virus in primary chick kidney cells, Arch. Virol. 52:101 (1976).
4. P.W. Choppin, and W. Stoeckenius, The morphology of SV5 virus, Virol. 23:195 (1964).
5. R.W. Compans, J. Content, and P.H. Duesberg, Structure of the ribonucleoprotein of influenza virus, J. Virol. 10:795 (1972).
6. R.W. Compans, K.V. Holmes, S. Dales, and P.W. Choppin, An electron microscopic study of moderate and virulent virus-cell interactions of the Parainfluenza Virus SV5, Virol. 30:411 (1966).
7. C.H. Cunningham, M.P. Spring, and K. Nazerian, Replication of avian infectious bronchitis virus in African green monkey kidney cell line VERO, J. gen. Virol. 16:432 (1972).
8. S. Dales, and H. Hanafusa, Penetration and intracellular release of the genomes of Avian RNA tumor viruses, Virol. 50:440 (1972).
9. J.F. David-Ferreira, and R.A. Manaker, An electron microscope study of the development of a mouse hepatitis virus in tissue culture cells, J. Cell Biol. 24:57 (1965).
10. H.J.A. Fleury, R.D. Sheppard, M.B. Bornstein, and C.S. Raine, Further ultrastructural observations of virus morphogenesis and myelin pathology in JHM virus encephalomyelitis. Neuropath. App. Neurobiol. 6:165 (1980).
11. D. Hamre, D.A. Kindig, and J. Mann, Growth and intracellular development of a new respiratory virus, J. Virol. 1:810 (1967).
12. R.W. Horne, A.P. Waterson, P. Wildy, and A.E. Farnham, The structure and composition of the Myxoviruses. 1. Electron

microscope studies of the structure of Myxovirus particles by negative staining techniques, Virol. 11:79 (1960).
13. D.A. Kennedy, and C.M. Johnson-Lussenberg, Isolation and morphology of the internal component of human coronavirus, strain 229E, Intervirol. 6:197 (1976).
14. A. Lucas, W. Flintoff, R. Anderson, D. Percy, M. Coulter, and S. Dales, In vivo and in vitro models of demyelinating diseases: I. Tropism of the JHM strain of murine hepatitis virus for cells of glial origin, Cell 12: 553 (1977).
15. M.R. Macnaughton, H.A. Davies, and M.V. Nermut, Ribonucleoprotein like structures from coronavirus particles, J. Gen. Virol. 39:545 (1978).
16. K. Nazerian, and C.H. Cunningham, Morphogenesis of avian infectious bronchitis virus in chicken embryo fibroblasts, J. gen. Virol. 3:469 (1968).
17. E.C.J. Norrby, and P. Magnusson, Some morphological characteristics of the internal component of Measles virus, Arch. ges. Virusforsch 17:443 (1964).
18. L.S. Oshiro, J.H. Schieble, and E.H. Lennette, Electron microscopic studies of coronavirus, J. gen. Virol. 12:161 (1971).
19. D.H. Pocock, and D.J. Garwes, The polypeptides of hemagglutinating encephalomyelitis virus and isolated subviral particles, J. gen. Virol. 37:487 (1977).
20. M.W. Pons, I.T. Schulze, and G.K. Hirst, Isolation and characterization of the ribonucleoprotein of influenza virus, Virol. 39:250 (1969).
21. E.S. Reynolds, The use of lead citrate at high pH as an electron-opaque strain in electron microscopy, J. Cell Biol. 17:208 (1963).
22. J.A. Robb, and C.W. Bond, Coronaviridae, in: "Comprehensive Virology", H. Fraenkel-Conrat and R. Wagner, ed., Plenum, New York (1979).
23. J.A. Robb, and C.W. Bond, Pathogenic murine coronaviruses. 1. Characterization of biological behavior in vitro and virus specific intracellular RNA of strongly neurotropic JHMV and weakly neurotropic A59V viruses, Virol. 94:352 (1979).
24. J.A. Robb, C.W. Bond, and J.L. Leibowitz, Pathogenic murine coronaviruses. 111. Biological and biochemical characterization of temperature-sensitive mutants of JHMV, Virol. 94:385 (1979).
25. B.H. Ruebner, T. Hirano, and R.J. Slusser, Electron microscopy of the hepatocellular and Kupffer cell lesions of mouse hepatitis with particular reference to the effect of cortisone, Amer. J. Path. 51:163 (1967).
26. D.A.J. Tyrrell, J.D. Almeida, C.H. Cunningham, W.R. Dowdle, M.S. Hoestad, K. McIntosh, M. Tajima, Y.L. Zakstelskaya, B.C. Easterday, A. Kapikian, and R.W. Bingham, Coronaviridae, Intervirol. 5:76 (1975).

27. P.K. Uppal, and H.P. Chu, An electron microscope study of the trachea of the fowl infected with avian infectious bronchitis virus, J. med. Microbiol. 3:643 (1970).
28. R.R. Wagner, Reproduction of Rhabdoviruses, in: "Comprehensive Virology", H. Fraenkel-Conrat and R. Wagner, eds., Plenum, New York (1975).
29. K. Watanabe, Electron microscopic studies of experimental viral hepatitis in mice. 1. Virus particles and their relationship to hepatocytes and Kupffer cells, J. Electron Micro. 18:158 (1969).
30. K.H. Witte, M. Tajima, and B.C. Easterday, Morphologic characteristics and nucleic acid type of transmissible gastroenteritis virus of pigs, Arch. ges. Virusforsch. 23:53 (1968).

GLYCOPROTEIN E1 OF CORONAVIRUS A59: A NEW TYPE OF VIRAL GLYCOPROTEIN

Heiner Niemann and Hans-Dieter Klenk

Institut für Virologie FB Humanmedizin
Frankfurter Str. 107
6300 Giessen

INTRODUCTION

Glycosylation of viral glycoproteins as a co- and posttranslational event has been studied in a large number of viral systems (for review see Klenk and Rott, 1980). From these data a general picture can be drawn:

In a first step the nascent polypeptide chain extending into the lumen of the rough endoplasmic reticulum (RER) is glycosylated by an *en bloc* transfer of the oligosaccharide from a dolichol-linked intermediate Dol-P-P-$(GlcNAc)_2$ Man_9 Glc_3. This glycosylation step requires a tripeptide-sequence (H_2N·Asn-X-Ser(Thr)·COOH) and the resulting carbohydrate-protein linkage is of the N-glycosidic type between N-acetylglucosamine and asparagine. During transport of the glycoprotein to smooth membranes the carbohydrate side chains become trimmed by specific glycosidases. After sequential removal of the glucoses, a varying number of mannose residues may be cleaved off to yield the generally heterogeneous "mannose rich" side chains, also found in glycoproteins of mature virions.

If trimming of the side chains proceeds to a $Man_5(GlcNAc)_2$-Asn-species, re-addition of N-acetylglucosamine, galactose, fucose, and neuraminic acid will occur to form various "complex type" side chains. This presumably takes place in the Golgi. From here the viral glycoproteins are transported to the plasma membrane where they are sequestered into budding virus particles.

In this paper we describe a new type of viral glycoprotein having a carbohydrate composition and characteristics hitherto unknown for viral glycoproteins.

MATERIALS AND METHODS

Virus and Cells

The A59 strain of murine coronavirus was grown in the 17 clone 1 line of spontaneously transformed Balb C 3T3 cells. Both the virus and the cell line were kindly provided by Dr. L. S. Sturman. Virus was radiolabeled by the addition of radioisotopes to the growth medium, reinforced Eagle's medium containing 10 % fetal calf serum, after the 1 hr adsorption period. Virus was harvested 30 hrs after infection, collected by centrifugation (2 hrs, 53 700 xg) and purified by isopycnic centrifugation on a 30 to 50 % (w/w) sucrose gradient.

SDS-polyacrylamide gel electrophoresis

Initially cylindrical gels containing 10 % polyacrylamide were employed essentially as described by Laemmli (1970).

For preparative isolation of radiolabeled glycoprotein E1 samples were prepared according to Sturman et al. (1980). Glycoprotein was recovered from crushed gels after freezing and thawing by elution with 0.1 % SDS, filtration through o.45 µm Millipore filter units and precipitation in 90 % aqueous acetone at 0° C. Preparations were then exhaustively dialysed against distilled water and lyophilized.

Isolation of E1 glycopeptides

Radiolabeled glycoprotein was digested with predigested pronase at 50° C in 1.0 M-Tris-chloride containing 10^{-4} M $CaCl_2$ at pH 8.0 for 48 hrs with a second addition of protease after 24 hrs. Insoluble degradation products were removed by centrifugation and the supernatant was extracted with chloroform/methanol (2/1). The upper phase containing essentially all the radioactive label was desalted by gel filtration on a Biogel P2 column (1x35 cm).

E1 glycopeptides were further fractionated by affinity chromatography on WGA-Sepharose 6B as described by Krusius and Finne (1978).

Release of carbohydrate by alkali-borohydride-treatment

Glucosamine labeled E1 was subjected to β-elimination conditions according to Carlson (1968). In short, lyophilized E1 was incubated in a solution containing 0.05 M NaOH and 1.0 M $NaBH_4$ at 45° C for 10 hrs. After cooling to room temperature excessive borohydrate was destroyed by the addition of glacial acetic acid to pH 5.0 and boric acid was chased by repeated evaporation with methanol. Aliquots were spotted onto Whatman 3 MM paper sheets and subjected to high voltage paper electrophoresis in pyridine-acetic acid-water (4/10/86) at pH

4.5. Electrophoresis was carried out at 35 V/cm for 6 hrs. The paper was then cut into 0.5 cm stripes and counted for radioactivity.

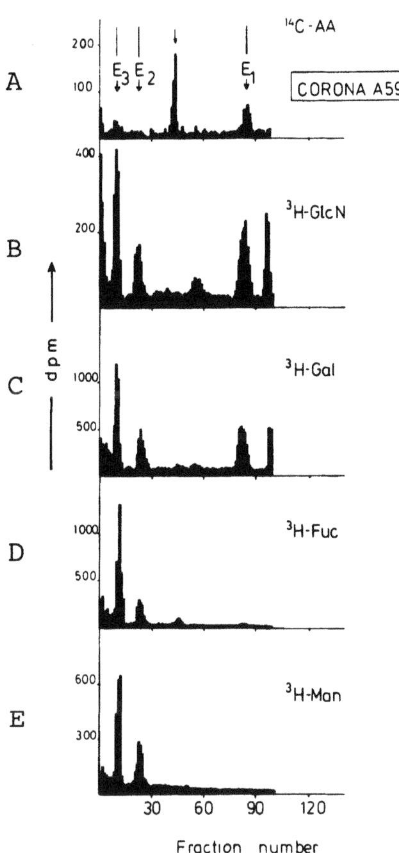

Fig. 1 Incorporation of radioactive markers into coronavirus A59 polypeptides

Coronavirus A59 was grown in spontaneously transformed Balb C 3T3 cells in the presence of ^{14}C amino acids (panel A) or radiolabeled sugars as indicated (panels B to E). Virus was harvested 30 hrs post-infection and analyzed on cylindrical 10 % polyacrylamide gels. Whereas E2 and E3 could be metabolically labeled with glucosamine, galactose, fucose, and mannose, E1 was only labeled with galactose and glucosamine.

Note that the incorporation of labeled amino acids into E2 and E3 is comparatively small indicating a numerical abundance of E1.

Sugar constituent analyses

All reagents were of ultrapure grade or freshly distilled. Desalted glycopeptides containing 5 - 10 µg of total sugar were hydrolyzed in 0.5 N H_2SO_4 in 90 % aqueous acetic acid at 80° C for 8 hrs, reduced and peracetylated as described by Stellner and Hakomori (1974).

Peracetylated alditol acetates were analyzed on a Finnigan model 4021 combined gas chromatograph mass spectrometer using a 25 m fused silica capillary column with Dexsil 410 as a stationary phase. Sugar ratios were calculated on the basis of the total reconstructed ion chromatograms.

RESULTS

Incorporation of radioactive sugars into viral glycoproteins

The polypeptide pattern of coronavirus A59 grown in the 17 clone 1 line of spontaneously transformed Balb C 3T3 cells was previously characterized in detail (Sturman, 1977; Sturman and Holmes, 1977; Sturman et al., 1980). Four size classes of polypeptide species were observed in SDS polyacrylamide gel electrophoresis: E1 (23 K), N (50 K), E2 (90 K), and E3 (180 K).

When coronavirus A59 was grown in the presence of ^{14}C-amino acid hydrolysate (Fig. 1A), label was mainly incorporated into the nucleocapsid protein N and into the low molecular weight glycoprotein E1 whereas E2 (and E3) were only poorly labeled. Panels B to E show the glycosylation pattern of A59 obtained by labeling with [6-^3H]glucosamine, [1-^3H]galactose, [2-^3H]mannose, and [1-^3H]fucose. All four sugar markers were incorporated into E2 (and E3), whereas E1 was labeled only with galactose and glucosamine. These labeling data cannot be explained on the basis of any structure or carbohydrate composition reported so far for viral glycoproteins. It should be noted that glucosamine label may be metabolically converted into galactosamine and neuraminic acid. A metabolical conversion of sugar label into amino acids on the other hand can be excluded, since under the described conditions no label was incorporated into the nonglycosylated N-protein.

In order to investigate, whether the presence of E1 with its abnormal labeling characteristics is unique for the murine coronavirus A59 or a rather general corona-specific phenomenon, we have also studied the glycosylation pattern of bovine coronavirus L9 grown in primary bovine fetal thyroid cells (J. Storz et al., this meeting). A corresponding low molecular weight glycoprotein comigrating with the murine E1 in SDS-polyacrylamide gel electrophoresis was found in the bovine virus. In analogy this glycoprotein

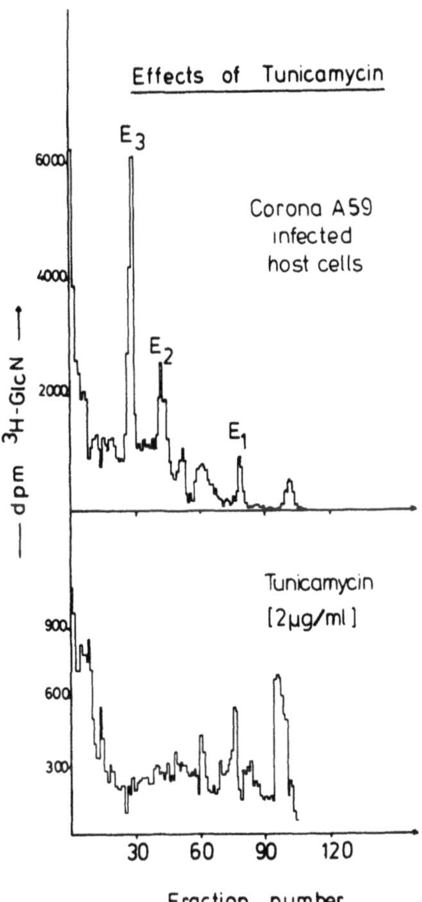

Fig. 2 Effects of tunicamycin

Upper panel: A59-infected 17 Cl 1 were labeled with ^{3}H-glucosamine. 20 hrs after infection cells were extracted with a buffer containing 6 M urea, 4 % SDS in 0.0625 M Tris-HCl at pH 6.7. The extract was analyzed on a 5 to 15 % polyacrylamide gradient gel.

Lower panel: same as above, but tunicamycin (2 µg/ml) was added after infection.

The glycosylation of E2 and E3 is inhibited under these conditions, whereas E1 is made in normal amounts. The virus titer dropped from 5×10^{7} PFU/ml in the control to 1×10^{2} PFU/ml in the supernatant ot tunicamycin-treated cells.

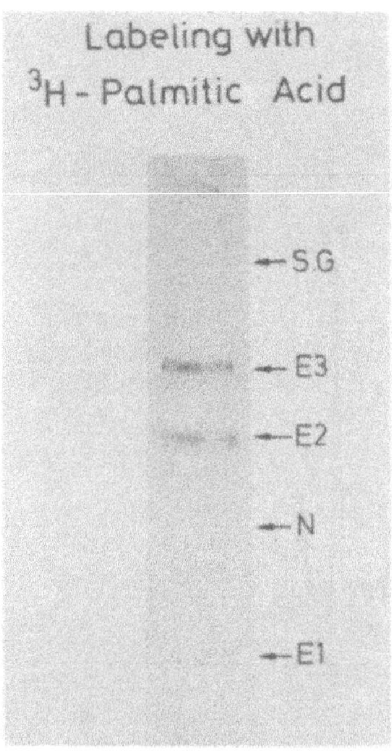

Fig. 3 Labeling with ^{3}H-palmitic acid

Coronavirus was grown in the presence of ^{3}H-palmitic acid (25 µCi/ml). Virus was harvested 18 hrs after infection. E2 and E3 are the only polypeptides showing incorporation of fatty acids. (S. G. indicates the begin of the separation gel).

could be labeled only with galactose and glucosamine but not with fucose and mannose. Furthermore this polypeptide readily aggregated to a 38K species when boiled in the presence of reducing agents as described for the murine glycoprotein E1 (Sturman, 1977).

Effects of tunicamycin

Tunicamycin is a drug known to inhibit the formation of dolichol-linked N-acetyl-glucosamine (Dol-P-P-(GlcNAc)), which serves as an acceptor in the formation of the dolichol-bound oligosaccharide Dol-P-P-$(GlcNAc)_2$ Man_9 Glc_3 (for review see Schwarz and Datema, 1980). In the first glycosylation event this oligosaccharide is then N-glycosidically linked to specific asparagine residues on nascent polypeptides in the RER. It was therefore of interest to study the effects of this drug on the glycosylation of E1. Figure 2 shows the viral glycoproteins in infected cells that were labeled with radioactive glucosamine for 18 hrs with or without tunicamycin. Production of infective virus particles was reduced by more than five log steps in the presence of tunicamycin. In this case glycosylation of E2 was completely inhibited, whereas E1 incorporated glucosamine label in normal amounts.

This again indicates that E2 is glycosylated in a different biochemical pathway from all the viral glycoprotein hitherto described (similar results were obtained by K. Holmes, personal communication).

Labeling with ^{3}H-palmitic acid

It was recently established that attachment of fatty acids to glycoproteins synthesized at membrane-bound ribosomes is another kind of posttranslational modification (Schmidt and Schlesinger, 1980). When A59 was grown in the presence of [9,10-^{3}H]palmitic acid label was only incorporated into E2 and E3 but not into E1 (Fig. 3). Although we do not know the absolute number of fatty acid residues per E2 molecule, the numerical abundance of E1 in the virus particle, which is indicated by the ratio of ^{14}C amino acid label incorporated into E1 and E2 (Fig. 1A) argues against any undetected presence of fatty acids in E1.

This finding also excludes a contamination of E1 with glycolipids.

Alkali-borohydride treatment of El

Carbohydrate side chains linked O-glycosidically to serine or threonine can be released from the polypeptide under alkaline and reducing conditions in a β-elimination reaction. Since this reaction is hindered when these amino acids are located at the termini of proteolytic peptides, β-elimination was carried out with undigested glucosamine labeled E1. The released products were analyzed by high voltage paper electrophoresis (Fig. 4). About 90 - 95 % of the carbohydrate label could be released under conditions established for the elimination of carbohydrate side chains from hog submaxillary mucin (Carlson, 1968). A considerable degradation of the elimination products is indicated by the fact that about 20 % of the label comigrated in electrophoresis with free N-acetylneuraminic acid. Control material which was only shortly exposed to alkaline and reductive conditions but then neutralized remained at the origin. N-glycosidic linkes are only slightly affected by this treatment as was shown for influenca virus glycoproteins (Keil et al., 1979).

Molecular weight and carbohydrate constituent analyses of E1 glycopeptides.

Glucosamine labeled glycoprotein E1 was digested with pronase and the degradation products were chromatographed on a calibrated Biogel P6 column (Fig. 5). A remarkable degree of heterogeneity of the eluted material was observed, partly due to a varying substitution of the side chains with neuraminic acid. After neuraminidase treatment (vibrio cholerae) or partial acid hydrolysis (1 % acetic acid, 80 min at 100° C) the molecular weight of the main glycopeptide fraction was reduced from about 2000 dalton to 1500 dalton.

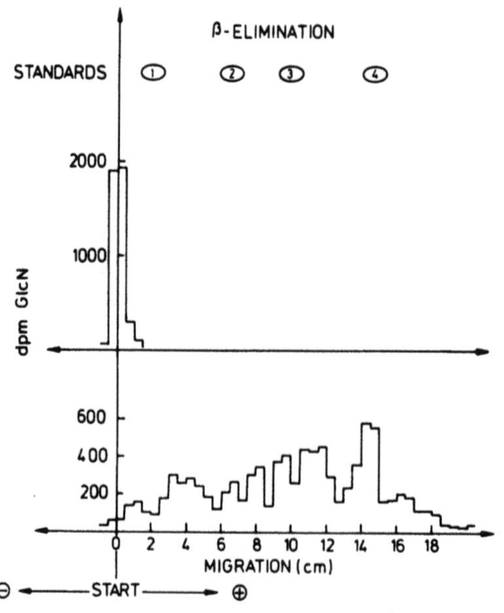

Fig. 4 β-Elimination reaction

^{3}H-glucosamine labeled E1 was treated with 1 M $NaBH_4$ in 0.05 N NaOH at 45° C for various length of time. The reaction products were analyzed by high voltage paper electrophoresis.

Upper panel: all sugar label remains at the origin, when E1 is shortly exposed to alkaline conditions but immediately neutralized.

Lower panel: E1 elimination products obtained after 10 hrs of incubation at 45° C. When ^{14}C-serine labeled E1 was treated similarly all radioactivity remained at the origin.

Standards applied: 1,2 porcine submaxillary mucin oligosaccharides, 3 neruaminyl-lactose, 4 N-acetyl-neuraminic acid.

Fig. 5 Elution pattern of El glycopeptides from a Biogel P6 column

^{3}H-glucosamine labeled E1 glycopeptides were applied to a Biogel P6 column (1 x 150 cm) and eluted with 0.02 % NaN_3 in water. The dark elution profile shows glycopeptides prior to neuraminidase treatment which elute at molecular weights of about 2200 to 1800 dalton. After enzymatic removal of neuraminic acid residues a reduction in molecular weight to about 1500 dalton for the main fraction is observed (white profile). About 30 % of the label elutes in the position of free N-acetyl-neuraminic acid.

For sugar constituent analyses further purification steps of the glycopeptides were necessary and involved extraction of pronase digest with chloroform/methanol (2/1) and affinity chromatography on a wheat germ agglutinin-Sepharose 6B column. 37 % of the radioactivity applied bound tightly to the column and could be specifically eluted with 0.1 M N-acetylglucosamine. Both the unbound and the bound fraction were desalted on Biogel P2 and subjected to sugar constituent analyses. Sugar derivatives were identified as peracetylated alditol acetates by combined gas chromatography-mass spectrometry.

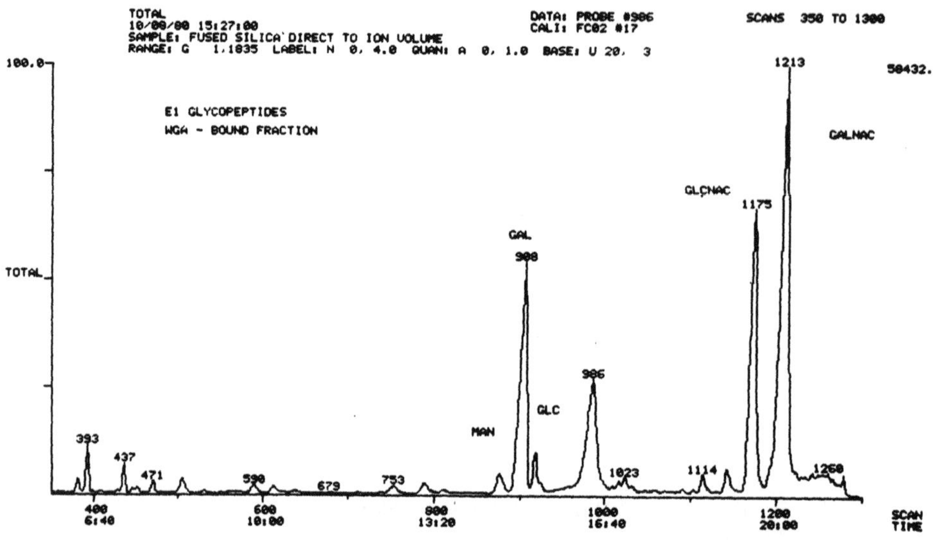

Fig. 6 Total reconstructed ion chromatogram of the alditol acetates obtained from E1 glycopeptides

The sugar constituents of the WGA-bound E1 glycopeptides containing about 5 µg of total sugar were hydrolyzed and converted into alditol acetates. Combined gas chromatographic-mass spectrometric analyses were carried out on a Finnigan model 4021 mass spectrometer equipped with a 25 m fused silica capillary column. A temperature program of 2° C/min from 150° to 230° C was applied after a 5 min delay of the starting temperature. Peaks were identified according to their retention time and their fragmentation.

Table 1 Sugar composition of E1 and E2 glycopeptides

Sugar Constituent	E1 WGA-bound %	E1 WGA-bound ratio	E1 WGA-unbound %	E1 WGA-unbound ratio	E2 %	E2 ratio
Fucose	0	0	0	0	3.5	0.47
Mannose	2.54	0.17	3.05	0.18	22.2	3.00
Galactose	28.87	2.00	17.02	1.00	21.3	2.87
Glucose	2.26	0.25	8.76	0.51	6.8	0.92
GlcNAc	28.73	2.01	15.73	0.92	46.3	6.27
GalNAc	59.50	4.21	68.87	4.04	0	0
Neuraminic Acid	+		+		+	

As summarized in table 1 both the unbound and the bound fraction of E1-glycopeptides contain negligible amounts of mannose. The absence of fucose is also consistant with the labeling data. Glucose is considered to be a contamination since no radioactive glucose was detected in hydrolysates of ^{3}H-galactose labeled glycopeptides by paper chromatography.

In comparison to the WGA-bound fraction the unbound fraction contains about the double amount of N-acetylgalactosamine. The carbohydrate composition of E2 glycopeptides (Table 1, right column) shows the presence of fucose and mannose. E2 carbohydrate side chains may thus very well represent the commonly found complex type side chains containing an internal mannose-trisaccharide core structure which is N-glycosidically linked to asparagine via a chitobiose-unit.

DISCUSSION

Coronavirus A59 contains three glycoprotein species: E1, E2, and E3. Whereas E2 (90 K) and E3 (180 K) can be metabolically labeled with [1-^{3}H]fucose, [2-^{3}H]mannose, [6-^{3}H]glucosamine, and [1-^{3}H]galactose, E1 (23 K) was shown to incorporate label only with the two latter markers. Using the same experimental approach a similar species corresponding to E1 was also found in a bovine transmissible gastroenteritis virus grown in bovine fetal thyroid cells. These coronavirus specific labeling characteristics of glycoprotein E1 are different from all other viral glycoproteins hitherto described.

Glycosylation of E1 is not inhibited by tunicamycin, indicating that different from other viral glyoproteins including coronavirus E2, dolichol-linked N-acetylglucosamine is not involved in the biosynthesis of E1 carbohydrates.

Furthermore, essentially all the carbohydrate could be released under alkaline conditions, supporting the concept of O-glycosidic linkages in E1. Absolute proof must await the identification of the amino acid counter part(s) in the carbohydrate protein linkage, experiments which are currently underway. Amino acid analyses of E1 glycopeptides have shown serine and threonine residues as prominent constituents. Sugar constituent analyses of E1 glycopeptides revealed galactose, N-acetylglucosamine, N-acetylgalactosamine, and neuraminic acid. This sugar profile is quite typical for mucin glycoproteins, which are known to contain O-glycosidic linkages between N-acetylgalactosamine and serine or threonine.

These findings raise the question as to whether glycoprotein E1 is synthesized by a different pathway involving different cellular compartments, as described in the introduction. In this context it is of interest that K. Holmes reported that by means of fluorescamine labeled antibodies E1 could only be detected in perinuclear regions of infected host cell, whereas E2 was found throughout the cytoplasm (Doller and Holmes, 1980). A novel biosynthetic pathway for the glycoprotein E1 is further substantiated by our finding that E1 in contrast to E2 could not be labeled with ^{3}H-palmitic acid. This posttranslational attachment of fatty acids has been reported for several membrane bound viral glycoproteins and has been localized to the Golgi.

REFERENCES

Carlson, D. M. (1968)
Structures and immunochemical properties of oligosaccharides isolated from pig submaxillary mucins.
J. Biol. Chem. 243, 616 - 626.

Doller, E. W., and Holmes, K. V. (1980)
80th Annual meeting of the Americal Society of Microbiology in Miami, 11 - 16th May 1980, T 190.

Keil, W., Klenk, H.-D., and Schwarz, R. T. (1979)
Carbohydrates of influenza virus. III. Nature of oligosaccharide-protein linkage in viral glycoproteins.
J. Virol. 31, 253 - 256.

Klenk, H.-D., and Rott, R. (1980)
Cotranslational and posttranslational processing of viral glycoproteins.
Current Topics in Microbiol. and Immunol. 90, 19 - 48.

Krusius, T., and Finne, J. (1978)
Characterization of a novel sugar sequence from rat-brain glycoproteins containing fucose and sialic acid.
Eur. J. Biochem. 84, 395 - 403.

Laemmli, U. K. (1970)
Cleavage of structural proteins during the assembly of the head of bacteriophage T4.
Nature (London) 227, 680 - 685.

Schmidt, M. F. G., and Schlesinger, M. J. (1980)
Relation of fatty acid attachment to the translation and maturation of vesicular stomatitis and sindbis virus membrane glycoproteins.
J. Biol. Chem. 255, 3334 - 3339.

Schwarz, R. T., and Datema, R. (1980)
Inhibitors of protein glycosylation.
Trends in Biochem. Sciences 5, 65 - 67.

Stellner, K., and Hakomori, S. I. (1974)
Methylation analysis of aminosugars: A few examples of determination of amino-sugar linkages in glycolipids.
In: Methodologie de la Structure et du metabolisme des glycoconjugues. Editions du Centre National de le Recherche Scientifique, 95 - 109.

Sturman, L. S. (1977)
Characterization of coronavirus: I. Structural protein: effectors of preparative conditions on the migration of protein in polyacrylamide gels.
Virology 77, 637 - 649.

Sturman, L. S., and Holmes, K. V. (1977)
Characterization of a coronavirus. II. Glycoproteins of the viral envelope: tryptic peptide analysis.
Virology 77, 650 - 660.

Sturman, L. S., Holmes, K. V., and Behnke, J. (1980)
Isolation of coronavirus envelope glycoproteins and interaction with the viral nucleocapsid.
J. Virol. 33, 449 - 462.

ACKNOWLEDGEMENT

This work was supported by the Deutsche Forschungsgemeinschaft Sonderforschungsbereich 47 (Virologie).

The excellent technical assistance of M. Rosing and S. Kühnhardt are gratefully acknowledged.We also thank Drs. R. Geyer and M. F. G. Schmidt for valuable discussion.

ANALYSIS OF THE FUNCTIONS OF CORONAVIRUS GLYCOPROTEINS BY DIFFERENTIAL INHIBITION OF SYNTHESIS WITH TUNICAMYCIN

Kathryn V. Holmes, Elizabeth W. Doller and James N. Behnke

Department of Pathology, The Uniformed Services University of the Health Sciences, Bethesda, Maryland 20014

INTRODUCTION

The virion associated polypeptides of the A59 strain of mouse hepatitis virus (MHV) have been studied extensively (Sturman, 1977; Sturman and Holmes, 1977; Sturman et al., 1980) and are described by Dr. Sturman in this symposium. The nucleocapsid polypeptide N is phosphorylated and has a molecular weight of 50K. Two glycoproteins are associated with the viral envelope. The peplomers are composed of the glycoprotein E2(MW ≃ 180K) which may be proteolytically cleaved to yield two molecules which both migrate with an apparent molecular weight of 90K. The glycoprotein E1 (MW ≃ 23K) is deeply embedded in the viral membrane with the small glycosolated portion protruding. We have studied the intracellular synthesis of these structural polypeptides of A59 in the 17 clone 1 line (17 Cl 1) of spontaneously transformed BALB/c 3T3 cells. A59 acts as a moderate virus in 17 Cl 1 cells causing limited cell fusion. Virus particles are shed from intact cells following a 6 to 7 hour latent period at 37°, and the yield of infectious virus at 24 hours is 10^8 to 10^9 PFU/ml.

This report focuses on the intracellular synthesis of the virion-associated polypeptides of A59. We have studied the effects on A59 polypeptides of tunicamycin (TM) which prevents the formation of N-glycosidic linkages to polypeptides. Incubation with tunicamycin blocks the synthesis and incorporation into A59 virions of the peplomeric glycoprotein E2, but does not affect synthesis or glycosylation of the membrane glycoprotein E1. This observation suggests that unlike E2 and all other glycoproteins of enveloped viruses which have been studied to date, E1 may not be an N-linked glycoprotein. E1 may be the first O-linked viral glycoprotein. Formation of O-glycosidic linkages to cellular polypeptides such as mucin does not require transfer of oligosaccharides from dolichol linked-intermediates and is not inhibited by tunicamycin. Thus, mouse hepatitis virus apparently utilizes two different host cell mechanisms for glycosylation of the envelope glycoproteins E1 and E2. We have made use of the differential effects of tunicamycin on E1 and E2 to characterize the functions of these two viral glycoproteins.

SYNTHESIS AND PROCESSING OF THE STRUCTURAL POLYPEPTIDES OF A59 VIRUS

The normal intracellular synthesis of the structural polypeptides of A59 will be described first to provide a comparison with that observed in the presence of tunicamycin. These results differ in part from published reports on the intracellular synthesis of polypeptides of the A59, JHM and MHV3 strains of MHV (Bond et al., 1979; Siddell et al., 1980; Anderson, 1979).

Initial studies of virus infected cells were done using 1 hour labeling periods at different times after infection. By 4 hours after infection E1, E2 and N could be detected. Only the 180K form of E2 was observed in intracellular labeling experiments. The relative amounts of E1 and E2 synthesized at various times after infection were constant but the synthesis of N was not correlated to that of the glycoproteins. N appeared to be made in relatively large amounts early, whereas the maximal rate of synthesis of the glycoproteins occurred late in the infectious cycle.

In order to detect possible precursors to the structural polypeptides and to follow the fate of newly synthesized polypeptides within the infected cells, pulse chase studies were done at various times after infection. Figure 1 shows control and MHV-infected 17 Cl 1 cells labeled 6 hours after virus inoculation with a 15 minute pulse of ^{3}H leucine followed by chase periods of up to 6 hours in excess unlabeled leucine. At the end of the 15 minute pulse all three of the viral structural polypeptides were detected. E2 was found only in the 180K form and E1 appeared as a 20K form which was not glycosylated (data not shown). No change in molecular weight of E2 was observed. Thus the glycosylation of E2 may be a cotranslational event. In contrast, E1 was first synthesized as a 20K nonglycosylated protein and then chased into higher molecular weight forms up to 23K. The 23K form of E1 was glycosylated (data not shown). Thus glycosylation of E1 is a post translational event which occurs rather slowly. Pulse chase studies at later times after infection showed that a small amount of the nucleocapsid protein N chased into lower molecular weight forms which were not incorporated into virions. Another viral protein X (MW $\simeq$ 17K) was detected about 2 hours after the pulse label. Since this polypeptide was not immunoprecipitable with anti-virion antibody, we do not yet know from which viral polypeptide it was generated.

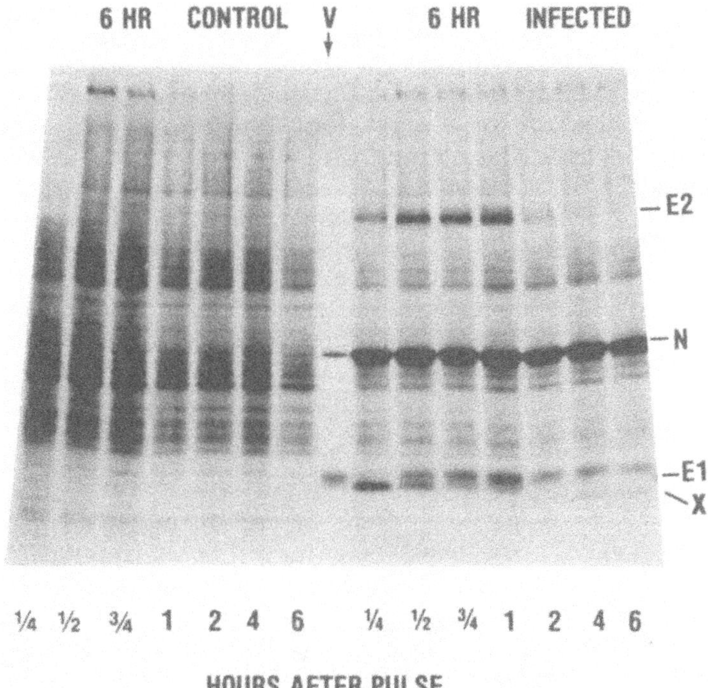

Fig. 1 Pulse chase study of control and A59 infected 17Cl 1 cells. Fluorograph of 5 to 20% polyacrylamide gradient slab gel with gradient purified A59 virion marker (V), and NP40 extracts of cells labeled for 15 min at 6 hrs after inoculation with 20μCi/ml ^{3}H leucine, and chased with excess cold leucine for the times indicated.

During the six hour chase period some labeled structural polypeptides were incorporated into virions which were released from the infected cells. The E2 synthesized 6 hours after infection was released from the cell in infectious virions within 2 hours after synthesis. Similarly the bulk of labeled E1 was released in virions within 2 hours. Both nonglycosylated and glycosylated forms of E1 were found in purified virions. No loss of the nucleocapsid protein N from the cells was detected. Apparently a large intracellular pool of N was synthesized early.

EFFECTS OF TUNICAMYCIN ON A59 GLYCOPROTEIN SYNTHESIS

When tunicamycin (TM) was added to cells 1 hour after virus inoculation and the cells were pulse labeled for 15 minutes with ^{3}H leucine at various times after infection, two surprising results were observed. First, glycosylation of E1 continued in the presence of TM, and second, the incorporation of ^{3}H leucine into E2 was prevented by TM. Figure 2 shows the effects of TM on synthesis and processing of MHV polypeptides labeled at 10 hours after infection during a 2 hour chase period. At 10 hours the chase of E1 and E2 into virions was somewhat slower than at early times after infection. Cells with TM synthesized less E1 than untreated cells but the processing of the 20K form of E1 to 23K due to glycosylation was detectable within ½ hour after labeling. The glycosylation of E1 in the presence of tunicamycin clearly shows that E1 is unlike other viral glycoproteins which have been studied to date and suggests that E1 may be an O-linked glycoprotein. Studies by Nieman and Klenk (personal communication) and Sturman (personal communication) which have been presented at this meeting show that the oligosaccharide side chains of E1 are different from those of E2 and that the carbohydrate composition of E1 is similar to that of O-linked glycoproteins. The significance of this unusual mechanism for glycosylation will be discussed below.

The presence of tunicamycin did not alter the synthesis of the N polypeptide. However, in TM both control and infected cells showed three new cellular polypeptide species of molecular weights between 70 and 93K.

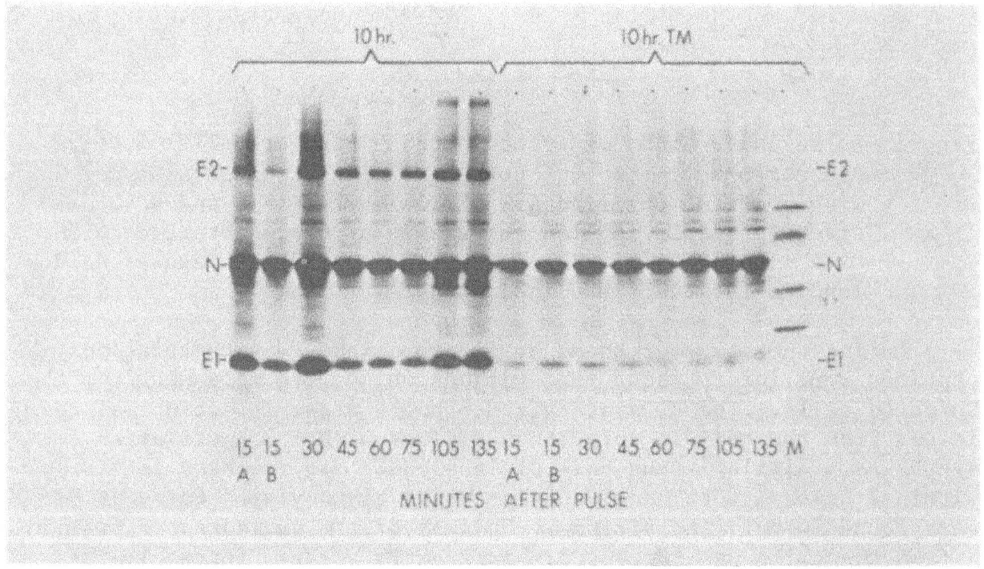

Fig 2. Effects of tunicamycin on A59 polypeptide synthesis. Fluorograph of 5 to 20% polyacrylamide gradient slab gel of NP40 extracts of A59 infected cells labeled for 15 min at 10 hrs after virus inoculation with 20μCi/ml ^{3}H leucine in the presence (TM) and absence of 0.5μg/ml of tunicamycin and then chased with excess cold leucine. A and B are replicate samples from identical plates and M is ^{14}C labeled molecular weight standards (30K, 46K, 69K and 92.5K).

In TM, synthesis of E2 was not detectable with the 15 minute pulse. Other viral glycoproteins such as the G protein of VSV are synthesized but not glycosylated in the presence of tunicamycin (Gibson et al., 1979). However, in TM, synthesis of the peplomeric glycoprotein of an oncorna virus was not detectable (Schwarz et al., 1976). It is possible that the E2 polypeptide was subject to rapid degradation if it was not glycosylated during translation. This degradation could occur either during or shortly after the

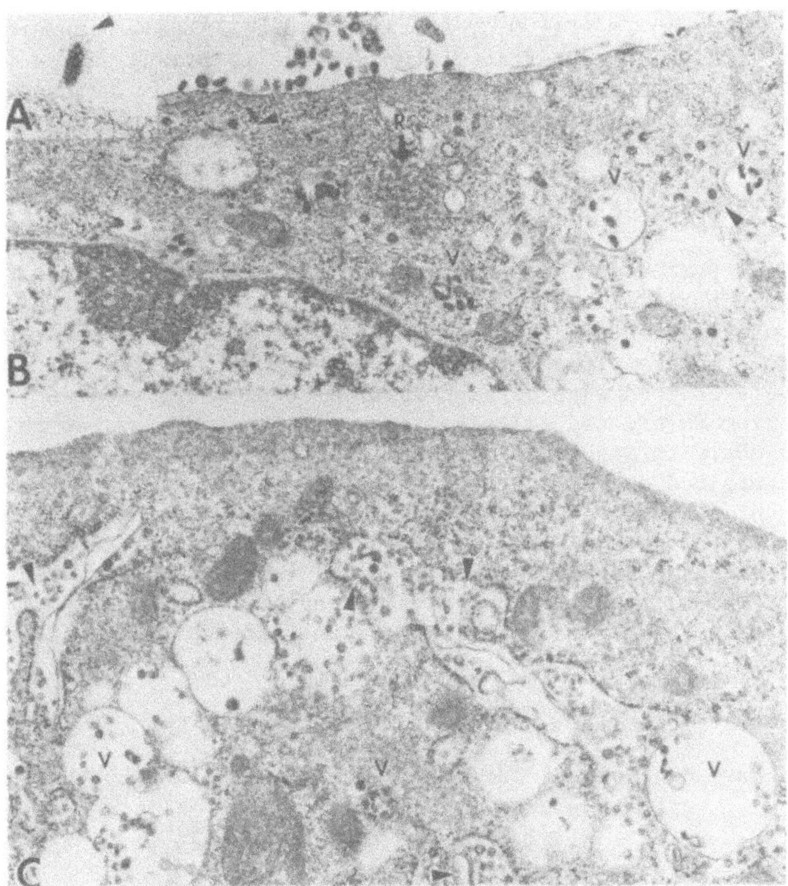

Fig 3. Effects of tunicamycin on virus maturation. 17 Cl 1 cells 24 hr after A59 infection (B) showed virions in RER (arrows), in smooth walled vesicles (V), and adsorbed to the plasma membrane and a reticular inclusion (R) in the cytoplasm. Insert (A) shows viral peplomers (arrow). TM treated cells (C) had virions in the RER, and smooth walled vesciles (V) but none on the plasma membrane. Arrows show long tubules in the RER. (A X60,000; B and C X23,000).

synthesis of the E2 polypeptide and could account for our failure to detect E2 in this pulse chase study (Klenk and Rott, 1980).

EFFECTS OF TUNICAMYCIN ON A59 VIRION FORMATION

The yield of infectious virus in the presence of tunicamycin was 0.1% of the yield in the absence of the drug at 24 hours. However transmission electron microscopic studies showed that virions are made in cells treated with TM (Fig. 3). A59 infected cells without TM (Fig. 3A and B) showed virions in the lumen of the rough endoplasmic reticulum (RER), in smooth walled vesicles (V) and adsorbed in large numbers to the plasma membrane by the tips of the peplomers. With TM (Fig 3C), A59 infected cells showed numerous virions in dilated cisternae of the RER and in smooth walled vesicles (V) but no virions adsorbed to the plasma membrane. In addition, numerous long tubules approximately 50nm in diameter were found in the lumen of the RER. Thus, virus particles were formed in TM and these virions migrated into smooth walled vesicles from which they could be discharged from the intact cells.

Virus particles released into the medium from intact TM treated cells were purified and concentrated by sucrose density gradient ultracentifugation and examined in negatively stained preparations (Fig. 4). Unlike virions purified from untreated infected cells which were covered with a thick layer of peplomers, virions released from TM treated cells had no surface peplomers. At this meeting, Dr. Sturman has shown that these virions from TM treated cells contained no E2, but showed normal ratios of E1 and N. The effects of tunicamycin on the replication of MHV are summarized in Table 1. The TM induced block in the synthesis of E2 does not prevent viral budding or the release of virions from infected cells. However, the released virions have no peplomers, contain no E2, are noninfectious, and cannot reabsorb to the surface of the infected cells.

FUNCTIONS OF THE GLYCOPROTEINS E1 and E2

We have made use of the differential inhibition by tunicamycin

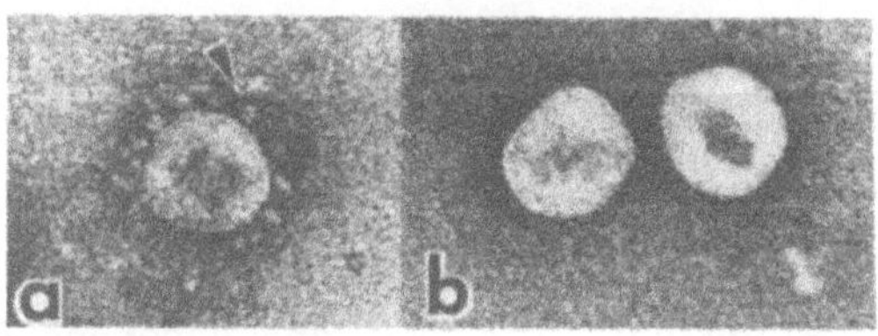

Fig 4. Effect of tunicamycin on virions. Virions purified from the medium over untreated cells (A) were covered with peplomers (arrow). No peplomers were seen on virions from TM treated cells (B) (X110,000).

Table 1. EFFECTS OF TUNICAMYCIN ON REPLICATION OF MHV

Yield of infectious virus decreased 1000X.

Synthesis of E2 blocked.

Synthesis and glycosylation of E1 not affected.

Virus budding continued.

Released virions contain N, E1 and RNA but no E2, are noninfectious and have no peplomers.

of the synthesis of the E1 and E2 glycoproteins of MHV and supporting data from other experiments to analyze the functions of the E1 and E2 glycoproteins. Our present concepts of the functions of E1 and E2 based on these studies are shown on Table 2.

That E2 is responsible for binding to susceptible cells is demonstrated by the inability of TM treated virions to bind to and infect cells and also by studies showing that binding of purified radiolabeled E2 to susceptible cells is prevented by pretreatment of the cells with concentrated MHV virions (data not shown).

The role of the peplomeric glycoprotein E2 in induction of cell fusion is suggested by the observation that tunicamycin, which prevents the synthesis of E2, also markedly reduces cell fusion in A59 infected L2 cells which are usually highly susceptible to fusion during replication of A59 (Fig. 5).

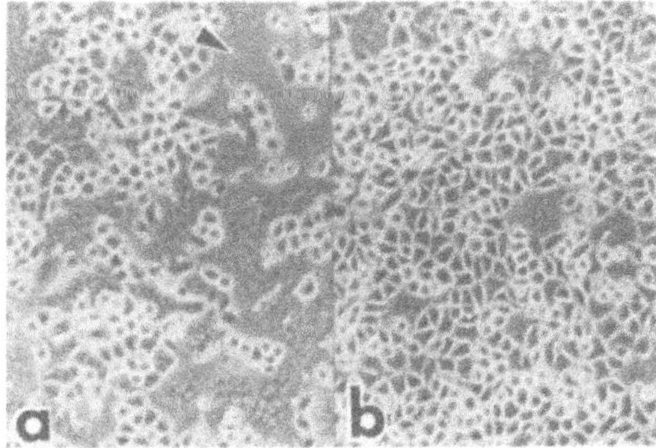

Fig 5. Inhibition of A59-induced cell fusion by tunicamycin. L2 cells 10 hours after inoculation were extensively fused (A). Arrow indicates area where syncytium has peeled off. Incubation of infected cells with 0.5μg/ml tunicamycin markedly reduced cell fusion (B).

Table 2. FUNCTIONS OF CORONAVIRUS GLYCOPROTEINS

E2, the peplomeric glycoprotein

1. Binding to susceptible cells.
2. Induction of cell fusion.
3. Induction of neutralizing antibody.

E1, the membrane glycoprotein

1. Determines location of viral budding.
2. Formation of viral envelope.

The role of E2 in cell fusion is also suggested by the observation that anti-E2 antibody but not anti-E1 antibody prevents fusion of MHV infected L2 cells (data not shown).

In neutralization tests anti-E2 antibody neutralized A59 virions more effectively than did anti-E1 antibody. These studies suggest that E2 is responsible for binding to receptors on susceptible cells and induction of cell fusion.

Immunofluorescent staining of MHV-infected cells with antibodies against purified E1 or purified E2 showed that these glycoproteins migrated differently within the infected cell (Doller and Holmes, 1980). Figure 6 shows MHV-infected 3T3 cells 8 hours after infection

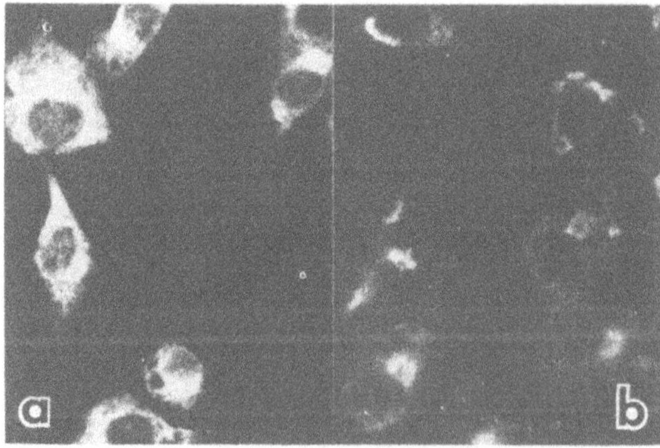

Fig 6. Localization of glycoprotein antigens. At 8 hrs after inoculation with A59, 17 Cl 1 cells were fixed with acetone and stained by the indirect fluorescent antibody technique with antibody to purified E2 (A) or antibody to purified E1 (B).

stained with anti-E2 or with anti-E1. Although the E2 antigen was distributed throughout the cytoplasm of the infected cells, the E1 antigen was restricted to tight clusters in the perinuclear area of the infected cells. This may correspond to the RER or Golgi apparatus of the infected cells. The localization of the E1 on these intracellular membranes may determine the site at which virions bud. It is possible that the restricted migration of E1 may be associated with the unusual glycosylation pattern of this glycoprotein. Perhaps E1 is glycosylated by the O-linked glycosylation pathway because it resembles cellular proteins which are localized in the RER or Golgi and which are glycosylated differently from the N-linked glycoproteins that rapidly disperse to the plasma membrane.

From the experiments showing formation of virions in the presence of tunicamycin it is clearly evident that E2 is not required for viral budding or for release of the virions from infected cells. Even in the TM-induced absence of E2 the formation of the viral envelope occurs in the intracytoplasmic membranes where E1 is localized and the nucleocapsid associates with the viral envelope normally. Thus, the E1 glycoprotein of this coronavirus appears to be functioning like the matrix or M proteins of other enveloped RNA viruses. However the matrix polypeptides of rhabdoviruses, paramyxoviruses, and orthomyxoviruses are not glycosylated.

Studies of E1 glycoprotein may serve as useful models for the synthesis, glycosylation and intracellular migration of cellular O-linked glycoproteins. The unique biochemical features of the E1 molecule may be responsible for important biological properties of coronaviruses such as budding from intracytoplasmic membranes and persistence of viral infection.

ACKNOWLEDGEMENTS

The authors are grateful for the excellent technical assistance of M. Kerchief and B. O'Neill. This work was supported by research grant R07403 from the Uniformed Services University of the Health Sciences. The opinions expressed in this report are the private views of the authors and should not be construed as official or as necessarily reflecting the views of the Uniformed Services University or the Department of Defense.

References

Anderson, R., Cheley, S., and Hayworth-Hatherell, E., 1979. Comparison of the Polypeptides of Two Strains of Mouse Hepatitis Virus, Virol., 97:492.

Bond, C.W., Leibowitz, J.L., and Robb, J.A., 1979. Pathogenetic

Murine Coronaviruses II. Characterization of Virus Specific Proteins of Murine Coronaviruses JHMV and A59V, Virol. 94:371.

Doller, E.W., and Holmes, K.V., 1980. Different Intracellular Transportation of the Envelope Glycoproteins E1 and E2 of the Coronavirus MHV. Abst. Amer. Soc. Microbiol., p 267.

Gibson, R., Schlesinger, S., and Kornfield, S., 1979. The Non-glycosylated Glycoprotein of Vesicular Stomatitis Virus is Temperature-sensitive and Undergoes Intracellular Aggregation at Elevated Temperatures. J. Biol. Chem., 254:3600.

Klenk, H-D., and Rott, R., 1980. Cotranslational and Posttranslational Processing of Viral Glycoproteins, Current Topics in Microbiol. Immunol., 90:19.

Schwarz, R.T., Rohrschneider, J.M., and Schmidt, M.F.G., 1976. Suppression of Glycoprotein Formation of Semliki Forest, Influenza, and Avian Sarcoma Virus by Tunicamycin, J. Virol., 19:782.

Siddell, S.G., Wege, H., Barthel, A., and ter Meulen, V., 1980. Coronavirus JHM: Cell Free Synthesis of Structural Protein p60, J. Virol., 33:10.

Sturman, L.S., 1977. Characterization of a Coronavirus I. Structural Proteins: Effects of Preparative Conditions on the Migration of Protein in Polyacrylamide Gels, Virology, 77:637.

Sturman, L.S., and Holmes, K.V., 1977. Characterization of a Coronavirus II. Glycoproteins of the Viral Envelope: Tryptic Peptide Analysis, Virology, 77:650.

Sturman, L.S., Holmes, K.V., and Behnke, J., 1980. Isolation of Coronavirus Envelope Glycoproteins and Interaction with the Viral Nucleocapsid, J. Virol., 33:449.

OLIGONUCLEOTIDE FINGERPRINTING OF THE RNA OF DIFFERENT STRAINS OF INFECTIOUS BRONCHITIS VIRUS

Jon P. Clewley, John Morser and Béla Lomniczi*

Department of Biological Sciences
University of Warwick
Coventry CV4 7AL

INTRODUCTION

Infectious bronchitis virus /IBV/, the prototype of the family coronaviridae[1] causes pathological conditions of the respiratory tract, the reproductive tract and the kidneys of chickens[2]. The disease was first described in the United States[3], but by the early sixties it had been identified all over the world. Early work showed that more than one serotype of IBV existed[4]. Since then a large number of strains have been isolated and attempts have been made to classify these strains using a serological approach. On the basis of immunofluorescence data, and virus neutralization tests carried out mostly with reference strains, at least eight serotypes[5] were established. However, in a study where large numbers of field strains were examined and compared to reference strains, it became apparent that it was not feasible to classify IBV isolates using a serological approach[6]. In an attempt to circumvent this problem strains were examined by cluster analysis using Euclidean distance as the measure of similarity and two main groups were established[7]. It was also found that twelve strains, fell into one or other of two categories of protein pattern differing in the mobility of a small glycoprotein on polyacrylamide gels[8,9]. It is of interest that reference strains placed in different groups by the cluster analysis also showed different protein patterns[8].

Under circumstances when live vaccine strains are used against a disease or when the relatively rapid emergence of new field strains

*Present address: Veterinary Medical Research Institute of the Hungarian Academy of Sciences, Budapest

Table 1. Description of IBV strains used for fingerprinting.

Serotype and strain designation	Symbol	Isolation Place	Isolation Year	Protein pattern[8]	Reference
1. Massachusetts					
Massachusetts 41	Mass 41	USA,Ma.	1941	M*	11
Connaught	Mass-C	USA	1954	M	12
Beaudette No.66579	Bea	USA	1937	M	13,14
927	927	England	1965-70	M	6
Houghton, HVI 140	HVI 140	England	1965-70	M	15
H120	H120	Holland	1956	M	17
2. Georgia					
SE 17	SE 17	USA,Ga.	1969	M	18
3. Connecticut					
Connecticut	Conn	USA, Co.	1951	C*	19
LED	LED	Hungary	1968	C	20
4. Delaware					
Holte	Holte	USA,Wisc.	1954	C	21
5. Iowa 97					
Iowa 97	Iowa 97	USA,Io.	1947	C	22
6. Australia T					
Australia T	Au T	Australia	1963	C	23
7. New Zealand A					
7533	NZ-A	New Zealand	1976	C	24

*Characterized by gp30 /M/ and gp28 /C/.

occurs /as in the case of infectious bronchitis/ a reliable method for strain identification is essential. The increasing understanding of the molecular biology of coronaviruses during the past few years prompted us to compare the RNAs of different IBV strains by oligonucleotide fingerprinting, which has been found to be useful in establishing the genetic basis of a serological classification of rhabdoviruses, picornaviruses, polioviruses, bunyaviruses, alfaviruses and retroviruses[10]. Previous studies have shown that viruses which cannot be antigenically differentiated usually give comparable but distinguishable oligonucleotide fingerprints. When few differences are seen the viruses are called variants of one another. In other cases where many differences occur between the fingerprints of

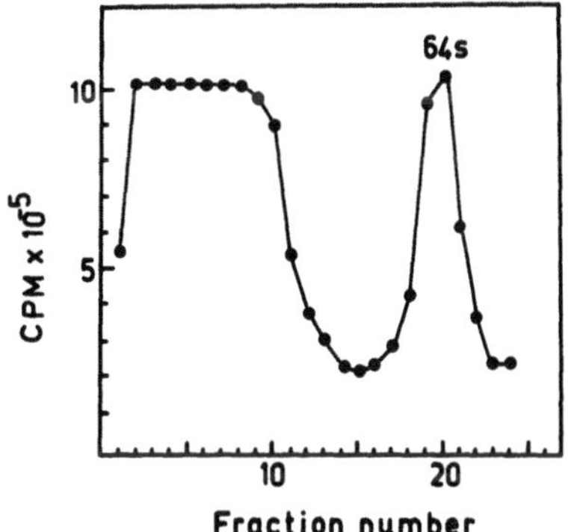

Fig. 1. 64s IBV RNA fractionated on sucrose gradient.

two isolates classified by other methods as the same virus type, the viruses are called varieties of the same type.

In this study the RNAs of strains of IBV belonging to the same serotype, and strains representing different serotypes have been compared by oligonucleotide fingerprinting.

MATERIALS AND METHODS

The identification code, year of isolation and geographical origin of the IBV strains used in this study are summarized in Table 1. The exact number of passages of the strains since their isolation is unknown but is probably in the order of ten to twenty. Strain Bea

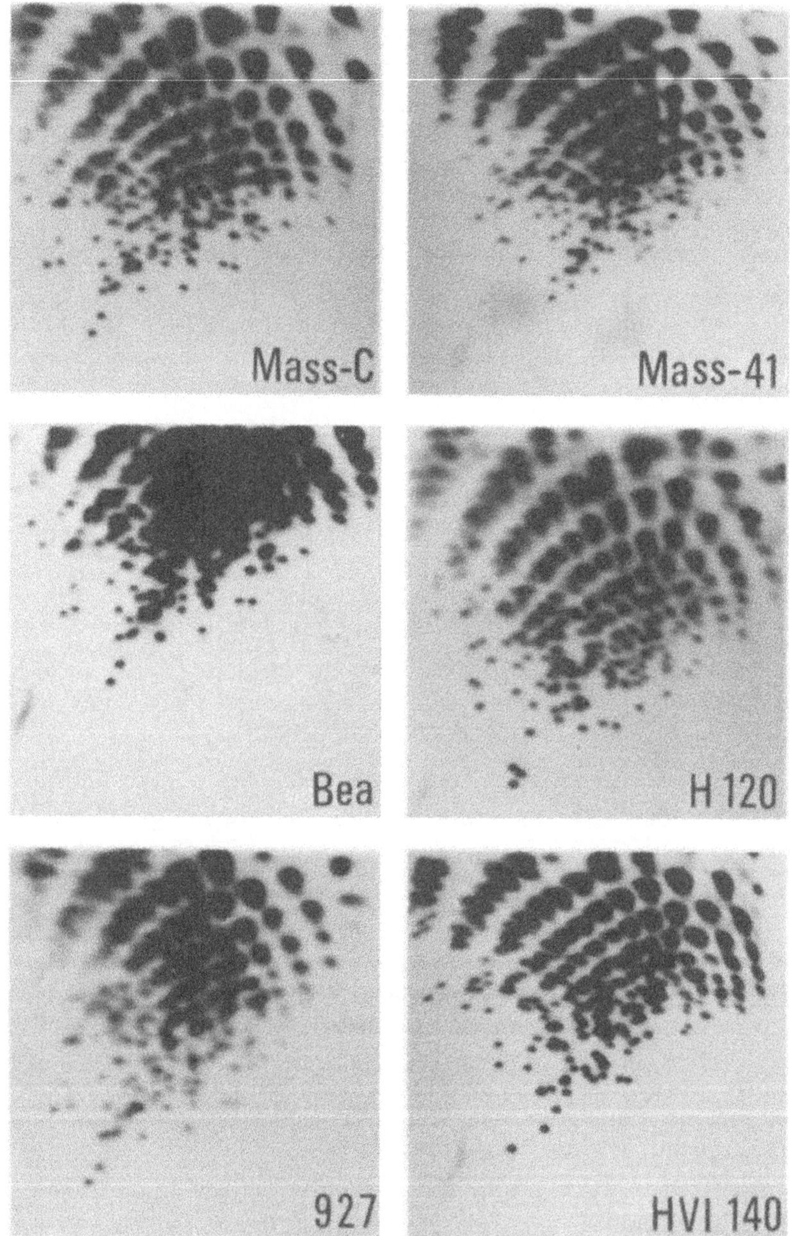

Fig. 2. Oligonucleotide fingerprints of RNA from six strains of IBV belonging to the Massachusetts serotype.

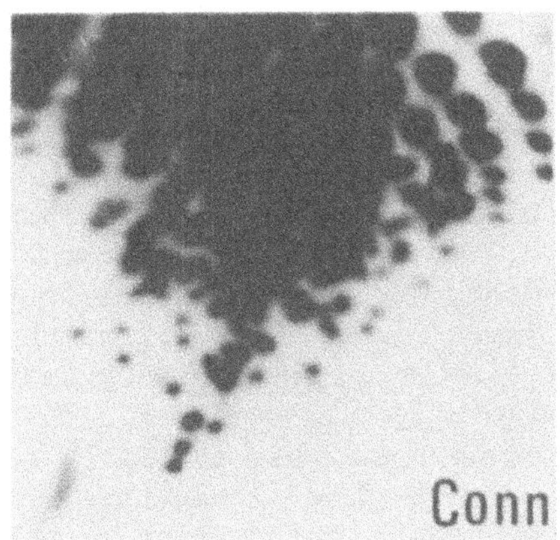

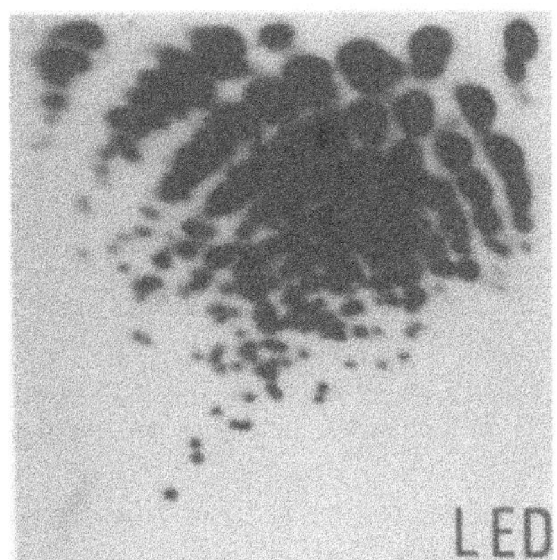

Fig. 3. Oligonucleotide fingerprints of RNA from two strains of IBV belonging to the Connecticut serotype.

is a highly passed strain, whose passage number is close to 300, for strain H120 the passage number is above 120 and for strain LED it is between 60 and 70.

IBV was grown in CEK cells as previously described[25].

^{32}P-labelled RNA was extracted from purified virus and fractionated on sucrose density gradients as described in detail earlier[25]. A typical profile of IBV RNA used for further analysis is shown on Fig. 1.

Labelled RNA precipitated from ethanol was digested with RNase T_1, and oligonucleotides were resolved on 2-dimensional gels, before visualization by autoradiography[26].

RESULTS

RNA was isolated from six strains of the Massachusetts serotype and fingerprinted /Fig. 2/. Three of the patterns obtained were obviously related to each other, showing only a few differences in their characteristic oligonucleotides. These were from strains Mass-C, Bea and 927, which are therefore variants of the same parental variety. The fingerprints of the other three strains are dissimilar to the extent that no common large oligonucleotides could be recognized. Thus Mass 41, HVI 140 and H120 represent other varieties of the Massachusetts serotype, and a total of 4 distinct varieties were identified in the 6 strains examined. These results show that oligonucleotide fingerprinting is much more incisive for strain differentiation than any methodology previously applied to IBV.

The relationships between viruses in the Connecticut serotype was investigated in a similar way. The reference strain Conn and a more recent isolate LED were compared and may have a few common spots, but their overall difference is conspicuous /Fig. 3/. Thus these represent different varieties within the Connecticut serotype.

The difference between the two major serotypes, Massachusetts and Connecticut was more rigorously investiagaed by co-electrophoresis of T_1 digests of their RNAs /not shown/. The majority /more than 70 per cent/ of the characteristic oligonucleotides did not co-electrophorese, suggesting that the viruses are only distantly related with little sequence homology. This is reflected in the differences that have been observed in the polypeptide composition of these viruses[8,9].

Representative viruses from five other serotypes were analysed by oligonucleotide fingerprinting in order to ascertain whether any have a significant degree of sequence homology. The fingerprints of three isolates from the Northern Hemisphere SE 17, Holte and Iowa 97 are shown in Fig. 4. There is no apparent relationship between these viral RNAs.

It was of interest to examine two strains from the Shouthern Hemisphere /NZ-A and Au T/ to determine whether it was possible to shed any light on the origin of these strains, since they were isolated later than Iowa 97 and Holte /see Table 1/. The fingerprints of these RNAs are shown in Fig. 5. As far as it is possible to tell NZ-A and Au T are unrelated to each other and to Iowa 97, Holte and

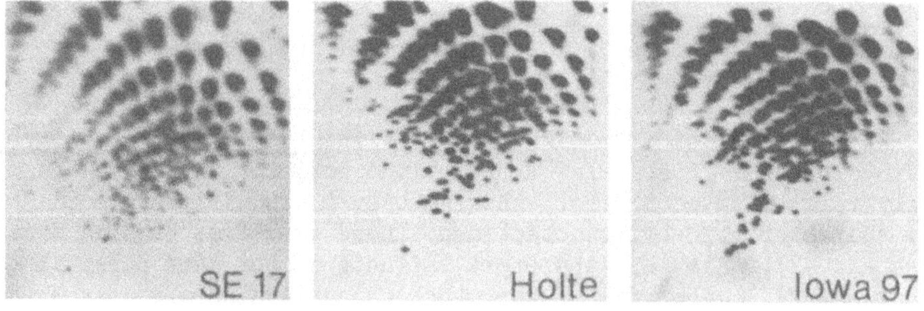

Fig. 4. Oligonucleotide fingerprints characteristic of the Georgia /SE 17/, Delaware /Holte/ and Iowa 97 serotypes of IBV, all of which are other Northern Hemisphere isolates.

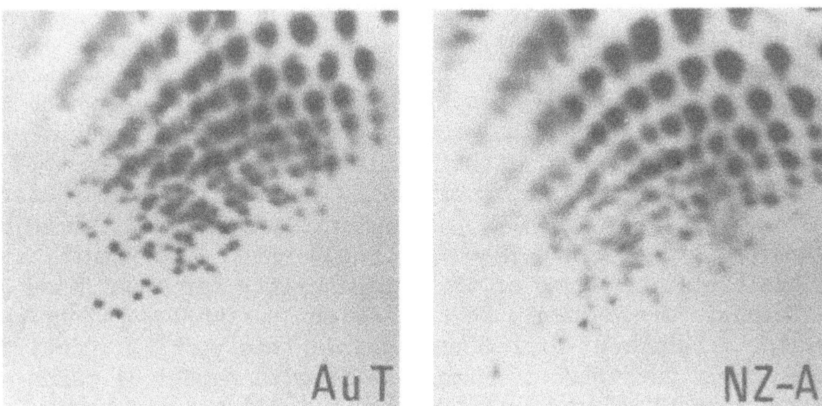

Fig. 5. Oligonucleotide fingerprints characteristic of Australia T /Au T/ and New Zealand A /NZ-A/ serotypes isolated in the Southern Hemisphere.

SE 17, suggesting that NZ-A was not derived from the Australian strain although New Zealand allowed the import of chickens from Australia before the NZ-A virus was isolated.

In addition, none of these five strains showed any obvious similarity with the two other major serotypes, Massachusetts and Connecticut.

DISCUSSION

We present here the T_1 oligonucleotide fingerprints of RNA prepared from 13 virus isolates. All these isolates were originally classified as IBV using pathological criteria. We have confirmed that all the viruses studied in this work have the virion density, genome size and protein profile expected for IBV /data not shown/. Nevertheless at least 11 different fingerprints were recognized. These were given by Mass 41, Mass-C, HVI 140 and H120 from the Massachusetts serotype, Conn and LED from the Connecticut serotype and five representatives of other serotypes, SE 17 from the Georgia serotype, Holte from the Delaware serotype, Iowa 97 from the Iowa 97 serotype, Au T from the Australia T serotype and NZ-A from the New Zealand A serotype. Thus different serotypes gave distinct fingerprints, but so did varieties within a serotype. Whether variants with similar fingerprints, such as Mass-C, Bea and 927 are antigenically closer to each other than to other varieties of the same serotype with different fingerprints is not yet established.

Further generalizations about the genetic basis of antigenic relationships among IBV isolates would be premature, and must await the introduction of more precise methods capable of recognizing subtle antigenic differences between strains.

One problem raised by this study is the question of which isolate should be considered the prototype virus of the Massachusetts serotype. Three of the viruses from the Massachusetts serotype characterized in this study, have virtually identical fingerprints. These are Mass-C, Bea and 927. These fingerprints differ substantially from the fingerprint of another virus which is currently regarded as the prototype virus of the Massachusetts serotype /Mass 41/. The differences are unlikely to have arisen during laboratory passage because the fingerprint of Bea produced in this work is identical to that previously published[25]. Thus the limited number of passage between these viruses /fewer than ten/ has not allowed the accumulation of sufficient mutations to change the pattern of characteristic oligonucleotides. This agree with results from other viruses[10]. Stern and Kenndey[27] have recently published a fingerprint of strain Beaudette /IBV 42/ obtained from the American Type Culture Collection which differs only slightly from the fingerprints we have obtained from Mass-C, Bea and 927. IBV 42 and strain Bea /No. 66579/ used by us, have been maintained as separate passage lines. Thus these four viruses are all variants of the same parental virus.

IBV was first recognized as a disease in the U.S.A. in 1931[3], but by the early sixties outbreaks had occurred all over the world. The viruses examined in this study were isolated over a period of years from widely separated geographical locations.

A great diversity among the fingerprints of these viruses all identified as IBV by other criteria indicates that considerable variation of the genome is possible. Fingerprint analysis provides information concerning theories of origin and spread of IBV. For example the NZ-A virus could be postulated to be derived from the Au T virus. This would seem reasonable since Au T was present in Australian chickens during the period in which these were imported into New Zealand. However fingerprint analysis of the virus subsequently isolated in New Zealand shows that it is not related to Au T. Therefore either the New Zealand virus has diverged very rapidly from Au T or it is derived from another source. This source, however, could not be any of the other viruses studied here because their fingerpints were also different.

Vaccines have been used prophylactically in attempts to control the disease caused by IBV. Some of these vaccines have been composed of live attenuated virus. When live vaccines are used there is an obvious danger that if the virus escapes, and if virulence is recovered, then the vaccine itself can actually be the cause of disease outbreaks. Two of the viruses used in this study /H120 and

Mass-C/ have been used as live vaccines. Mass-C was used as a vaccine in North America in the late fifties and early sixties. Subsequently /1965-70/ 927, whose fingerprint analysis showed to be very closely related to Mass-C, was isolated in England. Thus it is possible that 927 could be derived from escaped Mass-C virus, although at that time no live vaccine was licensed for use in England. Alternatively this variety of the Massachusetts serotype /Mass-C, Bea and 927/ has a wide temporal and geographical spread. In order to resolve this question, and others about the origin and spread of IBV varieties, further studies will be required following the evolution of IBV in the field.

SUMMARY

11 distinct oligonucleotide fingerprints were obtained in studies of the RNA of 13 isolates of IBV. Different serotypes had distinct fingerprints, but so did varieties within a serotype; allowing a greater degree of strain differentiation than was previously possible. Some conclusions can be drawn from the fingerprints concerning theories of origin and spread of IBV.

ACKNOWLEDGEMENTS

The authors wish to thank Professor D. C. Burke for his encouragement and interest. JPC was supported by a grant from C.R.C., JM by a M.R.C. programme grant awarded to Professor D. C. Burke and BL by Grants from the Royal Society, M.R.C. and E.M.B.O.

REFERENCES

1. D. A. J. Tyrell, D. J. Alexander, J. D. Almeida, C. H. Cunningham, B. C. Easterday, D. J. Garwes, J. C. Hierholzer, A. Kapikian, M. R. MacNaughton, and K. McIntosh, Coronaviridae: second report, Intervirol. 10:321 /1978/.
2. C. H. Cunningham, Avian infectious bronchitis, Adv. Vet. Sci. Comp. Med. 14:105 /1970/.
3. A. F. Schalk, and M. C. Hawn, An apparently new respiratory disease of baby chicks, J. Amer. Vet. Med. Ass. 78:413 /1931/.
4. M. S. Hofstad, Antigenic differences among isolates of avian infectious bronchitis virus, Amer. J. Vet. Res. 19:740 /1958/.
5. S. R. Hopkins, Serological comparisons of strains of infectious bronchitis virus using plaque-purified isolants, Avian Dis. 18:231 /1974/.
6. P. S. Dawson, and R. E. Gough, Antigenic variation in strains of avian infectious bronchitis virus, Arch. g. Virusforsch. 34:32 /1971/.

7. J. G. Darbyshire, J. G. Rowell, J. K. A. Cook, and R. W. Peters, Taxonomic studies on strains of avian infectious bronchitis virus using neutralization tests in tracheal organ culture, Arch. Virol. 61:227 /1979/.
8. E. Nagy, and B. Lomniczi, Polypeptide patterns of infectious bronchitis virus serotype fall into two categories, Arch. Virol. 61:341 /1979/.
9. M. S. Collins, and D. J. Alexander, Avian infectious bronchitis virus structural polypeptides: effect of different conditions of disruption and comparison of different strains and isolates. Arch. Virol. 63:239 /1980/.
10. J. P. Clewley, and D. H. L. Bishop, Oligonucleotide fingerprinting of viral genomes, in: " Newer Techniques in Practical Virology," C. R. Harvard, ed., Alan R. Liss Inc., New York /in press/.
11. H. Van Roekel, K. L. Balls, M. K. Clarke, O. M. Olesiuk, and F. G. Sperling, Infectious bronchitis. Mass. Agric. Exp. Stn. Bull. No. 460. /1950/.
12. S. B. Hitchner, and P. G. White, Groth-curve studies of chick embryo-propagated IBV. Poultry Sci. 34:590 /1955/.
13. F. R. Beaudette, and C. B. Hudson, Cultivation of the virus of infectious bronchitis. J. Amer. Vet. Med. Ass. 90:51 /1937/.
14. H. G. Purchase, C. H. Cunningham, and B. R. Burmaster, Identification and epizootiology of infectious bronchitis in a closed flock, Avian Dis. 10:111 /1966/.
15. J. W. Harkness, and C. D. Bracewell, Morphological variation among avian infectious bronchitis virus strains, Res. Vet. Sci. 16:128 /1974/.
16. J. Hoekstra, and B. Rispens, Infectieuze bronchitis bij pluimvee. I. Laboratorium-experimenten met een sterkwerkende entstam, Tijdschr. Diergeneesk. 85:398 /1960/.
17. G. Bijlenga, Het infectieuze bronchitis virus bij kiuken in Nederland, aangetoond mit behulp von ei-enting, dierexperimenteel onderzoek en serumneutralisatie-proveven, Tijdschr. Diergeneesk. 81:43 /1956/.
18. S. R. Hopkins, Serological and immunological properties of a recent isolate of infectious bronchitis virus, Avian Dis. 13: 356 /1969/.
19. E. L. Jungherr, T. W. Chomiak, and R. E. Luginbuhl, Immunologic differences in strains of infectious bronchitis virus, Proc. 60th Ann. Meeting U.S. Livestock San. Ass. Chicago. 203 /1956/.
20. B. Lomniczi, and L. Stipkovits, Isolation of the virus of infectious bronchitis, Magy. Áo. Lapja 23:600 /1968/.
21. R. W., Winterfield and S.B. Hitchner, Etiology of an infectious nephritis-nephrosis syndrome of chickens, Amer. J. Vet. Res. 23:1273 /1962/.
22. M. S. Hofstad, and H. W. Yoder, Jr., Avian infectious bronchitis – Virus distribution in tissues of chickens. Avian Dis. 10:230 /1966/.

23. R. B. Cummings, Infectious avian nephrosis /uraemia/ in Australia, Austral. Vet. J. 39:145 /1963/.
24. J. E. Lohr, Serological differences between strains of infectious bronchitis virus from New Zealand, Australia and the United States, Avian Dis. 20:478 /1976/.
25. B. Lomniczi, and I. Kennedy, Genome of infectious bronchitis virus. J. Virol. 24:99 /1977/.
26. J. P. Clewley, J. Gentsch, and D. H. L. Bishop, Three unique species of snowshoe hare and LaCrosse bunyviruses. J. Virol. 22:459 /1977/.
27. D. F. Stern, and S. I. T. Kennedy, Coronavirus multiplication strategy. I. Identification and characterization of virus-specified RNA. J. Virol. 34:665 /1980/.

CORONAVIRUS CELL-ASSOCIATED RNA-DEPENDENT RNA POLYMERASE

Douglas E. Dennis and David A. Brian

Department of Microbiology
The University of Tennessee
Knoxville, Tennessee 37916

INTRODUCTION

Infectious, single-stranded, nonsegmented, polyadenylated, genomic RNA has been demonstrated for the avian infectious bronchitis virus (Lomniczi and Kennedy, 1977; Schochetman et al., 1977), the mouse hepatitis virus (Lai and Stohlman, 1978; Wege et al., 1978), and the transmissible gastroenteritis virus (TGEV) of swine (Brian et al., 1980), three members of the coronavirus family. These properties alone would characterize these coronaviruses as positive-strand viruses and place them in category IV of the Baltimore Scheme (Baltimore, 1971). By analogy with the picornaviruses and togaviruses that have been characterized, also belonging to category IV of the Baltimore scheme, one would not expect to find an RNA-dependent RNA polymerase as part of the virion, but would expect to find such an enzyme in infected cells. In this paper we report that we are unable to detect an RNA-dependent RNA polymerase in purified virions, but we do find it associated with apparent membrane structures in infected cells between 4 and 6 h postinfection, a time when the rate of viral RNA synthesis is maximal. The [^{3}H]UMP-incorporating activity probably represents coronaviral- specified RNA-dependent RNA polymerase since (a) the activity was 10- to 100-fold greater than any similar activity in uninfected cells, (b) the activity was insensitive to actinomycin D, (c) the product was destroyed by RNase but not by DNase, (d) the activity was associated with an apparent replication complex that had sedimentation properties the same as cytoplasmic structures containing virus-specific RNA. In addition, the enzyme required the presence of all four ribonucleoside triphosphates, and Mg^{++} at approximately 5 mM concentration, for maximal activity. The enzyme was associated with cytoplasmic membrane-like structures. In an effort to determine the coronaviral specificity of the *in vitro* polymerase products, we examined the molecular weight, strandedness, (i.e., whether the RNA is single or double stranded), and polyadenylation of the *in vitro* polymerase products and compared these to the same properties for intracellular virus-specific RNA. Cells pulse-labeled with [^{3}H] uridine between 4 and 6 h post-infection contained five major species of single-stranded, polyadenylated RNA with apparent molecular weights of 6.8-, 3.15-, 1.40-, 0.94-, and 0.66 x 10^6 and seven minor species of single-stranded RNA with apparent molecular weights of 6.2-, 1.55-, 1.05-, 0.64-, 0.39-, 0.34- and 0.24 x 10^6 all of which were polyadenylated except for the 1.55 x 10^6 molecular weight species. When the membrane complex containing the viral RNA polymerase and endogenous template were used for the *in vitro* synthesis of RNA, three species of single-stranded, nonpolyadenylated RNA were made. These electrophoretically comigrated with three of the species made *in vivo* and they had molecular weights of approximately 3.15-, 1.40-, and 0.66 x 10^6. TGEV therefore apparently replicates as a positive-strand virus which employs a cell-associated, but not virion associated, RNA-dependent RNA polymerase for the synthesis of viral RNA. The virus also apparently replicates by synthesizing multiple mRNA species, and the synthesis of these species appears to be associated with membranous cytoplasmic structures.

MATERIALS AND METHODS

Cells, Virus, and Virus Purification

The epithelioid swine testicle cell line, (ST), developed by McClurkin (1966) was used as previously described (Brian et al., 1980). Clone 116 of the Purdue strain of swine TGEV was cloned again again by us and stocks were used between passages 3 and 6 as previously described (Brian et al., 1980).

TGEV was grown and purified as previously described (Brian et al., 1980). Essentially, supernatant fluids were collected at 18 to 20 h p.i, clarified by centrifugation at 10,000 x g for 10 min, layered onto an 18 ml continuous 20-60% (wt/wt) sucrose gradient, made up in, TNE (0.01 M Tris-hydrochloride [pH 7.5] - 0.1 M NaCl - 1.0 mM EDTA), and virus was isopycnically sedimented by centrifugation at 90,000 x g for 4 h at 4°C in a Sorvall AH-627 rotor. Virus was then pelleted at 150,000 x g for 2 h in a Sorvall AH-650 rotor.

RNA Polymerase Assay

The assay for virion-associated RNA-dependent RNA polymerase was one optimized by Huang et al.(1970), for the VSV-associated enzyme. In a standard reaction, 50 µl of purified virus, suspended to a concentration of 0.5 mg/ml in reticulocyte standard buffer (RSB) (0.01 M Tris hydrochloride (pH 7.4) - 0.01 M NaCl - 0.0015 M $MgCl^2$), was assayed in a 300 µl solution (total volume) containing 50 mM

Tris-hydrochloride (pH 7.3); 5.3 mM magnesium acetate; 100 mM sodium chloride; 3.3 mM 2-mercaptoethanol 830 μg Triton N-101 per ml; 0.83 μM [5-^{3}H] UTP (4.4 x 10^7 cpm/pmole) or 2.20 mM [8-^{3}H] GTP (1.65 x 10^7 cpm/pmole); 0.67 mM each of ATP, CTP, and GTP (or UTP when [^{3}H]GTP was used). The amount of labeled substrate incorporated into product in 30 min at 33°C was measured by collecting the product on membrane filters (Amicon, 0.45 μm) after precipitation with 5% trichloroacetic acid - 0.05 M sodium pyrophosphate at 0°C. Dried filters were counted by scintillation spectrophotometry.

The assay for cell-associated RNA-dependent RNA polymerase was a modification of that described by Polatnick and Arlinghaus (1967). In a standard reaction, 50 μl of sample, suspended to a protein concentration of 5 to 10 mg per ml in 0.25 M sucrose - 0.0015 M $MgCl_2$ - 40 μg dextran sulfate per ml - 0.28% (wt/wt) deoxycholate, was assayed in a 200 μl solution (total volume) containing: 50 mM Tris-hydrochloride (pH 8.0); 5 mM magnesium acetate; 10 mM phosphoenolpyruvic acid; 40 μg phosphoenol pyruvate kinase per ml; 17.5 mM 2-mercaptoethanol; 20 μg actinomycin D per ml; 1.25 M [5-^{3}H] UTP (4.4 x 10^7 cpm/pmole) or 3.30 μM [8 ^{3}H] GTP (1.65 x 10^7 cpm/pmole); 0.5 mM each of ATP, CTP, and GTP (or UTP when [^{3}H]GTP was used). The amount of labeled substrate incorporated into product in 60 min at 37°C was measured by collecting the product on membrane filters as described above.

Subcellular Fractionation

Batches of 2- to 8 x 10^8 cells (representing 1 to 4 confluent roller bottle cultures) were treated as described in individual experimental protocols with regard to infection and radioisotopic labeling. At the designated times, cells were drained and washed 5 times with ice cold TN buffer (0.01 M Tris-hydrochloride (pH 7.4)-0.14 M NaCl). All further steps were done at 0-4°C. Cells were scraped into TN buffer and pelleted by centrifugation at 500 x g for 5 min. Cells were resuspended in 5-10 ml of a 0.3 M sucrose solution, allowed to swell for 10 minutes, and then disrupted using 15 strokes in a tight fitting glass Dounce homogenizer. Cellular disruption and nuclear breakage were monitored by light microscopy. The suspension was centrifuged at 650 x g for 7 min and the pellet which contained nuclei and other large debris was designated the nuclear fraction. The resultant supernatant was then centrifuged at 13,000 x g for 20 minutes, conditions known to pellet mitochondria, endoplasmic reticulum, cytoplasmic membranes and other membranous organellar structures. This pellet was designated the post-nuclear fraction. The resultant supernatant was designated the soluble fraction and was either analyzed directly for measurement of trichloroacetic acid-precipitable radioactive material, or was further treated with 10% polyethylene glycol to form a precipitate which was then resuspended and analyzed for enzymatic activity.

Extraction of RNA

Total cytoplasmic RNA was extracted by the method of Erickson et al. (1973). RNA was extracted from the pelleted postnuclear fraction or from the *in vitro* reaction mixture by the SDS-proteinase K-phenol method that we have previously described (Brian et al., 1980).

Agarose Gel Electrophoresis and Fluorography

The method of Lerach et al. (1977) was used to analyze RNA by electrophoresis in agarose gels. RNA samples were heated in 2.2M formaldehyde-50% (wt/wt) formamide-0.018M Na_2HPO_4-0.002M NaH_2PO_4, for 5 min. at 60°C immediately prior to electrophoresis. Electrophoresis buffer was 2.2M formaldehyde-0.0018M Na_2HPO_4-0.002M NaH_2PO_4. Slab gels of 0.75% agarose were used with a horizontal apparatus of 11 x 13 cm dimensions. Gels were 6 mm thick. Electrophoresis was carried out using 50 volts of constant voltage with a current of approximately 50mA. Upon termination of electrophoresis, gels were dehydrated in two sequential baths of 10 volumes of methanol for 2.5 h each. Methanol was then blotted from the gels using filter paper until the gels were approximately 1.5 mm thick at which time they were treated with Enhance (New England Nuclear, Boston, Mass.) and dried in a slab gel drier under vacuum and low heat. Gels were fluorographed by the method of Laskey and Mills (1975).

Materials

[^3H] uridine (8 Ci/mole) was obtained from Schwartz/Mann. [5,6-^3H]UTP (40 Ci/mmole) and [8-^3H] GTP (15 Ci/mmole) obtained from ICN Chemical and Radioisotope Division were in a 50% ethanol solution. The ethanol was removed by lyophilization and the nucleoside triphosphate was dissolved in the reaction medium. Cellular and viral RNA marker species were prepared as previously described (Brian et al., 1980).

RESULTS

Absence of RNA-Dependent RNA Polymerase in Purified TGEV

To examine the possibility that TGEV does possess a viron-associated RNA-dependent RNA polymerase, semi-purified and purified viral preparations were examined using an RNA polymerase optimized for vesicular stomatitis virus-associated enzyme. Table 1 illustrates that no RNA polymerase activity could be found in purified TGEV. At no time could polymerase activity be detected when a variety of different protocols were used (data not shown). The assay as employed for the detection of cell associated enzyme was also used, but modified to include detergent, and no enzyme activity could be detected (data not shown).

Table 1. Absence of RNA polymerase in purified TGEV.

Experiment	$[^3H]$UMP incorporation (fmole/mg protein/hr) VSV	TGEV
1[a]	62	0.01
2[b]	49	0.01
3[c]	49	0.02

[a]Approximately 10^{10} pfu of virus was partially purified from 800 ml of tissue culture fluid and assayed directly. Tissue culture fluid harvested from cells at 24 h p.i. was clarified at 13,000 x g for 20 min and virus was pelleted from the supernatant at 90,000 x g for 2 h through an 8 ml barrier of 20% sucrose (wt/wt) made up in TNE.

[b]Approximately 10^{10} pfu of virus was purified from 800 ml of supernatant fluids as described in the text, except that virus was first concentrated by sedimentation onto a 60% (wt/wt) sucrose cushion before resuspension and isopycnic sedimentation. Purified virus was pelleted and stored at -80°C for 1 week prior to assay.

[c]Approximately 10^{10} pfu of virus was purified from 800 ml of supernatant fluids as described in the text, except that virus was first concentrated by polyethylene glycol precipitation before resuspension and isopycnic sedimentation. For polyethylene glycol precipitation, clarified supernatant was made 10% final concentration with polyethylene glycol (6000) - 0.1 M NaCl-0.001 M EDTA, held at 0°C for 0.5 h with constant stirring, and the precipitate was pelleted at 1500 x g for 40 min at 0°C. The pellet was resuspended by Dounce homogenization prior to isopycnic sedimentation. In each experiment, virus was resuspended and assayed as described in the text.

Kinetics and Site of In Vivo RNA Synthesis

For the purpose of optimizing chances of detecting an active cell-associated RNA-dependent RNA polymerase, studies were made to determine the interval, within the 20 h growth cycle of the virus (Brian et al., 1980), during which viral RNA was synthesized at a maximal rate, and to determine the site of RNA synthesis during this time. The interval was determined by pulse-labeling infected cells with $[^3H]$uridine in the presence of actinomycin D (Fig. 1). The rate of RNA synthesis was found to be maximal between 4 and 6 hours postinfection. Mock-infected cells showed no such increase throughout the 20 h period indicating that the observed RNA synthesis is induced by the viral infection and probably represents virus-specific RNA synthesis. To determine the site of viral RNA synthesis, infected cells were pulse-labeled at 5 h postinfection with $[^3H]$uridine in

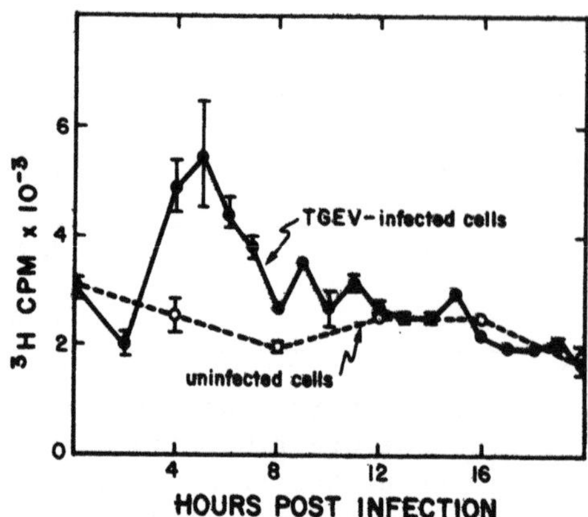

Fig. 1. Kinetics of viral RNA synthesis. Cells in 30 mm plates were infected simultaneously with TGEV at a multiplicity of 10 pfu/cell, or mock infected with balanced salt solution, and refed with medium containing 2% fetal calf serum. At 1 hour pior to labeling, actinomycin D was applied to the cells at a concentration of 0.1 μg/ml and kept there for the duration of the RNA labeling period. 4 μCi [^{3}H]uridine was added per plate at the indicated time postinfection for a 1 hr pulse. Periods were timed from the beginning of virus adsorption. Duplicate cultures were used for each time point. Acid precipitable radioactivity was determined for each culture.

the presence of actinomycin D, immediately fractionated into nuclear, postnuclear, and soluble fractions, and the fractions were analyzed for acid-precipitable radioactivity (data not shown). Infected cells incorporated 50 times more labeled uridine than did uninfected cells. The postnuclear fraction of the infected cells contained 80% of the total radioactivity. The postnuclear fraction of infected cells contained 50 times more radioactivity than the postnuclear fraction from uninfected cells. We concluded therefore that the viral RNA synthesizing structures were contained in the postnuclear fraction and this fraction was selected for further study of a viral RNA polymerase activity.

RNA Polymerase Activity in the Infected Cells

When we sought an RNA polymerase activity in the postnuclear fraction, 10 to 100-fold greater activity was found over any similar activity detectable in the postnuclear fraction from uninfected cells (Table 2).

Table 2. RNA polymerase activity in the sedimentable postnuclear fraction of TGEV-infected cells.[a]

Origin of postnuclear fraction	$[^3H]$UMP incorporation	
	cpm/assay/hr	fmole/mg protein/hr
Uninfected cells	122	2.5
Infected cells	6385	145

[a]Separate roller cultures, each containing 2 x 10^8 cells, were infected at a multiplicity of 10 pfu/cell or mock infected with a balanced salt solution, and refed with medium containing 2% fetal calf serum. At 5 h p.i., cells were scraped from the bottle and fractionated as described in the text. The postnuclear fraction was assayed for RNA polymerase as described in the text. Each assay was done in triplicate and the number shown represents the arithmetic mean of the three assays.

Characteristics of the Enzyme Activity

The $[^3H]$UMP incorporating activity was characterized with respect to the properties listed in Table 3. The polymerizing activity was reduced by 25% in the absence of Mg^{++}, and was reduced by 85% when Mn^{++} was substituted for Mg^{+}. The activity therefore apparently requires Mg^{++}. No other divalent cations were tested. The polymerizing activity was reduced by only 2% in the absence of 2-mercaptoethanol so a reducing agent is apparently not required for full activity. Enzymatic activity was not diminished when phosphoenol pyruvate and phosphoenol pyruvate kinase were omitted from the reaction mixture. An ATP generating system is evidently not required for activity. This may be evidence that ATPases which are normally present in crudely prepared postnuclear fractions were adequately removed by pelleting the postnuclear preparation through 20% sucrose. The presence of 20 µg actinomycin D per ml in the reaction failed to inhibit $[^3H]$UMP incorporation and therefore precludes the possibility that the product was made from a DNA template. Because there was decreased activity in the absence of all three supplementary nucleoside triphosphates when $[^3H]$UMP was used as the labeled compound, there is apparently a template requirement for the activity. It is therefore unlikely that we were merely detecting a polyuridylic acid synthetase activity. When dependence on individual nucleoside triphoshates was measured, we observed a complete dependence on ATP, but very little or no dependence on CTP and GTP. We are unable to explain these latter observations. When $[^3H]$GTP was used as the labeled nucleoside triphosphate a substantial dependence on each of the supplementary

Table 3. Characteristics of the RNA polymerase activity.[a]

Sample	[^{3}H]UMP or [^{3}H]GMP incorporation (fmole/mg protein/hr)	% of complete reaction
Complete reaction[b]	137	100
minus Mg^{++}[bd]	103	75
minus Mg^{++}, plus 2 mM Mn^{++}[bd]	20	15
minus 2-mercaptoethanol[b]	134	98
minus PEP and PEP kinase[b]	142	104
minus actinomycin D[b]	142	104
minus ATP[b]	13	9
minus CTP[b]	113	82
minus GTP[b]	123	90
minus ATP, CTP, and GTP[b]	3	2
minus dextran sulfate[b]	175	127
200 µg/ml dextran sulfate[be]	129	94
heated product plus DNase[bf]	137	100
heated product plus RNase[bg]	37	27
complete reaction[c]	286	100
minus ATP[c]	123	43
minus UTP[c]	87	31
minus CTP[c]	29	10
minus ATP, UTP, and CTP[c]	6	2
uninfected cell postnuclear fraction[c]	6	2

[a]The assay was performed as described in the text on a postnuclear fraction prepared in the following manner. Cells were lysed and and the nuclear fraction was removed as described. The supernant from the nuclear pellet was made 17 ml total volume by the addition of 0.3 M sucrose and layered onto a 20 ml cushion of 20% sucrose (wt/wt)-0.01 M Tris-hydrochloride (pH 7.4) in a 38 ml centrifuge tube. The pellet formed by centrifugation at 60,000 x g for 1.5 h at 4°C in a Sorvall AH-627 rotor was drained and resuspended in a solution of 0.01 M Tris-hydrochloride (pH 8.0) - 0.0015 M $MgCl_2$ - 40 µg dextran sulfate 500 (Sigma) per ml - 0.28% (wt/wt) sodium deoxycholate to a final protein concentration of 5-10 mg/ml.
[b][^{3}H]UTP was used.
[bc][^{3}]HGTP was used.
[d]The postnuclear fraction was resuspended in 0.25 sucrose - 0.28% (wt/wt) - sodium deoxycholate.
[e]At the end of the 60 min reactions, the entire mixture was heated at 100° for 2 min, cooled to 37°C and treated with 50 µg DNase I (Worthington) per ml for 15 min at 37°C.
[f]At the end of the 60 min reaction, the entire mixture was heated at 100° for 2 min, cooled to 37°C and treated with 20 µg RNase A (Sigma) per ml and 20 units T1 RNase (Sigma) per ml for 15 min at 37°C
nucleoside triphosphates was observed. These observations can most

readily be explained by the dependence of the activity on a template. Since the enzyme was not inhibited by actinomycin D, we conclude that the template was RNA. The heat denatured product was resistant to DNase but was 73% degraded by a mixture of pancreatic and T_1 RNases. We therefore conclude that the product was RNA.

When concentrations of Mg^{++} were used in 5 mM increments above 0 mM, a maximal activity of 325 fmole [^{3}H]UMP incorporation/mg protein/hour was observed at 5 mM concentration (data not shown). Increased concentrations above 5 mM caused an apparent aggregation within the reaction mixture which had the appearance of a precipitate. This may have been the cause of the inhibition at the higher concentrations. The rate of [^{3}H]UMP incorporation at 37°C increases rapidly for the first 10 min and then decreases by more than 50% to remain constant for at least 50 min. (data not shown). For studies in which the RNA product was analyzed reaction times were normally held to less than 15 minutes to minimize the liklihood of RNase degradation.

Apparent Membrane Association of the Polymerase

Viral RNA synthesizing complexes, of both positive-strand picornaviruses and togaviruses, and negtive-strand myxoviruses and rhabdoviruses, are found to have an intimate association with cytoplasmic membranous structures. These structures usually have buoyant densities of 1.20 g/cm^3 or less in sucrose gradients. We have found that the postnuclear fraction of TGEV-infected cells, pulse-labeled with [^{3}H]uridine in the presence of actinomycin D, can be resolved by isopycnic sedimentation on sucrose gradients into structures with buoyant densities of 1.15 and 1.19 g/cm^3 (data not shown). Material from each of these fractions contains virus-specific RNA, and therefore a membrane-association of the TGEV-RNA synthesizing apparatus is suggested. When the postnuclear fraction prepared in the same way was sedimented on a rate zonal sucrose gradient, the TGEV-specific RNA sedimented in one peak apparently as part of a complex having an average sedimentation coefficient of approximately 500S. This complex also contained the RNA-dependent RNA polymerase activity (data not shown). In an attempt to verify the membrane association of the polymerase, the postnuclear fraction of TGEV- infected cells prepared as described above, was treated with the nonionic detergent deoxycholate and sedimented on a rate zonal gradient in the presence of deoxycholate (Fig. 2). The TGEV-specific RNA now sediments as one peak with a sedimentation coefficient of approximately 230S. The detergent apparently destroyed a membrane association. When an unlabeled postnuclear fraction was sedimented on a rate zonal gradient in the presence of deoxycholate, two peaks of polymerase activity were resolved (Fig. 2). These peaks had sedimentation coefficients of approximately 600S and 160S, suggesting again that the detergent had destroyed a membrane association. As yet, we have no direct proof that the enzyme is associated with membranes.

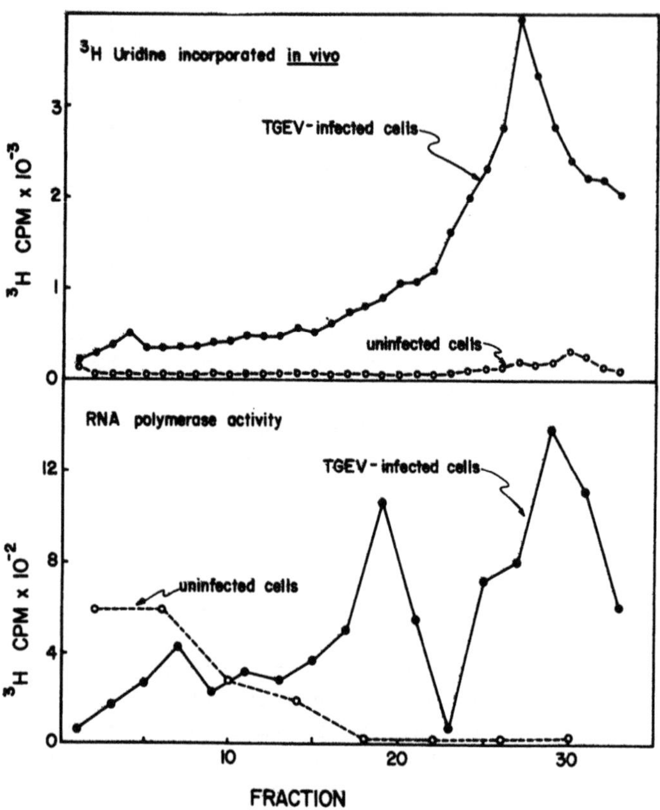

Fig. 2. Rate zonal sedimentation of deoxycholate-solubilized postnuclear fraction. a) 2 x 10^8 cells in roller culture were infected at a multiplicity of 10 pfu/cell and an identical culture was mock infected with a balanced salt solution. At 3 h p.i., timed from the beginning of the adsorption period, actinomycin D was added to make a final concentration of 1.0 µg/ml. At 5 h p.i., 100 µCi [^{3}H]uridine was added per culture and cells were incubated for 0.5 h at 37°C. Cells were then fractionated as described in the text except that the postnuclear fraction was resuspended in 0.25 M sucrose - 0.0015 M $MgCl_2$ and immediately made 1% (wt/wt) with sodium deoxycholate. The solubilized postnuclear fraction was then sedimented on a 15 to 40% (wt/wt) sucrose gradient which contained 1% (wt/wt) final concentration sodium deoxycholate. Sedimentation was at 23,500 x g for 1.5 h at 4°C in a Sorvall AH-627 rotor and the gradients were fractionated and analyzed for acid precipitable radioactivity. b) 2 x 10^8 each of infected and uninfected cells were treated and fractionated as described in part a) except that they were not isotopically labeled. The postnuclear fractions were sedimented on rate zonal gradients containing 1% (wt/wt) sodium deoxycholate in parallel with the gradients described in part a). Indicated fractions of the gradient were assayed for [^{3}H]UMP-incorporating activity. Sedimentation is from right to left.

Virus Specific RNA in Infected Cells.

To characterize the in vitro polymerase products and to determine their viral specificity, RNA extracts of infected cells, the postnuclear fraction of infected cells, and in vitro polymerase products, were examined on a comparative basis. All preparations were from cells between 4 and 6 h postinfection. To examine the RNA species made during this interval of time infected cells were labeled with [^{3}H] uridine in the presence of actinomycin D and the RNA was extracted from whole cells by the method of Erickson et al., 1973, and examined under denaturing conditions by electrophoresis on agarose gels (Fig. 3). Five major species having apparent molecular weights of 6.8-, 3.15-, 1.40-, 0.94-, and 0.66 x 10^6 were seen. In additon, 3 minor species having apparent molecular weights of 6.2-, 1.55-, and 1.05 x 10^6 were also seen. No RNA could be observed in extracts from uninfected cells even though the total rate of RNA synthesis under these conditions was 3% of that in infected cells. To determine whether the RNA species found in the postnuclear fraction were the same as those extracted from whole infected cells, infected cells were

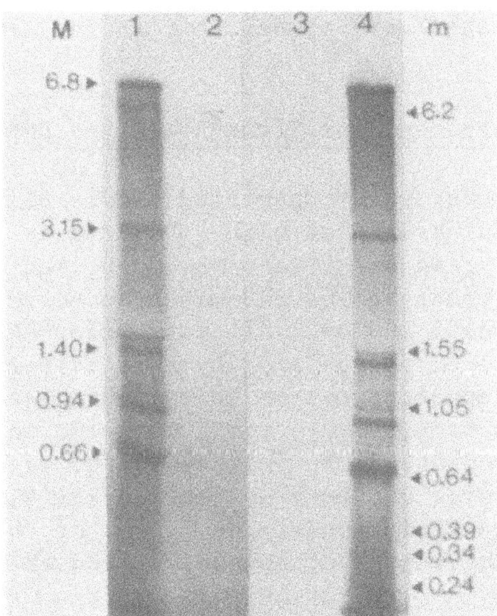

Fig. 3. Electrophoresis of intracellular RNA on denaturing agarose gel. Cells were infected with TGEV or mock infected and radiolabeled with [^{3}H]uridine using the conditions discribed in Fig. 2. (1) RNA extracted from infected whole cells. (2) RNA extracted from uninfected whole cells. (3) RNA extracted from the postnuclear fraction of uninfected cells. (4) RNA extracted from the postnuclear fraction of infected cells. M and m indicate the molecular weight (X10^{-6}) of the major and minor species respectively.

pulse-labeled with [^{3}H] uridine at 5 h postinfection in the presence of actinomycin D and the postnuclear fraction was prepared. RNA was extracted and analyzed by electrophoresis under denaturing conditions on agarose gels (Fig. 3). Five major RNA species were found which had the same electrophoretic mobilities as the five major species extracted from whole cells. In addition, there were seven minor species, three of which migrate the same as the three minor species in whole cell extracts. The minor species had apparent molecular weights of 6.2-, 1.55-, 1.05-, 0.64-, 0.39-, 0.34-, and 0.24 x 10^6 molecular weight. Molecular weights were estimated by extrapolation and interpolation from a plot of molecular weight vs relative mobility for known single-stranded RNA markers. The 6.8 x 10^6 molecular weight species comigrated with TGEV virion RNA. Approximately 5% of the total radioactivity was observed as unresolved species migrating with 4S RNA.

Single-Stranded Nature of Intracellular Virus-Specified RNA

All RNA species extracted from infected cells were single-stranded as judged by their sensitivity to digestion with RNase T_1 in 0.3M NaCl (Fig. 4). It is possible that double-stranded replicative intermediates were present but in too few numbers to be detected by this method.

Polyadenylation of Intracellular Virus-Specified RNA.

To determine whether virus-specified RNA is polyadenylated, infected cells were pulse-labeled with [^{3}H] uridine at 5 h postinfection in the presence of actinomycin D, and RNA was extracted from the postnuclear fraction and chromatographed on oligo (dT)-cellulose (Figures 4 and 5). All five major RNA species and six minor RNA species were polyadenylated by this criterion. The 1.55 x 10^6 molecular weight appeared not be be polyadenylated. In addition, some of the 6.8-, 1.40-, and 0.66 x 10^6 molecular weight species appeared not to be polyadenylated as well. The nonpolyadenylated species may be minus-strand RNA's, or they may reflect incomplete transcription of the 3' end of the molecule. Alternatively, they may represent molecules from which the 3' end was lost by breakage.

Viral RNA Species Synthesized During the In Vitro Polymerase Reaction

In order to make a direct comparison between RNA species made *in vitro* and those made *in vivo*, both were analyzed by electrophoresis on the same agarose slab gel following denaturation (Figures 4 and 5). By these analyses, two *in vitro* transcripts with apparent molecular weights of 1.40-, and 0.66 x 10^6 and a possible third transcript with an apparent molecular weight of 3.15 x 10^6 were observed. In addition a broad band of material with a molecular

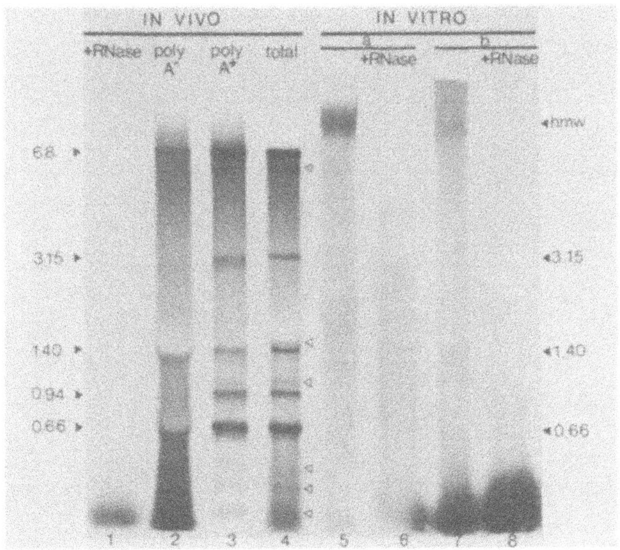

Fig. 4. RNase susceptibility of intracellular TGEV-specific RNA and in vitro polymerase products. The radiolabeled postnuclear fraction of infected cells was prepared as described in Fig. 2. The RNA was extracted and electrophoresed on denaturing agarose gels after the following treatments. (1) Digestion with 20 units T_1 RNase per ml - 0.3 M NaCl for 1h at 37°C. (2) and (3), oligo(dT)-cellulose chromatography using the procedure we have previously described (Brian et al., 1980). (4) No treatment. Radiolabeled in vitro reaction products from two separate experiments (a and b) were extracted as described in the text and electrophoresed after the following treatments. (5) No treatment. (6) RNase digestion as described in (1). (7) No treatment. (8) RNase digestion as described in (1).

weight of greater than 6.8×10^6 was observed. This is designated as high molecular weight (hmw) RNA. Digestion of the in vitro products with T_1 RNase in 0.3M NaCl demonstrates that all but the hmw RNA species are single stranded (Fig. 4). Oligo (dT)-cellulose chromatography of the in vitro products reveals that the 1.40- and 0.66×10^6 molecular weight species are apparently not polyadenylated (Fig. 5).

DISCUSSION

Our results indicate that the TGEV virion does not possess an RNA-dependent RNA polymerase but that the virus induces an enzyme of this type during intracellular replication. The absence of this enzyme(s) on the virion along with an infectious, single-stranded,

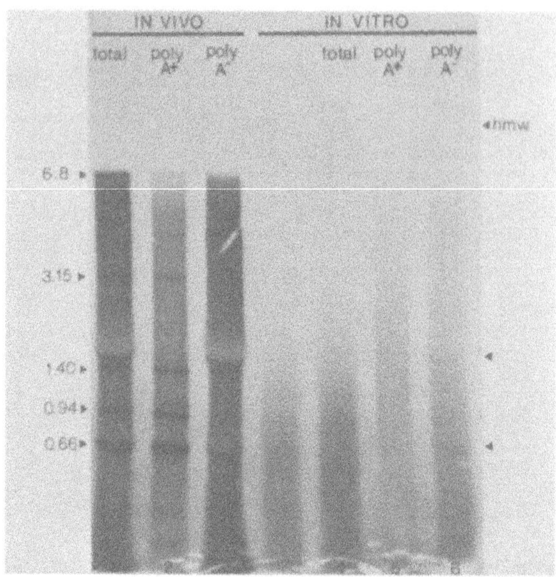

Fig. 5. Polyadenylation status of intracellular TGEV-specific RNA and in vitro polymerase products. The radiolabeled postnuclear fraction of infected cells was prepared as described in Fig. 2. The RNA was extracted and electrophoresed on denaturing agarose gels after the following treatments: (1) No treatment. (2) and (3), chromatography on oligo(dT)-cellulose using the previously described procedure (Brian et al., 1980). Radiolabeled in vitro reaction products were extracted as described in the text and electrophoresed after the following treatments: (4) No treatment. (5) and (6), chromatography on oligo(dT)-cellulose.

RNA genome are properties shared by picornaviruses and togaviruses. Many features of the coronavirus enzymatic activity are shared by the picornavirus and togavirus counterparts. Maximal activity requires Mg^{++} and the presence of all nucleoside triphosphates. The enzyme is apparently part of a membrane associated replication complex as judged by the bouyant density of the complex. Treatment of the complex with a nonionic detergent changes the sedimentation coefficient of the complex and further suggests a membrane-association.

One unique feature of coronavirus replication which contrasts sharply with the replicational schemes of picornaviruses and togaviruses is that apparent multiple mRNA species are employed during coronavirus replication (Stern and Kennedy, 1980). We demonstrate that a similar scheme is apparently true for the replication of TGEV as well.

While a cell-associated RNA-dependent RNA polymerase is undoubtedly used in the replication of the genomic RNA (i.e., synthesis of the minus-strand) as well as transcription of the genomic RNA and mRNA species (i.e., synthesis of the positive-strands), no effort was made in our studies to separate the two activities. Several attempts to demonstrate double-stranded forms of RNA from infected cells were not successful suggesting that perhaps negative-strand species were present in only very small numbers or possibly positive and minus strands were loosely associated in the replicative forms and were thus separated during RNA extraction. The only possible double-stranded candidates were the high molecular weight RNA species observed after nuclease treatment of _in vitro_ transcripts suggesting that perhaps the _in vitro_ polymerase reaction favors the production of minus-strand species which then anneal to readily present positive strand species during the incubated reaction. This interpretation is supported by the fact that the sizes of the _in vitro_ transcripts are the same as nonpolyadenylated _in vivo_ species found, namely 3.15-, 1.40- and 0.66 x 10^6, and at least two of the _in vitro_ products appear nonpolyadenylated.

It is of interest to note that while every major and almost every minor virus-specific intracellular RNA species identified appears to be polyadenylated, three abundant species appear to be nonpolyadenylated as well. These have molecular weights of approximately 6.8-, 1.40- and 0.66 x 10^6. These may represent genomic and subgenomic minus-strand RNA species or alternatively they may be mRNA species with poly(A) tracts too short to anneal to the oligo (dT) cellulose.

REFERENCES

Baltimore, D., 1971, Expression of animal virus genomes, _Bacteriol. Rev._, 35:235.

Brian, D.A., Dennis, D. E., and Guy, J. S., 1980, Genome of porcine transmissible gastroenteritis virus, _J. Virol._, 34:410.

Erikson, E., Erikson, R. L., Henry, B., and Pace, N. R., 1973, Comparison of oligonucleotides produced by RNase T1 digestion of 7S RNA from avian and murine oncornavriuses and from uninfected cells, _Virology_, 53:40.

Huang, A. S., Baltimore, D. A., and Bratt, M. A., 1971, Ribonucleic acid polymerase in virions of Newcastle disease virus: comparison with the vesicular stomatitis virus polymerase. _J. Virol._, 7:389.

Lai, M.M.C. and Stohlman, S. A., 1978, RNA of mouse hepatitis virus. _J. Virol._, 26:236.

Laskey, R.A. and Mills, A. D., 1975, Quantitative film detection of ^3H and ^{14}C in polyacrylamide gels by fluorography. _Eur.J. Biochem._, 56:335.

Lehrach, H., Diamond, D., Wozney, J., and Boedtker, H, 1977, RNA molecular weight determinations by gel electrophoresis under denaturing conditions, a critical review, Biochemistry, 16:4743.

Lomniczi, B. and Kennedy, I., 1977, Genome of infectious bronchitis virus, J. Virol. 24:99.

McClurkin, A. W. and Norman, J. O., 1966, Studies on tranmissible gastroenteritis of swine II. Selected characteristics of a cytopathogenic virus common to five isolates from transmissible gastroenteritis. Cn. J. Comp. Med. Vet. Sci., 30:190.

Polatnick, J. and Arlinghaus, R. B., 1967, Foot-and-mouth disease virus-induced ribonucleic acid polymerase in baby hamster kidney cells, Virology, 31:601.

Schochetman, G., Steven, R. H., and Simpson, R. W., 1977. Presence of infectious polyadenylated RNA in the coronavirus avian bronchitis virus, Virology, 77:772.

Wege, H., Muller, A. and Ter Meulen, V, 1978, Genomic RNA of the murine coronavirus JHM, J. Gen. Virol., 41:217.

ON ENTEROPATHOGENIC BOVINE CORONAVIRUS

J. Storz[2], G. Kaluza[1], H. Niemann[1] and R. Rott[1]

Institut für Virologie, Justus-Liebig-Universität Giessen, D-6300 Giessen, Germany[1] and the Department of Microbiology, College of Veterinary Medicine and Biomedical Sciences, Colorado State University, Fort Collins, Colorado, USA[2].

INTRODUCTION

Cornonaviruses cause severe and economically important intestinal infections in newborn calves which become manifest as enteritis with diarrhea and additional clinical consequences. Studies concerning the pathogenesis of enteropathogenic bovine coronavirus (EBC-virus) enteritis have led to a better understanding of morphological alterations of the intestinal tract as well as of the individual cells, helping to explain the functional disorders observed with this disease (for references see Storz and Rott, 1980). Relatively little is known, however, about structural details of the virus and about the biochemical events of EBC-virus replication,principally a result of the difficulties encountered in growing the virus in tissue culture. After we succeeded in adapting EBC-virus strain L-9 isolated by Mebus et al. (1973) to grow in bovine fetal thyroid or brain cells in reasonable amounts it became possible to study some of the many unanswered questions. As a beginning, efforts were made to determine optimal growth conditions in order to provide an in vitro source for viral antigen. In addition, biochemical analysis of the virus was undertaken.

DISTRIBUTION OF EBC-VIRUS IN HUMANS AND CALVES

In a sero-epidemiological survey in certain regions of Germany we used immunodiffusion with an alkali extract of infected bovine fetal thyroid cells or the serum neutralization test for the assay of antibodies.

TABLE 1

Frequency of Antibodies against Enteropathogenic Bovine Coronavirus in Man and Cattle

Serum group	Number positive* per total tested	Percent of positive sera
Cattle from Bavaria	62/97	67
Cattle from Hesse	113/192	61
Cattle Mü 1978	8/12	66
Cattle Mü 1979	0/7	0
Cattle Ma	3/5	60
Cattle HKR	2/8	25
Calf (for tissue culture)	2/3	
Fetal Calf	0/5	
Human (blood bank)	7/100	7
Human (hospital)	9/36	25
Students (from Colorado)	8/26	31
Laboratory personnel	4/8	50

*tested by immunodiffusion

The results are demonstrated in Table 1. About 60% of randomly selected bovine sera were positive for EBC-virus. Antibodies were also found in two out of three batches of calf serum purchased for tissue culture purposes. Fetal calf serum never contained antibodies to EBC-virus (Storz and Rott, 1980).

EBC-virus-specific antibodies could also be demonstrated in human sera. This was true for blood samples obtained from the local blood bank and in particular for sera from the clinics of the university of Giessen where respectively 7% or 25% sera gave positive reactions in the immunodiffusion test. Lines of identity were formed when the positive human sera were alternated with positive bovine sera. All positive serum samples had a very high antibody content with neutralization indices of 3 and more. The results with human antibodies were confirmed by immunofluorescence and immune electron microscopy (Storz and Rott, 1981). Studies with fluorescent antibodies already implied an antigenic relationship between the human coronavirus strain OC43 and a bovine strain (Pedersen et al., 1978).

These findings clearly demonstrate that infections with EBC-virus or a closely related virus are wide spread in cattle and in humans. The high titers in human sera indicate that the virus must be capable of replicating in human. One should therefore be aware of the possibility that the infection is of clinical importance. Whether the same virus strain infect man as well as cattle or whether the demonstration of antibodies is merely due to similarities in the antigenic structure in two different species-specific virus strains is not yet known. There is, however, evidence that EBC-virus can be transmitted from calves to man with ensuing gastroenteritis (Storz et al., 1981). The high content of neutralizing antibodies and the electron microscopic findings that the antibodies bind to the viral peplomers suggest that the reactive antigen is a glycoprotein of the viral envelope. The general experience that viral glycoproteins are strain-specific antigens could support the assumption that the same virus strain, which has a stable antigenic structure, infects either species.

GROWTH AND STRUCTURE OF EBC-VIRUS

In bovine fetal thyroid and bovine fetal brain cells EBC-virus induces only mild cytopathic changes. As in other coronavirus infections, virus titers begin to increase after a lag period of about 4 hours to reach a maximum of about 10^6 PFU/ml at 20 - 25 hours after infection. Cell-associated virus titers rise faster than released virus titers. Principally 5 size classes of viral polypeptide species were observed in virus particles and infected cells analyzed by SDS polyacrylamide gel electrophoresis: gp 23, p50, gp65, gp90 and gp180.

In spite of similar growth characteristics in these two cell types, analyses by polyacrylamide gel electrophoresis revealed differences in virus structure. These differences mainly concern the high molecular weight glycoproteins gp 180 and gp 90 (Fig. 1). After multiplication in fetal brain cells gp 180 is the dominant glycoprotein while in EBC-virus grown in fetal thyroid cells gP 90 is much more prominent. A precursor relationship between gp 180 and gp 90 may exist, but it remains to be seen whether the differences in the proportion of these two structural components has any biological significance. The small differences in the molecular weights of gp 65 might be due to host cell specific variations in the size of the oligosaccharide side chains. The smallest glycoprotein, the gp 23, apparently corresponds to the glycoprotein E1 of the murine coronavirus A 59. In contrast to gp 180, gp 90 and gp 65, which could be metabolically labeled with glucosamine, galactose, mannose and fucose, gp 23 was only labeled with radioactive glucosamine and galactose (Fig. 2). It therefore represents a new type of viral glycoproteins which appears to be common in several coronaviruses (see Niemann and Klenk, this volume).

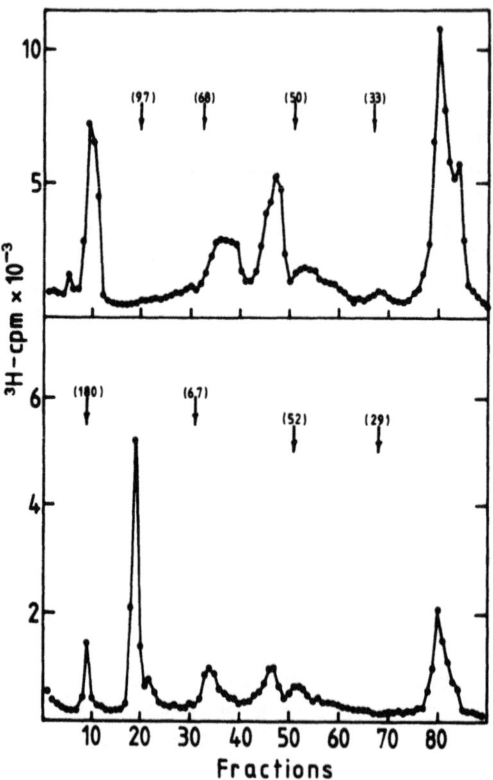

Fig. 1. Polyacrylamide gel electrophoresis of enteropathogenic bovine coronavirus strain L-9 grown in bovine fetal brain (upper panel) or thyroid cells (lower panel).

Virus was labeled with a mixture of tritiated leucine and valine and harvested 30 hours after infection. Clarified infectious culture medium (200 µl) was mixed at 4° C with a bovine convalescent serum (5 µl); 12 hours later an antibovine IgG serum from rabbits was added, 4 hours later the precipitates were washed and then subjected to 10% polyacrylamide gels. Markers were ^{14}C-labeled Semliki Forest virus proteins (upper panel) or Vesicular stomatitis virus proteins (lower panel) extracted from infected cells.

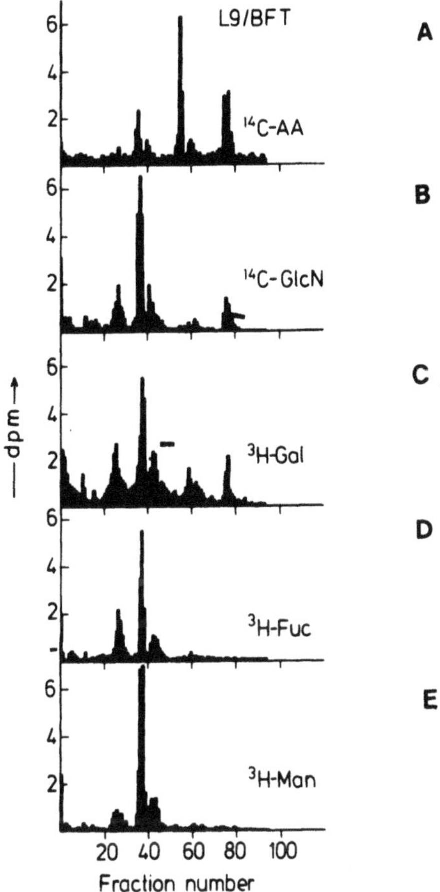

Fig. 2. Incorporation of radioactive markers into bovine coronavirus strain L-9 polypeptides.

Coronavirus L-9 was grown in primary bovine fetal thyroid cells in the presence of ^{14}C-amino acids (panel A) or radiolabeled sugars as indicated (panels B to E). Virus was harvested 30 hours after infection and analyzed on 5 to 15% SDS-polyacrylamide slab gels.

Whereas gp 180 and gp 90 and gp 65 could be labeled with glucosamine, galactose, mannose, and fucose, gp 23 was only labeled with galactose and glucosamine (for details see Niemann and Klenk, this volume).

ACTIVATION OF BIOLOGICAL PROPERTIES OF EBC-VIRUS BY TRYPSIN TREATMENT

In analogy to our experiences with myxoviruses (for review see Klenk and Rott, 1980) the enhancement effect of trypsin on virus replication was tested (Storz et al., 1981). As can be seen in Fig. 3 the presence of 10 µg of trypsin/ml in the culture medium indeed enhanced virus yield in bovine fetal thyroid cells by about 1 log unit. This is also the case when virus has been grown in bovine fetal brain cells. The hemagglutinin released into the culture medium appeared earlier and the concentration was increased by several factors in trypsin-treated, infected cell culture.

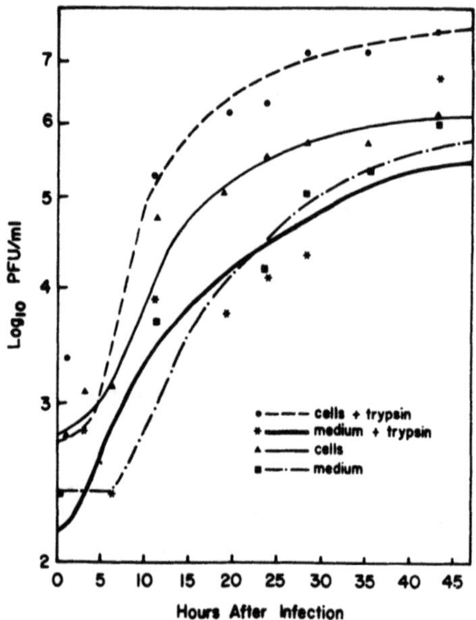

Fig. 3. Growth curve of bovine coronavirus strain L-9 in bovine fetal thyroid cells in the absence or presence of 10 µg trypsin per ml culture medium.

Under these conditions, syncytium formation could be observed 12 - 18 hours after infection. The number of polykaryons, which usually contained up to 20 nuclei each, increased with incubation time, however, their total size remained relatively small. Not all cells of a monolayer were recruited into polykaryons in trypsin-treated cell cultures. In the absence of the enzyme syncytia are not formed (Fig. 4).

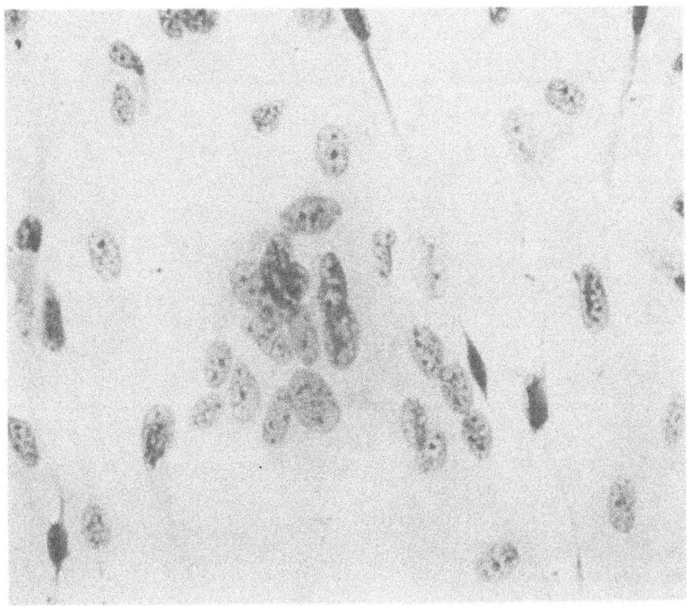

Fig. 4. Cell fusion in L-9 infected bovine fetal brain cells in the presence of 10 μg trypsin per ml culture medium.

A further consequence of trypsin treatment of infected cell cultures was the appearance of clearly visible plaques 3 days after plating, while in the absence of trypsin only turbid and tiny plaques could be observed, reaching a measurable size of about 1 mm in diameter 6 days after infection. In contrast, in the presence of 10 μg trypsin/ml overlay the maximal plaque size of 5 mm was reached already on day 4 (Fig. 5). The plaque number depended directly on the virus dilution.

If virus was pretreated with trypsin or trypsin was present only during viral adsorption, plaque enhancement and cell fusion was not observed. This could mean that a change in the structure of the newly synthesized glycoproteins rather than a change on the cell surface is responsible for the trypsin effect. Formation of syncytia in the presence of a protease is also reminiscent of the situation in ortho- and paramyxoviruses where the viral fusion factors must be activated by proteolytic cleavage (for review see

Klenk and Rott, 1980). However, the precise site of proteolytic attack in EBC-virus infection remains to be detected.

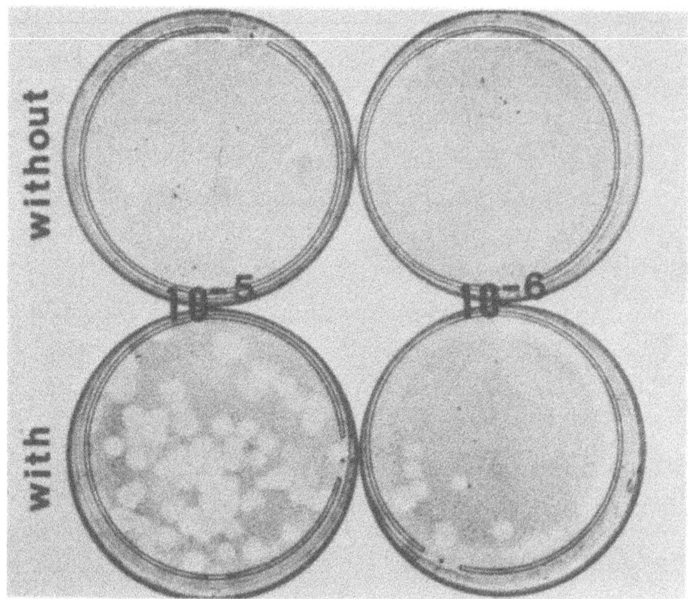

Fig. 5. Plaques induced by enteropathogenic coronavirus strain L-9 in bovine fetal thyroid cells 6 days after plating in the absence (without) or 4 days after plating in the presence (with) of 10 μg trypsin per ml of overlay.

The enhancing effect of trypsin on EBC-virus replication *in vitro* mimics the situation *in vivo* where in the intestinal tract ample amounts of trypsin and other proteases are present and may be an essential factor for massive virus multiplication and the clinical expression of cell destruction.

ACKNOWLEDGMENT

The work was supported by the Deutsche Forschungsgemeinschaft (Sonderforschungsbereich 47) and the Alexander von Humboldt-Stiftung under a special German Government Cooperation Programme between the Federal Republic of Germany and the United States of America, Senior Scientist Award to J. Storz.

REFERENCES

Klenk, H.-D., and Rott, R.
Cotranslational and posttranslational processing of viral glycoproteins.
Current Topics Microbiol. Immunol. 90, 19-48.

Mebus, C. A., Stair, E. L., Rhodes, M. B., and Twiehaus, M. J. (1973)
Neonatal calf diarrhea: Propagation, attenuation, and characteristics of a coronavirus-like agent.
Am. J. Vet. Res. 34, 145-150.

Pederson, N. C., Ward, J., and Mengeling, W. L. (1978)
Antigenic relationship of the feline infectious peritonitis virus to coronaviruses of other species.
Arch. Virol. 58, 45-53.

Storz, J., and Rott, R. (1980)
Über die Verbreitung der Coronavirusinfektion bei Rindern in ausgewählten Gebieten Deutschlands. Antikörpernachweis durch Mikrodiffusion und Neutralisation.
Dtsch. tierärztl. Wschr. 87, 249-288.

Storz, J., and Rott, R. (1981)
Reactivity of antibodies in human serum with an enteropathogenic bovine coronavirus.
Med. Microbiol. Immunol., in press.

Storz, J., Rott, R., and Kaluza, G. (1981)
Enhancement of plaque formation and cell fusion of an enteropathogenic coronavirus by trypsin treatment.
Infect. Immun., in press.

POLYPEPTIDE STRUCTURE OF BOVINE ENTERITIC CORONAVIRUS: COMPARISON BETWEEN A WILD STRAIN PURIFIED FROM FECES AND A HRT 18 CELL ADAPTED STRAIN

Jacques Laporte and Patrick Bobulesco

INRA, Station de Recherches de Virologie et d'Immunologie,
Route de Thiverval, 78850 - Thiverval-Grignon, France

Structural proteins of many of the members of the coronaviridae have been already studied (for reviews see 1). The variety of their number and size, the variability in the data can be accounted for by the different methods used in purification of the virions, protein dissociation and detection on polyacrylamide gel. Furthermore the origin of the virus from animal or from cell cultures can possibly play a role in the difference observed for the same virus.

For these reasons we compared in the same purification and polyacrylamide SDS gel conditions structural polypeptide patterns of a wild strain of Bovine Enteritic Coronavirus (BECV - Strain ws-) stained by coomassie brilliant blue and of the same HRT 18 cell adapted strain (F15) as revealed by autoradiography.

Virus

BECV-ws was produced on gnotobiotic calf as previously described (2). Diarrheic feces were harvested and clarified, after three fold dilutions by low speed centrifugation. This BECV-ws multiplies spontaneously with very high efficiency in HRT 18 cells ; this line established from human rectum adenocarcinoma presents some properties of the differentiated brush border cell of the intestinal villi. Titers obtained are very high (5×10^7 TCID 50/ml virus strain F15). The virus produced had the characteristic of BECV : shape, spikes, density 1.19, hemadsorption and hemagglutination of Rat erythrocytes.

^{14}C aminoacid labelled BECV-F15 was produced in 7 day old HRT 18 cell monolayers maintained in 2 % foetal calf serum RPMI medium containing 2 µCi/ml ^{14}C protein hydrolysate (C.E.A.) for three days. After freezing and thawing the virus suspension was clarified and titrated (starting material 60 ml at 17 x 10^7 PFU/ml).

Purification of the virus.

5 ml of virus suspension are layered onto a 20 % to 45 % wt/wt sucrose gradient and centrifuged in a SW 27 Beckman rotor for 90 min at 25,000 rpm, 4°C. The virus band is collected and pelleted after dilution in water (SW 50 Beckman rotor for 90 min., 45,000 rpm, 4°C). The pellet is then resuspended in distilled water and layered onto a 20 % to 60 % wt/wt sucrose gradient and centrifuged in a SW 27 rotor for 17 hrs at 25,000 rpm 4°C.

Fractions are collected and O.D. at 254 nm monitored (Isco U.A. 5 density gradient fractionator). Refractive index are read on Carl Zeiss refractometer, and radioactivity counted.

Polyacrylamide gel electrophoresis of virus polypeptides.

Purified virus fractions from linear sucrose gradients were treated with 3 % sodium dodecyl sulfate, 5 % 2-mercaptoethanol at 100°C for 1.5 min. A trace amount of bromophenol blue dye was added to the reduced polypeptides which were then electrophoresed in slab gels using the discontinuous SDS-gel system of Laemmli (3). After the run the slabs were stained in 0.1 % (wt/vol) Coomassie brilliant blue in acetic acid-methanol-water (5:40:55), analyzed for material absorbing at 620 nm on a Philips densitometer and when necessary processed for autoradiography.

The molecular weights of BECV specific proteins were determined by comparing their electrophoretic mobilities in polyacrylamide gels with proteins of known molecular weights (Calibration proteins for SDS electrophoresis Boehringer) : trypsin inhibitor from soybean (21,500), bovine serum albumin (68,000), RNA polymerase from E. Coli : subunit (39,000), subunit (155,000), subunit (165,000).

RESULTS

The polypeptide patterns obtained for BECV-ws and BECV-F15 are presented in figure 1 a, b.

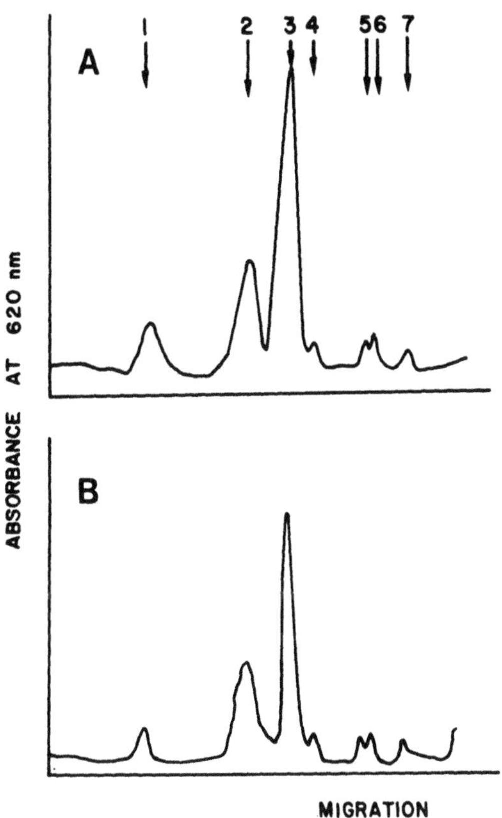

Figure 1.

It clearly shows that they are very similar in the number of peaks and in polypeptide sizes : 125,000, 65,000, 50,000, 45,000, 36,000, 34,000 and 28,000 daltons. VP_{50} is the major protein.

From these results we can conclude that this BECV isolate is composed of seven polypeptides, that adaptation to HRT 18 cells does not induce modifications in the structure of the virion and that the same purification and PAGE methods give the same results or by staining of protein bands or by autoradiography. Nevertheless our results are different from those published on Enteropathogenic Bovine Coronavirus Strain Ly 138 (4).

Literature cited:

(1) GARWES D.J. (1979) Structure and physicochemical properties of coronaviruses. Colloque INSERM Entérites virales. Vol. 90, 141-162.

(2) GOUET, Ph., CONTREPOIS, M., DUBOURGUIER, H.C., RIOU, Y., SCHERRER, R., LAPORTE,J.,VAUTHEROT, J.F., COHEN, J. and L'HARIDON, R. (1978) The experimental production of diarrhoea in axenic and gnotoxenic calves with enteropathogenic E. coli, rotavirus, coronavirus, and in a combined infection of rotavirus and E. coli. Ann. Rech. Vet. 3, 420-430.

(3) LAEMMLI, V.K. (1970) Cleavage of structural proteins during the assembly of the head of bacteriophage T 4. Nature (London) 227, 680-685.

(4) HAJER, I. and STORZ, J. (1979) Structural polypeptides of the Enteropathogenic Bovine Coronavirus Strain Ly 138 Arch. of Virology 59, 47-57.

THE AVIAN CORONAVIRUS MULTIPLICATION STRATEGY

David Stern*, Loyd Burgess*, Steve Linesch and
Ian Kennedy

Department of Biology, University of California, San
Diego, La Jolla, CA 92093; *The Salk Institute,
La Jolla, CA 92097

INTRODUCTION

Infectious bronchitis virus (IBV), the prototype of the coronavirus family, possesses a single-stranded polyadenylated RNA genome. This genome consists of a single polynucleotide chain with an estimated molecular weight of between 6 and 9 x 10^6,[1,2,3,4]. Since the genome is infectious, i.e., it is of positive polarity,[5] it must encode both the structural proteins of the virus particle and non-structural polypeptides some or all of which function in the infected cell to replicate the virus genetic material and to transcribe viral mRNA.

Our initial approach in elucidating the coronavirus multiplication strategy has been to examine the nature of the virus-specified RNA species synthesized in primary chicken embryo kidney (CEK) cells infected with IBV. We have described 6 major virus-specified RNAs,[6]. These species comprise RNA F, which is indestinguishable from the viral genome and 5 smaller RNAs, A, B, C, D and E, which have apparent molecular weights of 0.8 x 10^6, 0.9 x 10^6, 1.3 x 10^6, 1.5 x 10^6 and 2.6 x 10^6 respectively. Ribonuclease T_1 fingerprinting demonstrated that these subgenomic RNAs constitute a nested set such that the nucleotide sequence of each RNA is contained within all of the larger RNA species. In addition, all of these RNAs are polyadenylated and are therefore likely to be viral mRNAs.

In the present report we show that these subgenomic RNA species share a common 3' end and that all the RNAs extend inward from the 3' end of the genome. We also describe experiments to determine the number and nature of the structural proteins of IBV and to elucidate the mechanism of synthesis of these proteins in the infected cell.

METHODS

The several methods used in the present work have been described in detail elsewhere.[1,6,7,8]

RESULTS AND DISCUSSION

Sequence relationships between the subgenomic RNAs and the viral genome

In order to determine the nucleotide sequence relationship between the 5 subgenomic RNAs and the viral genome we prepared genomic RNA (trace labeled with ^{32}P-orthophosphate) from purified virus particles, cleaved it with alkali under limiting conditions, fractionated the cleavage products on sucrose gradients and from the gradients selected 7 pools of increasing size from about 8S to about 40S. These pools were then separately chromatographed over oligo(dT)-cellulose to select those fragments which contained 3' terminal sequences and then these pools of 3' terminal fragments were digested with ribonuclease T_1, labeled with polynucleotide kinase and ^{32}P-γ-ATP and fingerprinted. From these fingerprints a partial 3' to 5' oligonucleotide spot order was deduced. The spots were divided into groups according to which pool _first_ included each spot. Seven groups of oligonucleotides were defined in this way, with each group consisting of the 5' oligonucleotides unique to the corresponding pool. This data is illustrated in Fig. 1 (narrow lines). Pool 1 contained the smallest fragments, so the oligonucleotides in this pool were those closest to the 3' end of the genome and are designated "group 1". The next larger fragments were found in pool 2, which contained the group 1 oligonucleotides as well as a new set. Since pools 1 and 2 differed only at the 5' end, the oligonucleotides specific to pool 2 are located to the 5' side of the group 1 oligonucleotides and these additional oligonucleotides are termed "group 2". The other 5 groups were identified and designated in an exactly analogous fashion. The spot order data were internally consistent in the sense that each fingerprint included all the spots found in fingerprints of smaller pools. When the oligonucleotide fingerprints of each of the 5 IBV subgenomic RNAs A to E were compared with the group spot order it was clear that the intracellular RNAs could be interpolated into the spot order (Fig. 1; heavy lines). Since the spot order pools are a nested series of fragments differing only at their 5' ends, the intracellular RNAs must also form a similar series, with each member of the set sharing a 3' end common to all the intracellular RNA species including the genome. Within the resolution of the data the intracellular RNA species appear to be colinear with the genome, but we cannot rule out the occurrence of small sequence

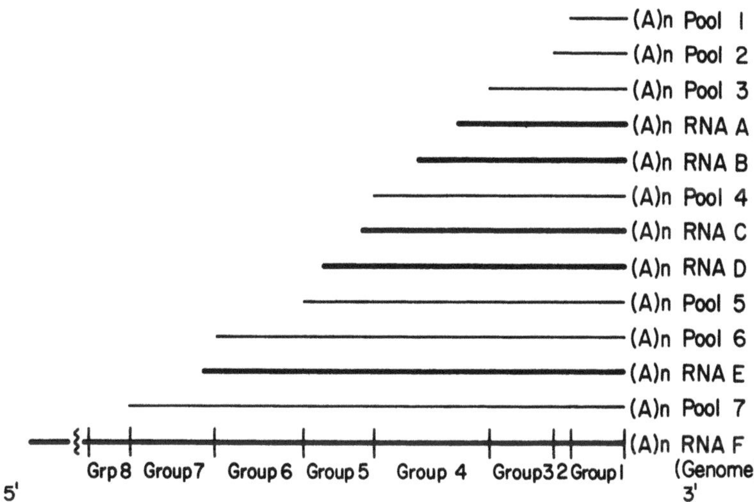

Fig. 1. Sequence relationship between the 5 intracellular IBV RNAs (drawn in heavy line) and the RNA fragment pools derived from the genome by alkali treatment (drawn in narrow line). Distances from the 5' end of group 8 to the 3' end of group 1 are drawn approximately to scale.

rearrangements such as might result from RNA splicing.

Synthesis of IBV structural proteins

There is general agreement in the literature that the coronaviruses contain 3 major structural polypeptides. These comprise two glycoprotein species with molecular weights of about 100,000 and 30,000 respectively and an internal phosphorylated protein with a molecular weight of about 50,000 (for example, see 9 and review in 3). In addition different laboratories have reported the presence of up to 8 minor polypeptide species. An autoradiograph of the ^{35}S-methionine labeled polypeptides of highly purified IBV is shown in Fig. 2. We routinely observe 8 polypeptides labeled 1 to 8 in Fig. 1. Labeling with ^{3}H-mannose and ^{32}P-orthophosphate and determination of the apparent molecular weight provides the following information on these polypeptides. Polypeptides 1 and 2 are glycoprotein species with apparent molecular weights of 90,000 and 84,000 respectively (hereafter termed gp90 and gp84). Polypeptide 3 is a phosphoprotein of molecular weight 51,000 (hereafter termed pp51). Polypeptide 4 has a molecular weight of 36,000 (hereafter termed p36). Polypeptide 5 is a glycoprotein with an apparent molecular weight of 31,000 (hereafter termed gp31) and polypeptides 6, 7 and 8 appear to be unmodified polypeptides with molecular weights of 28,000, 23,000 and 14,000 respectively

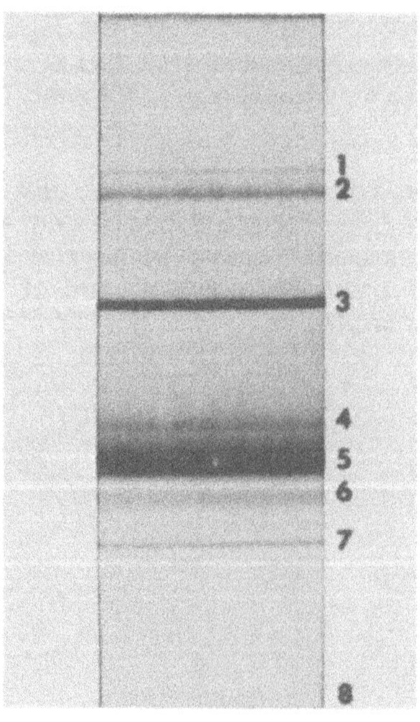

Fig. 2. Structural polypeptides of IBV. IBV grown in CEK cells in the presence of ^{35}S-methionine was purified by sucrose and renograffin gradient centrifugation, disrupted using SDS, reduced and alkylated and the resultant polypeptides fractionated by polyacrylamide gel electrophoresis. The origin of electrophoresis is at the top of the autoradiograph.

(hereafter termed p28, p23 and p14). Preliminary tryptic peptide mapping of these proteins show that gp90, gp84, pp51, gp31 and p14 are probably all unique polypeptides. By contrast the maps of p36, gp31, p28 and p23 strongly suggest that these four polypeptides all share common amino acid sequences. Of these structural polypeptides only pp51 and gp31 can unequivocally be seen in infected cells. In addition, two other polypeptides, unique to infected cells, are reproducibily seen. These are denoted p165 and p42 in Fig. 3. Clevland mapping clearly shows that p42 is related to pp51. As yet no information is available on the amino acid sequence of p165. A kinetic analysis of the synthesis of these intracellular virus-specified proteins show that they are all synthesized coordinately from the earliest time of detection ($\sim$ 3 h post-infection) to the end of the viral multiplication cycle. In an attempt to determine if any of the intracellular proteins are fashioned from high molecular weight precursors we used short pulse and pulse-chase conditions. These experiments, together with experiments using TPCK and amino acid analogues to prevent proteolytic cleavage[10] all failed to identify any high moelcular precursor to either pp51 or gp 30. From these data we conclude that pp51 and the polypeptide chain of gp30 are primary gene products. However since we have not succeeded in identifying gp90, gp84 or p14 in infected cells their synthesis may involve polyprotein processing. The complex relationship between p36, gp31, p28 and p23 must also be clarified.

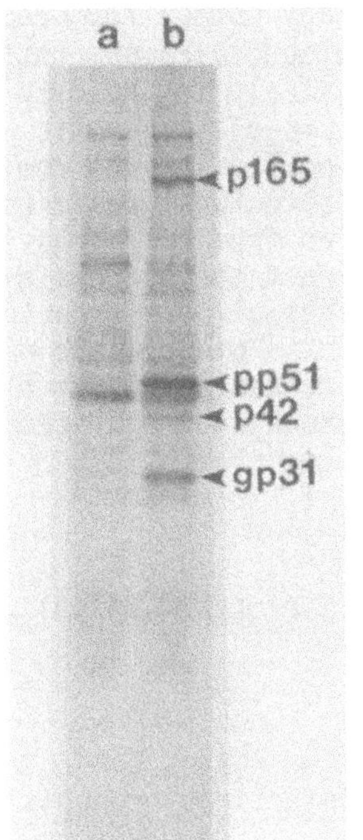

Fig. 3. Polypeptides synthesized in cells infected with IBV. CEK cells either mock infected (lane a) or infected with IBV (lane b) were labeled with ^{35}S-methionine for 1/2 h at 7 h post-infection.

Since each of the 5 intracellular virus-specified RNAs contain unique 5' nucleotide sequence information relative to the next smallest RNA species the most likely hypothesis for the translation of these RNAs is that they all function as monocistronic mRNAs and that expression of each one is limited to translation of its unique 5' nucleotide sequence. This hypothesis is consistant not only with our own studies on the intracellular synthesis of pp51 and gp30 but is strongly supported by the observations of Siddell et al.,[11] who showed that cells infected with the murine coronavirus JHM contain two mRNA species sedimenting at 17S and 19S and that the former of these is translated *in vitro* to give a 60,000 dalton protein (the equivalent of pp51) whilst the latter is translated *in vitro* to give a 23,000 dalton protein which is seen both in infected cells and virions. If the 17S and 19S RNA species correspond to IBV RNAs A and B, which would be congruent with the sedimentation coefficients, the translation results would agree with a non-overlapping translation scheme, with the two RNAs of similar size coding for proteins which differ greatly in size. This concept of a non-overlapping translation scheme would also be in accord with the observation that internal initiation of translation of eukaryotic mRNAs generally does not occur,[12]. For example, the internal translation initiation site in the alphavirus genome is cryptic and is only functional in 26S RNA which, like the IBV RNAs, contain nucleotide sequence information from the 3' end of the viral genome,[13]. Indeed the multiplication strategy of IBV and the alphaviruses share many common features. Both are positive-strand RNA-containing enveloped viruses, both appear to replicate extensively if not exclusively in the cytoplasm of the cell and both direct the synthesis of subgenomic RNA(s) whose nucleotide sequence(s) is/are located inward from the 3' end of the genome and which code for the structural proteins of the virus particle . The coronaviruses differ from the alphaviruses however, in that whereas the alphaviruses direct the synthesis of a single subgenomic mRNA which directly encodes all the structural proteins, the coronaviruses direct the synthesis of separate mRNAs for each of their structural proteins. The mechanism by which these several transcriptive events are performed and regulated should prove to be of particular interest.

ACKNOWLEDGEMENTS

This work was supported by grants for N.S.F. (#PCM 19388) and N.I.H. (# RO1 AI 15087) to S.I.T.K.

REFERENCES

1. B. Lomniczi and I. Kennedy, Genome of infectious bronchitis virus, *J. Virol*. 24:99 (1977).

2. M.R. MacNaughton and M.H. Madge, The characterization of the virion RNA of avian infectious bronchitis virus, FEBS Letters 77:311 (1977).
3. J.A. Robb and C.W. Bond, Coronaviridae, in: "Comprehensive Virology,"H. Frankel-Conrat and R.R. Wagner, eds., Plenum Press, New York.
4. G. Schochetman, R.H. Stevens and R.W. Simpson, Presence of infectious polyadenylated RNA in the coronavirus avian bronchitis virus, Virology 77:772 (1977).
5. B. Lomniczi, Biological properties of avian coronavirus RNA, J. Gen. Virol. 36:531 (1977).
6. D.F. Stern and S.I.T. Kennedy, Coronavirus multiplication strategy I. Identification and characterization of virus-specified RNA, J. Virol. 34:665 (1980).
7. D.F. Stern and S.I.T. Kennedy, Coronavirus multiplication strategy II. Mapping the IBV intracellular RNA species to the genome, J. Virol., in press.
8. L. Burgess, D.F. Stern, S. Linesch, B. Sefton and S.I.T. Kennedy, The coronavirus multiplication strategy. III. Synthesis of the virion structural proteins, in preparation.
9. L.S. Sturman, K.V. Holmes and J. Behnke, Isolation of coronavirus envelope glycoproteins and interaction with the viral nucleocapsid, J. Virol. 33:449 (1980).
10. M.J. Morser, S.I.T. Kennedy and D.C. Burke, Virus-specified polypeptides in cells infected with Semliki Forest virus, J. Gen. Virol. 21:19 (1973).
11. S.G. Siddell, H. Wege, A. Barthel and V. terMeulen, Coronavirus JHM: cell-free synthesis of structural protein p60, J. Virol. 33:10 (1980).
12. M.F. Jacobson and D. Baltimore, Polypeptide cleavages in the formation of poliovirus proteins, Proc. Natl. Acad. Sci. USA 61:77 (1968).
13. S.I.T. Kennedy, Sequence relationships between the genome and the intracellular RNA species of standard and defective-interfering Semliki Forest virus, J. Mol. Biol. 108:491 (1976).

INTRACELLULAR PROTEIN SYNTHESIS AND THE *IN VITRO* TRANSLATION OF CORONAVIRUS JHM mRNA

Stuart Siddell, Helmut Wege, Andrea Barthel and Volker ter Meulen

Institute of Virology, University of Würzburg, FRG

1. Introduction

The genome of the murine coronavirus JHM is a single-stranded, non-segmented RNA with a molecular weight of 5.4 - 6.7 x 10^6. The genomic RNA is infectious and at least one third is polyadenylated (Lai and Stohlman, 1978; Wege et al., 1978). The virion contains six proteins, four of which are glycosylated (Wege et al., 1979; Siddell et al., 1981b), including high and low molecular weight glycoproteins and a phosphorylated nucleocapsid protein of 60,000 molecular weight (Stohlman and Lai, 1979; Siddell et al., 1981a). Associated with purified virions is a protein kinase activity which specifically phosphorylates pp60 *in vitro* (Siddell et al., 1981a).

Information on the replication of JHMV is relatively incomplete. The synthesis and processing of JHMV proteins in infected cells, the genesis of genomic and subgenomic viral RNA, and the translation products of viral mRNA are all areas currently under investigation (Anderson et al., 1979; Bond et al., 1979; Siddell et al., 1980, 1981b; Wege et al., 1981). In this communication we report on the synthesis of polypeptides in JHMV infected cells and the *in vitro* translation of coronaviral mRNA in cell-free systems.

2. Materials and Methods

The following methods used here have been described previously. JHM virus and virus stocks were obtained and propagated on Sac (-) cells and virions were labelled with 35 S methionine and purified as described (Siddell et al., 1980). Cells were infected, labelled with 35 S methionine and cell or cytoplasmic lysates were prepared as described (Siddell et al., 1981b). The preparation of anti JHM serum in rabbits and immunoprecipitation procedures have been described (Siddell 1980; 1981b). The procedures for the preparation of cytoplasmic polyadenylated RNA and polysomal RNA from infected cells, sucrose-formamide gradient centrifugation and the translation of RNA in nuclease treated rabbit reticulocyte lysates or L cell lysates is described (Siddell et al., 1980). Samples were electrophoresed on discontinuous 15 % SDS/polyacrylamide gels (Laemmli, 1970) and the procedures for staining, drying and autoradiography of gels is described (Smith et al., 1974). Tunicamycin was obtained as a gift from Dr. R. Hamill, Lilly Research Laboratories, Indianapolis.

3. Results

Under our conditions cells infected with JHMV at a MOI of 5 TCID 50/cell start to release infectious virus 4 to 6 hours after infection. The cytopathic effect of JHMV is characterized by the formation of syncytia leading to a totally fused monolayer which is evident by approximately 10 hours after infection. After 12 hours of infection the cell monolayer starts to detach from the petri dish.

3.1. Virion proteins

The 35 S-methionine-containing proteins of purified JHMV are shown in Fig. 1. The virion is comprised of six major proteins which are designated by their molecular weight and whether or not they are glycosylated (Wege et al., 1979; Siddell et al., 1981b).

3.2. Intracellular protein synthesis

Fig. 2 shows the pulse labelling of cells for 15 minutes with 35 S-methionine at different times after infection. At late times in infected cells it is possible to detect the synthesis of three major (150 K, 60 K and 23 K) and three minor (65 K, 30 K and 14 K) polypeptides. The synthesis of the 30 K species is sometimes difficult to detect and the 150 K polypeptide is reproducibly resolved as a doublet.

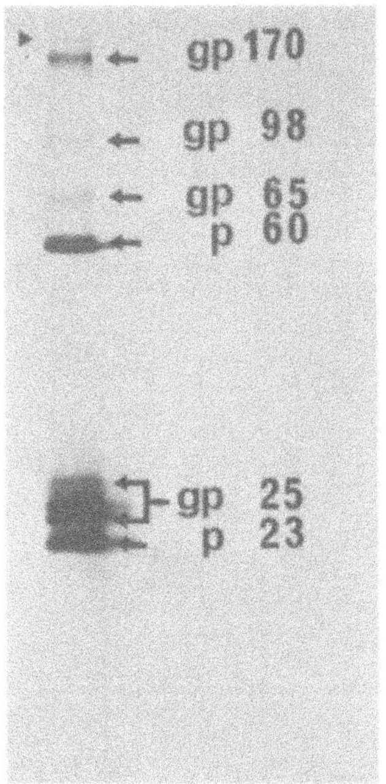

Fig.1: Structural proteins of JHMV. JHM virions were labelled with 35 S-methionine and purified as described in Siddell et al. (1980). Virus was mixed with an equal volume of electrophoresis sample buffer and heated to 37 °C for 2 minutes before electrophoresis.

To investigate any relationships between these intracellular polypeptides and the virion proteins, a 35 S-methionine pulse labelled cytoplasmic lysate was immunoprecipitated with serum directed against purified virions and the immunoprecipitate co-electrophoresed with labelled virus (Fig. 3, tracks V and pulse). This experiment shows that the three major intracellular species, 150 K, 60 K and 23 K and one minor species, 65 K, are specificlly immunoprecipitated (immunoprecipitation of infected lysates with control serum were negative).

These species are therefore related to virion proteins. The 65 K, 60 K and 23 K species comigrate with the virion proteins gp 65, p 60 and p 23. The 150 K species does not comigrate with a virion protein. The intracellular species of 30 K and 14 K which are not precipitated are assumed to be polypeptides which are not present in purified virions. The minor band migrating slightly faster than the 60 K species is generated during the immunoprecipitation procedure and is presumed to be a degredation product, most probably of nucleocapsid protein.

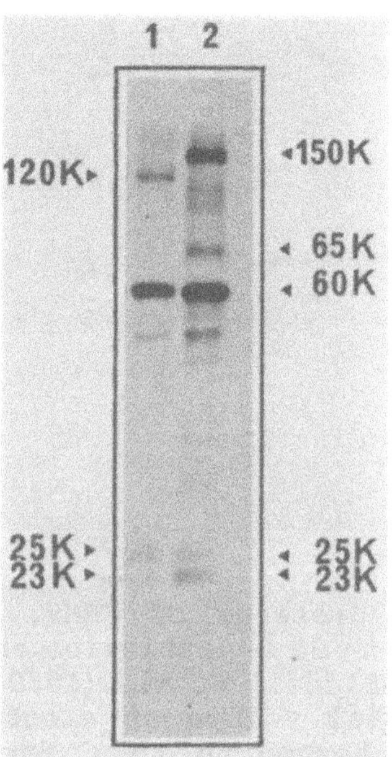

Fig.2: Polypeptides synthesized in JHMV-infected cells. Sac (-) cells were infected with JHMV and labelled for 15 minutes at the times indicated in medium containing 10 µCi/ml 35 S-methionine, and lysates were prepared and electrophoresed as described in Siddell et al., 1981b. M. Mock-infected, MW. Molecular Weight markers.

Fig. 3 also shows the immunoprecipitation with the same antiserum of cytoplasmic lysates pulsed with 35 S-methionine and then chased in the presence of an excess of methionine for various periods of time. During the chase period, the 150 K and 23 K species are processed and two new immunoprecipitable species of 98 K and 25 K appear. Also a small amount of material of 170 K and material which remains at the origin of the gel appear during the chase period. As we have shown (Siddell et al., 1981b) that boiling purified virions in

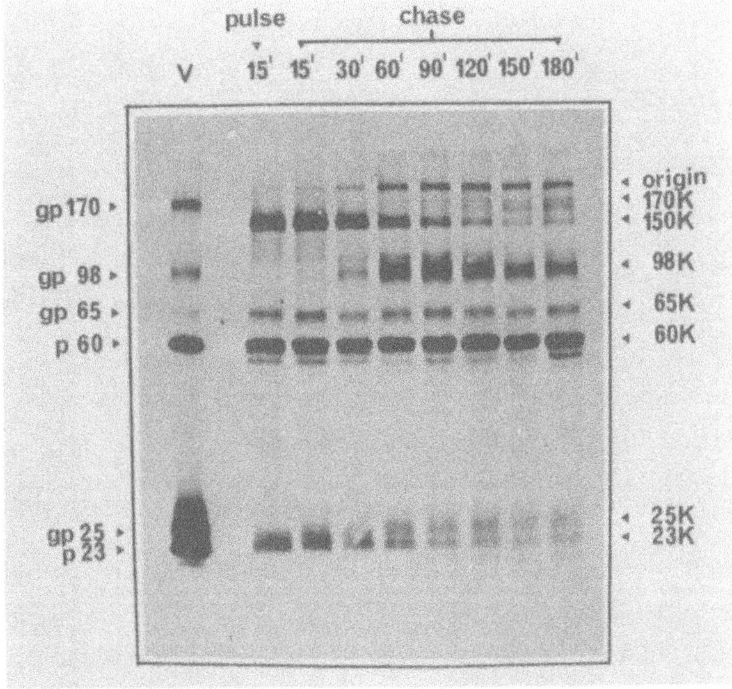

Fig.3: Pulse-chase labelling of JHMV-infected cells and immunoprecipitation of cytoplasmic lysates with anti-JHM serum. Sac (-) cells were infected with JHMV, pulse-labelled 9 hours after infection in medium containing 10 µCi/ml 35 S-methionine and chased with medium containing unlabelled methionine as described in Siddell et al., 1981b. Cytoplasmic lysates were prepared and aliquots immunoprecipitated with anti-JHM serum and electrophoresed. Purified virus (V) was prepared as described in Fig. 1.

electrophoresis sample buffer caused the disappearance of gp 170 and the appearance of material at the gel origin, we repeated this experiment without boiling the immunoprecipitated proteins. Under these conditions no radioactivity appears at the gel origin during the chase period but instead the intracellular species of 170 K is enhanced (data not shown). The intracellular species of 170 K, 98 K and 25 K which arise during the chase period comigrate with virion proteins gp 170, gp 98 and gp 25.

The effect of tunicamycin on the synthesis of JHMV proteins is illustrated in Fig. 4. When infected cells are pulse labelled for 1 hour with 35 S-methionine

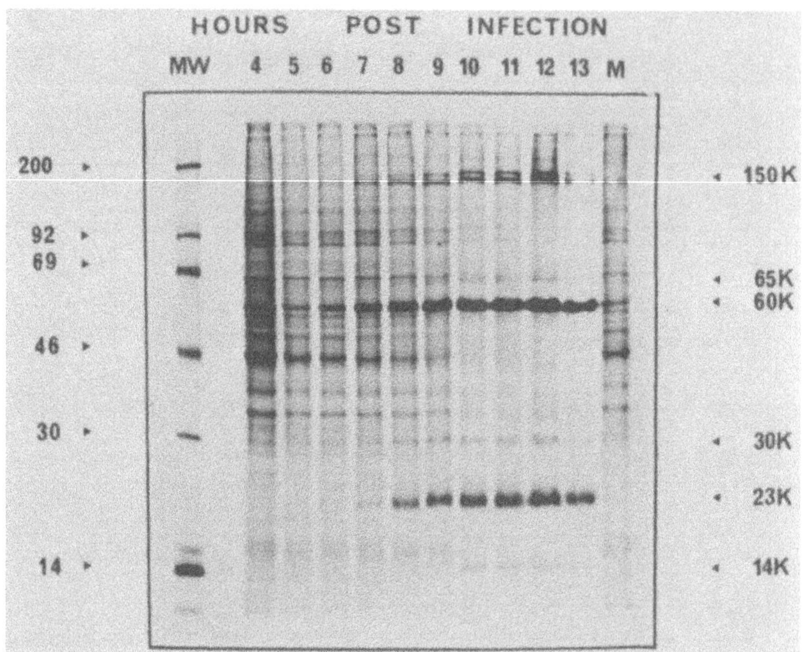

Fig.4: The effect of tunicamycin on JHMV polypeptide synthesis. Sac (-) cells were infected with JHMV and labelled 9 hours after infection for 1 hour in the presence (1) or absence (2) of tunicamycin (1 µg/ml). Cells labelled in the presence of tunicamycin were pretreated for 2 hours with the drug, at the same concentration. Cytoplasmic lysates were prepared, immunoprecipitated with anti JHM serum and the precipitates electrophoresed as described in Siddell et al., 1981b.

and a cytoplasmic lysate immunoprecipitated with anti-JHM serum, polypeptides of 150 K, 98 K, 65 K, 60 K, 25 K and 23 K are detected (track 2). In cells incubated with medium containing 1 µg/ml of tunicamycin during and for 2 hours previous to the labelling period, a different pattern is seen (track 1). The 150 K, 98 K and 65 K species are no longer detected and a new species of 120 K is found. The synthesis of the 60 K, 25 K and 23 K proteins is not affected by tunicamycin treatment.

3.3. In vitro translation

In cells infected with JHMV pulse labelling with 3 H uridine in the presence of actinomycin D reveals the synthesis of 9 RNAs. These range in size from 0.62×10^6 to 6.67×10^6, the size of JHMV genomic RNA. All these

RNAs are single stranded and at least a proportion of each is polyadenylated (Wege et al., 1981). To investigate whether these species function as mRNA we have isolated poly-A- containing RNA from infected cells, translated it in vitro and compared the products with JHM polypeptides by electrophoresis and immunoprecipitation. Furthermore we have size fractionated the translational activities in order to

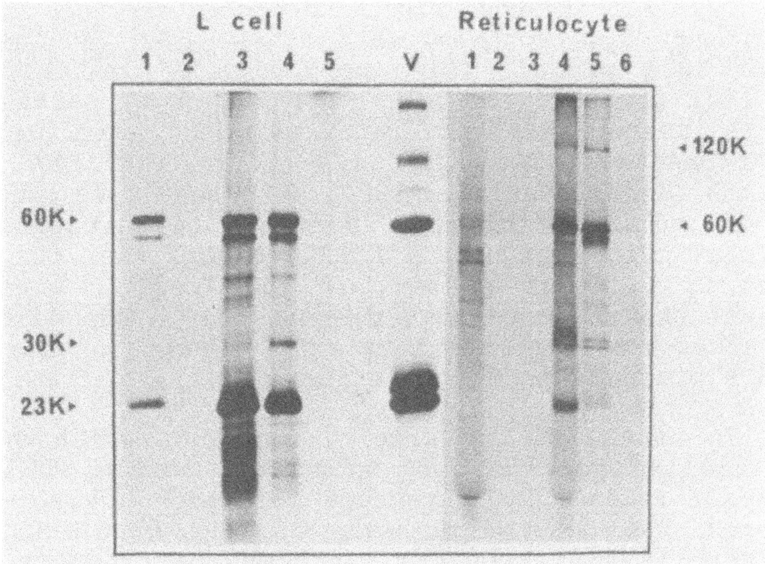

Fig.5: Polyacrylamide gel analysis of proteins made in vitro in response to cytoplasmic poly A RNA or polysomal RNA from JHMV infected cells. Cytoplasmic poly A RNA and polysomal RNA was isolated, translated in vitro, electrophoresed directly or immunoprecipitated with anti JHM serum and electrophoresed as described in Siddell et al., 1980. Purified virus (V) was prepared as described in Fig. 1. L cell translates, (5) no added RNA, (4) cytoplasmic poly A RNA, (3) polysomal RNA. Immunoprecipitation of (4) with preimmune serum (2) or with anti-JHM serum (1). Reticulocyte translates, (1) cytoplasmic poly A RNA from uninfected cells. Immunoprecipitation of (1) with anti JHM serum (2) or pre immune serum (3). (4) cytoplasmic poly A RNA from JHMV infected cells. Immunoprecipitation of (4) with anti JHM serum (5) or preimmune serum (6).

correlate individual mRNAs with their translation products.

Fig. 5 shows the translation of cytoplasmic poly A RNA from infected cells in L cell and rabbit reticulocyte lysates (tracks L4 and R4). Amongst the major products are polypeptides with molecular weights of 23 K, 60 K and 120 K which are specifically immunoprecipitable with anti-JHM serum (tracks L1 and 2 and R5 and 6). The 23 K and 60 K products coelectrophorese with virion p23 and p60 respectively (track V) whilst the 120 K product has no virion counterpart. Also synthesized in these translations are a major 30 K product (seen most clearly in L4) and a minor 14 K product (see also Fig. 6 A or C) neither of which is immunoprecipitable with anti-JHM serum. We have also translated RNA released from infected cell polysomes (Siddell et al., 1980). The result is shown in track L3 and is essentially identical to that obtained with total cytoplasmic poly A RNA, except that the 30 K product is made, if at all, in much reduced amounts. Polysomal RNA and total cytoplasmic poly A RNA directed the synthesis of approximately equal amounts of the 60 K and 23 K products in the experiment .

To establish the size of the RNAs which encode the viral polypeptides we sedimented poly A RNA from infected cells on sucrose-formamide gradients, recovered RNA from fractions of the gradients and translated it in vitro. Fig. 6 shows the products made in the L cell system (A and C) and the reticulocyte lysate (B) in response to unfractionated RNA (total) and RNA sedimenting between about 12S and 45S (A and B) or 17S to 22S (C). The RNA encoding the 60 K product sediments at about 17S, that encoding the 23 K product at 19S and that encoding the 14 K product at 21S (C). The RNAs encoding the 120 K and 30 K products sediment faster, at about 27 S and 29 S respectively (B and A).

4. Discussion

The protein composition of JHMV described here is in agreement with earlier reports (Wege et al., 1979). It also conforms to the pattern which appears to be emerging as characteristic of coronaviruses, namely 5 to 8 proteins, including high and low molecular weight glycoproteins and a 50 to 60 K phosphorylated nucleocapsid protein (Sturman et al., 1977; Sturman and Holmes, 1977; Bond et al., 1979; Siddell et al., 1981 a,b; Cavanagh, 1981; Garwes and Pocock, 1975; Pocock and Garwes, 1977; MacNaughton, 1980).

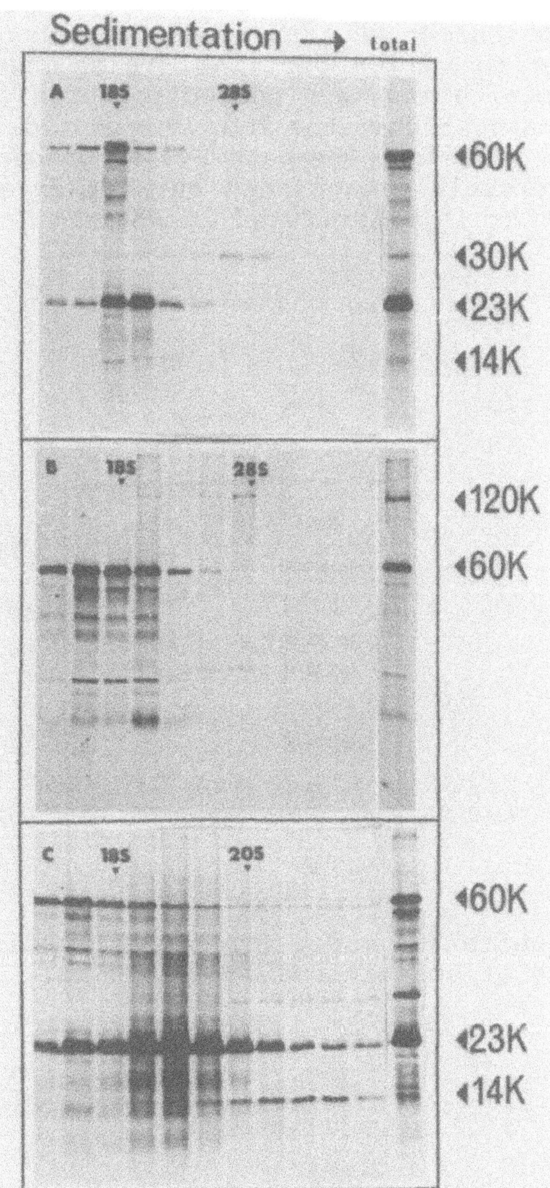

Fig 6: In vitro translation of fractioned poly A RNA from JHMV infected cells. Poly A RNA was sedimented on sucrose formamide gradients, recovered from fractions of the gradients and translated in a L cell lysate (A and C) or a reticulocyte lysate (B). The products were electrophoresed directly (A and C) or immunoprecipitated with anti JHM serum and electrophoresed (B).

In infected cells four polypeptides are synthesized which can be identified by immunoprecipitation as related to virion proteins. Pulse chase labelling, immunoprecipitation and coelectrophoresis with virion proteins suggest that the four polypeptides give rise to all virion proteins. The pathways of processing have yet to be rigorously established but our interpretation of these results is illustrated in Fig. 7.

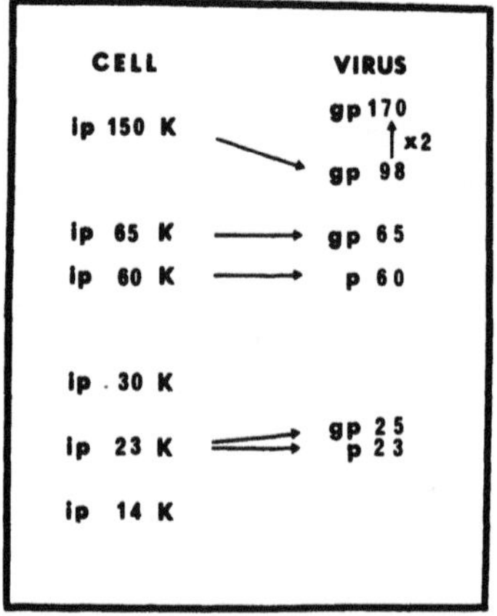

Fig.7: A tentative model for the synthesis and processing of coronavirus JHM proteins.

The intracellular 65 K, 60 K and 23 K polypeptides are incorporated into virions as gp 65, pp60 and p23. The intracellular 150 K polypeptide is processed to a 63 K species which is not incorporated into virions (unpublished data) and a 98 K species and its 170 K dimer, both of which are incorporated into virions, as gp 98 and gp 170 respectively. In the low molecular weight region the intracellular 23 K species is glycosylated to produce the 25 K polypeptide which is incorporated into the virus as gp 25. Tunicamycin inhibits the glycosylation (and consequent processing) of the 150 K species. The 120 K species synthesized in tunicamycin treated cells is presumed to be the polypeptide core of the 150 K protein. The glycosylation of the intracellular 65 K species also appears to be inhibited by tunicamycin but no core protein has yet been found. In contrast tunicamycin does not prevent the glycosylation of the 23 K species to yield gp 25. These conclusions, although tentative, are supported by the electrophoresis of intracellular polypeptides on two-dimensional (NEPHGE or IEF) PAGE (Siddell et al., 1981b) and in vitro translation studies (Siddell et al., 1980). Our tryptic peptide mapping studies which are in progress are also consistent with this interpretation of the data, and additionally confirm that the 30 K and 14 K species identified as putative non-structural proteins are unrelated to virion polypeptides (unpublished data).

The translation of RNA from JHMV infected cells provided some of the first evidence for the existence of multiple subgenomic coronavirus mRNAs (Siddell et al., 1980). Analysis of RNA from murine and avian coronavirus infected cells indicates there to be the genomic sized RNA and possibly up to 8 subgenomic RNAs which could function as mRNAs (Stern and Kennedy, 1980a,b, Wege et al., 1981, van der Zeijst, 1981). We have attempted to demonstrate directly the mRNA function of these RNAs by in vitro translation. Our results suggest that amongst the translation products of total cytoplasmic poly A RNA are polypeptides which give rise to all structural proteins of JHMV. The only exception is gp 65, an in vitro counterpart for which we have not yet identified. The in vitro synthesis of precursors to pp60 and p23 (and therefore as postulated gp 25) has been confirmed by electrophoresis, immunoprecipitation and tryptic peptide mapping (Siddell et al. 1980; unpublished data). In vivo experiments with tunicamycin suggest that the non-glycosylated form of the intracellular 150 K species has a molecular weight of 120 K. This corresponds to an in vitro product immunoprecipitable with anti JHM serum and we conclude this species to be related to the intracellular 150 K protein and as postulated gp 98 and gp 170 in the virion.

Additionally, we have shown that the mRNAs encoding the virion polypeptides are subgenomic, as are those encoding the 30 K and 14 K putative non-structural proteins. This conclusion is based on the sedimentation of mRNA activities in sucrose formamide gradients. To correlate these activities with the subgenomic RNA species identified in infected cells we have analysed on gels 32 P labelled RNA after recovery from gradients. The expected relationship was found in that larger RNA sedimented faster, i.e. RNA 1, 45 - 50S; RNA 2, 30S; RNA 3, 28S; RNA4 and 5, 21 - 22S; RNA 6, 19S and RNA 7, 17S, although the sedimentation of the larger RNAs is slower than may have been expected.

Taken together the data allows us tentatively to identify the majority of subgenomic JHM mRNAs and their translation products which is shown in Fig. 8.

RNA	SIZE ($x10^{-6}$)	SIZE (S)	TRANSLATION PRODUCT
1	6.67	45-50	not identified
a	4.7		not identified
2	3.42	30	30 K ▸ ns
3	2.76	28	120 K ▸ gp170/98
b,4,5	1.19-1.5	21-22	14 K ▸ ns
6	0.93	19	23 K ▸ p23/gp25
7	0.62	17	60 K ▸ pp60

Fig.8: Tentative coding assignments for coronavirus JHM subgenomic mRNAs.

At the moment we have detected only one translational activity sedimenting at about 21S, i.e. that encoding the 14 K protein. As two major and one minor RNA species sediment at about this value we cannot conclude which of these three RNAs encodes this protein or if the remaining two RNAs act as mRNA. We have also found no translational activity at the sedimentation value of the minor RNA a, nor have we identified any translation product for the intracellular genomic sized RNA 1. As the translation of the mRNAs encoding all major virion proteins has been demonstrated it seems most likely that RNA 1, if functional, encodes a non-structural protein(s).

The size of the murine coronavirus subgenomic mRNAs and their translation products, together with the known sequence arrangement of coronavirus IBV intracellular RNAs (Stern and Kennedy, 1980 a, b) is consistent with a replication strategy which involves multiple subgenomic mRNAs. Translation studies show that each mRNA functions monocistronically, although additional coding sequences are present in all but the smallest mRNA. This strategy appears to be particularly flexible in that it allows firstly for the control of viral protein synthesis at both transcriptional and translational levels and secondly the possibility to spatially separate the translation and post translational modification of different viral polypeptides into different cellular compartments.

Acknowledgement
We thank Helga Kriesinger for typing the manuscript. This research was supported by Deutsche Forschungsgemeinschaft Me 270/18.

References

Anderson, R., Cheley, S. and Haworth-Hatherell, H., (1979). Comparison of polypeptides of two strains of murine hepatitis virus. Virology 97, 492-494.

Bond, C.W., Leibowitz, J.L., and Robb, J.A., (1979). Pathogenetic murine coronaviruses. II. Characterization of virus specific proteins of murine coronaviruses JHMV and A59V. Virology 94, 371-384.

Cavanagh, D. (1981). Structural polypeptides of coronavirus IBV. Journal of General Virology, in the press.

Garwes, D.J. and Pocock, D.H. (1975). The polypeptide structure of transmissible gastroenteritis virus. Journal of General Virology 29, 25-34.

Laemmli, U.K., (1970). Cleavage of structural proteins during the assembly of the head of bacteriophage T4. Nature (London) 227: 680-685.

Lai, M.M.C. and Stohlman, S.A. (1978). RNA of mouse hepatitis virus. Journal of Virology 26:236-248.

Macnaughton, M.R. (1980). The polypeptides of human and mouse coronaviruses. Archives of Virology 63, 75-80.

Pocock, D.J. and Garwes, D.H. (1977). The polypeptides of haemagglutinating encephalomyelitis virus and isolated subviral particles. Journal of Virology 37, 487-499.

Siddell, S.G., Wege H., Barthel, A. and ter Meulen, V. (1980). Coronavirus JHM: Cell-free Synthesis of Structural protein p60. Journal of Virology 33, 10-17.

Siddell, S.G., Barthel, A. and ter Meulen, V. (1981a). Coronavirus JHM. A virion-associated protein kinase Journal of General Virology, in the press.

Siddell, S.G., Wege, H., Barthel, A. and ter Meulen, V. (1981b). Coronavirus JHM. Intracellular protein synthesis. Journal of General Virology, in the press.

Smith, A.E., Wheeler, T., Glanville, N. and Kääriäinen, L. (1974). Translation of Semliki Forest virus 42S RNA in a mouse cell-free system to give virus coat proteins. European Journal of Biochemistry 49, 101-110.

Spaan, W.J.M., Rottier, P.J.M., Horzinek, M.C. and van der Zeijst, B.A.M. (1981). Isolation and identification of virus specific mRNA's in cells infected with mouse hepatitis virus (MHV-A59). Virology, in the press.

Stern, D.F. and Kennedy, S.I.T. (1980a). The coronavirus multiplication strategy. I. Identification and characterization of virus-specified RNA. Journal of Virology 34, 665-674.

Stern, D.F. and Kennedy, S.I.T. (1980b). Coronavirus Multiplication Strategy. II. Mapping the avian infectious bronchitis virus intracellular RNA species to the genome. Journal of Virology 36, 440-449.

Stohlman, S.A. and Lai, M.M.C. (1979). Phosphoproteins of murine hepatitis viruses. Journal of Virology 32, 672-675.

Sturman, L.S. (1977). Characterization of a coronavirus. I. Structural proteins: effect of preparative conditions on the migration of protein in polyacrylamide gels. Virology 77, 637-649.

Sturman, L.S. and Holmes, K.V. (1977). Characterization of a coronavirus. II. Glycoproteins of the viral envelope: tryptic peptide analysis. Virology 77, 650-660.

Wege, H., Müller, A. and ter Meulen, V. (1978). Genomic RNA of the murine coronavirus JHM. Journal of General Virology 41, 217-227.

Wege, H., Wege, H., Nagashima, K., and ter Meulen, V. (1979). Structural polypeptides of the murine coronavirus JHM. Journal of General Virology 42, 37-47.

Wege, H., Siddell, S.G., Sturm, M. and ter Meulen, V. (1981). Coronavirus JHM. Characterization of intracellular viral RNA, Journal of General Virology, in the press.

MESSENGER RNAs OF MOUSE HEPATITIS VIRUS A59: ISOLATION AND CHARACTERIZATION, TRANSLATION IN XENOPUS LAEVIS OOCYTES OF RNAs 3, 6 and 7, UV TARGET SIZES OF THE TRANSCRIPTION TEMPLATES

Bernard A.M. Van der Zeijst, Marian C. Horzinek, Liesbeth Jacobs, Peter J.M. Rottier and Willy J.M. Spaan

Institute of Virology, Veterinary Faculty
State University, Yalelaan 1, 3508 TD Utrecht
The Netherlands

INTRODUCTION

At present, ten strains of murine coronaviruses have been isolated (Table 1). These viruses usually cause fatal hepatitis. A very interesting property of at least strains MHV-3, MHV-4 (JHM) and MHV-A59 is, however, that they may cause demyelination of the central nervous system or lead to other chronic neurological diseases(Table 1). Before these neurological disorders can be understood at the molecular level, more basic information about the structure and replication of murine coronaviruses is needed.

We have chosen to study mouse hepatitis strain MHV-A59. Here we report that in cells infected with this virus six subgenomic mRNAs are found in addition to the 5.6 x 10^6 molecular weight genome-sized RNA. The sum of the molecular weights of these subgenomic RNAs is almost twice that of the genome, indicating that sequence homologies should exist between the subgenomic MHV-A59 RNAs.

Direct evidence that at least three of these RNAs are functional mRNAs was obtained by microinjection into Xenopus laevis oocytes. The molecular weights of the proteins coded for by these RNAs are in agreement with our working hypothesis on the replication of MHV-A59 in which two points are central. First, the nucleotide sequence of each subgenomic RNA should be identical with the 3'-part of the genome i.e. each RNA contains a 5'-terminal sequence extension with respect to the next smaller one. Second, the expression of the genome-sized RNA and the subgenomic RNAs occurs by the translation of only that 5'-terminal part of the RNA, not present in the next smaller RNA; internal initiation of translation does not occur.

Finally, we have used UV transcription mapping to determine the target size of the template of the MHV-A59 RNAs. The conclusion of these studies is that the transcription of the MHV-A59 RNAs is initiated independently.

ISOLATION AND IDENTIFICATION OF VIRUS-SPECIFIC mRNAs IN INFECTED CELLS

Kinetics of virus growth and virus-specific RNA synthesis

Infection of murine cells with MHV may induce the production of endogenous retroviruses. Sac(-) cells were chosen as host cells for MHV-A59 since these cells are defective in the synthesis of retroviral proteins (31). This cell line does not form confluent monolayers, however, and is therefore less suitable for plaque-titration; mouse L cells were employed for this purpose, with highly reproducible results.

We wanted to study the replication of MHV-A59 under single cycle conditions. Immunofluorescence showed that all cells became infected at a multiplicity of 10 PFU/cell, so we have used this MOI in all further experiments. To obtain high titered stocks needed for these one-step growth experiments, the virus was concentrated and purified (24).

The kinetics of virus release into the medium are shown in Fig. 1A. Virus production was complete at 10 h p.i. by which time the cells had formed syncytia. About 50% of the infectivity remained cell-bound at 10 h p.i. Since we wished to use actinomycin D in most experiments, virus growth in cells incubated with 1 µg/ml actinomycin D and in untreated cells was compared. No significant dif-

Table 1. Strains of Mouse Hepatitis Virus (MHV)

Virus strains	Isolation	Chronic neurological disease
MHV-1	ref. 5	
MHV-2	ref. 16	
MHV-3	ref. 4	ref. 29
MHV-4 (JHM)	ref. 3	ref. 6, 7, 8, 11, 14, 15, 32
MHV-A59	ref. 12	ref. 17
MHV-S/CDC	ref. 9	
MHV-S	ref. 19	
MHV-LS	ref. 20	
H747	ref. 16	
EHF 210	ref. 16	

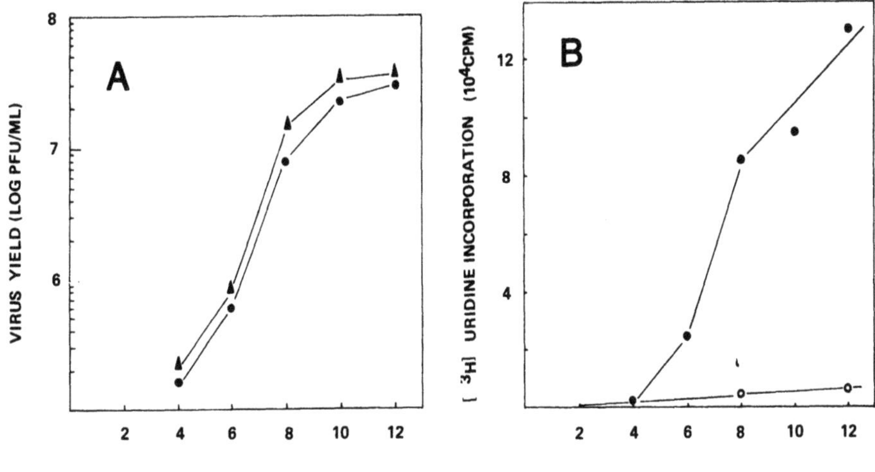

Fig. 1. Growth kinetics of MHV-A59 in Sac(-) cells (A). The cells were infected at a MOI of 10 PFU/cell and incubated in the absence of actinomycin D (▲) or this drug was added 1 h p.i. (●). In the latter case the kinetics of the synthesis of viral RNA were also measured by following the incorporation of ^{3}H-uridine added to the medium at 2 h p.i. The results are shown in (B). (o) mock-infected; (●) infected. For more details see ref.24.

ference in final virus yield or in kinetics of virus growth was observed (Fig. 1A). The synthesis of intracellular virus-specific RNA was measured by labeling cells with ^{3}H-uridine in the presence of actinomycin D. The synthesis of virus-specific RNA started at 4 h p.i. and continued until at least 12 h p.i. (Fig. 1B). At this time infection usually caused a 20-fold stimulation of the ^{3}H-uridine incorporation over the background in mock-infected cells.

Analysis of intracellular MHV-A59-specific RNA; isolation of poly(A)-containing RNA species

To determine the species of virus-specific RNA formed in Sac(-) cells, infected cells were labeled with ^{3}H-uridine in the presence of actinomycin D between 6 and 8 h p.i. At the end of this period total RNA was extracted from the cells, denatured with glyoxal and dimethylsulfoxide, and analyzed by agarose gel electrophoresis. Several virus-specific RNA species were found in infected but not in mock-infected cells (Fig. 2A, lane 1 and 2). The virus-specific RNA species were further characterized by oligo(dT)-cellulose chromatography. Forty eight percent of the material was found to bind the column. This material was eluted and analyzed by electrophoresis in an agarose gel. It contained all seven virus-specific RNA species (Fig. 2A, lane 3).

Since these RNAs contain poly(A), it is likely that they are mRNAs. The apparent molecular weights of the RNAs were in millions: 5.6 (RNA1), 4.0 (RNA2), 3.0 (RNA3), 1.4 (RNA4), 1.2 (RNA5), 0.9 (RNA6) and 0.6 (RNA7). Fig. 2A shows that purification of the RNAs using oligo(dT)-cellulose leads to sharper bands, except for RNA1. This RNA remains present as a broad and diffuse band. This could be due to the presence of A-U base pairs which are not denatured with glyoxal. Therefore we have used agarose gels containing 6 M urea for electrophoresis. By comparing lane 2 and 4 from Fig. 2 it is clear that the presence of urea indeed results in sharper bands, especially for RNA1. Therefore, we have used urea-containing gels in all subsequent experiments. Using this system we have compared the intracellular virus-specific RNAs to virion RNA. The largest RNA comigrated with the viral genome (Fig. 2B).

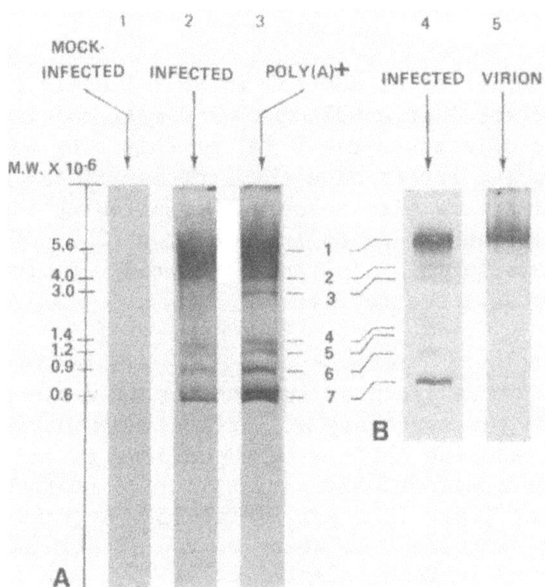

Fig. 2. Electrophoresis of glyoxal-dimethylsulfoxide denatured MHV-A59 specific intracellular RNA in an agarose gel without urea (A). Total RNA from mock-infected cells, labeled in the presence of actinomycin D, was run in lane 1, RNA from infected cells in lane 2. Equivalent amounts of RNA, obtained from about 10^5 cells, were analyzed. RNA extracted from Sindbis virus and rRNAs from Sac(-) cells were used as markers to calculate the molecular weights. Poly(A)-containing RNA was isolated by oligo(dT)-cellulose chromatography from a portion of the same material as run in lane 2. This material was run in lane 3. In (B) RNA isolated from purified virus and virus-specific RNA from cells were compared by electrophoresis in the same urea-containing gel. Other details are given in ref. 24.

There were two possible sources of artifacts we wanted to exclude, namely a) that defective interfering (DI) particles had accumulated in our virus stocks and b) that the smaller RNA species were degradation procucts of the genome sized 5.6×10^6 dalton RNA. To exclude a) the virus was plaque-purified twice before virus stocks were prepared by infecting Sac(-) cells at low MOI's (24). Moreover, RNA extracted from virions grown in a replicate culture of cells that made the 7 virus-specific RNAs, contained only one species of RNA, with a mass of 5.6×10^6 daltons (Fig.2B); if DI particles had been formed, smaller RNAs would have been found. The following control experiments to test b) were carried out: Sac(-) cells were infected with MHV-A59 as described above; actinomycin D was added but no ^{3}H-uridine. Just before lysis of the cells ^{3}H-uridine-labeled MHV-A59 was added and RNA was extracted from the mixture and analyzed. Virion RNA was not degraded in the extract of infected cells. In another experiment Sac(-) cells were infected with Sindbis virus and the cells were labeled between 6 and 8 h p.i. in the presence of actinomycin D. RNA was extracted and analyzed in the same way as described for MHV-A59 intracellular RNA. Only the well known 42S and 26S RNA species (10) were found.

Isolation of virus-specific polyribosomes and analysis of mRNAs

To obtain more direct evidence for a messenger function of the seven RNAs, we have looked at virus-specific mRNAs present in polyribosomes. The postnuclear supernatants from control cells and virus-infected actinomycin D-treated cells labeled with ^{3}H-uridine were analyzed by sedimentation in isokinetic sucrose gradients (Fig. 3). As expected, no ^{3}H-uridine was incorporated into RNA from mock-infected cells. In gradients loaded with lysates from infected cells two peaks were present: one with material sedimenting from 80-200 S and another at about 230 S. To determine whether the RNA sedimenting in the gradient was ribosome-associated, EDTA was added to the cell extract before analysis. The slower sedimenting material was EDTA-sensitive and remained at the top of the gradient. Treatment with EDTA did not alter the sedimentation of the bulk of the material present in the 230 S peak, indicating that this RNA was not polyribosome-associated (Fig. 3).

RNA extracted from every fourth gradient fraction was analyzed by electrophoresis in an agarose gel (Fig. 4). Seven virus-specific RNA species were detected throughout the sucrose gradient; they had the same apparent molecular weights as the intracellular RNAs described above. The mRNA species released with EDTA and the RNA present in the EDTA-resistant peak were also analyzed. The EDTA-resistant material contained only one RNA species of 5.6×10^6 daltons It is likely therefore that this material consists of subviral ribonucleoprotein. A small portion of this RNA species (9% determined by microdensitometry of a fluorograph) together with all of the six smaller RNAs were found at the top of the gradient after

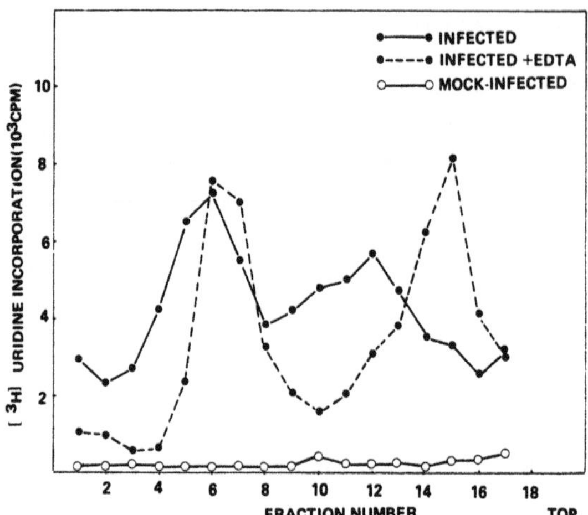

Fig. 3. Sucrose gradient analysis of polysomes containing viral mRNA. Cytoplasmic fractions from infected (•—•) and mock-infected (o—o) cells treated with actinomycin D and labeled with ^{3}H-uridine were compared. EDTA was added to a lysate of infected cells and this material was also run (•--•). For more experimental details:see ref.24.

EDTA-treatment. It can be concluded that all RNA species are indeed mRNAs.

TRANSLATION OF MOUSE HEPATITIS VIRUS A59 SUBGENOMIC RNAs IN XENOPUS LAEVIS OOCYTES

To test directly whether the MHV-A59 subgenomic RNAs are functional messengers, we have purified the virus-specific RNAs induced in Sac(-) cells upon infection with MHV-A59 and presented them to a suitable translation system. The *Xenopus laevis* oocyte system was selected since it is known to translate large-sized messenger RNAs with high fidelity and without premature termination as is often the case in cell-free systems (22); it also carries out the posttranslational modifications of the protein products, if necessary (1).

Isolation of virus-specific intracellular RNAs

Since the reaction with glyoxal will affect the proper functioning of RNAs as messengers, preparative separation for translational purposes was performed using a 1% agarose-6M urea horizontal slab gel but omitting the glyoxal dimethylsulfoxide treatment. It is clear from Fig. 5A that the virus-specific RNAs of MHV-A59 infected Sac(-) cells labeled with ^{3}H-uridine in the presence of actinomycin D were separated in this gel system in a similar way as after glyoxal denaturation. Agarose gels containing 6M urea melt upon heating for

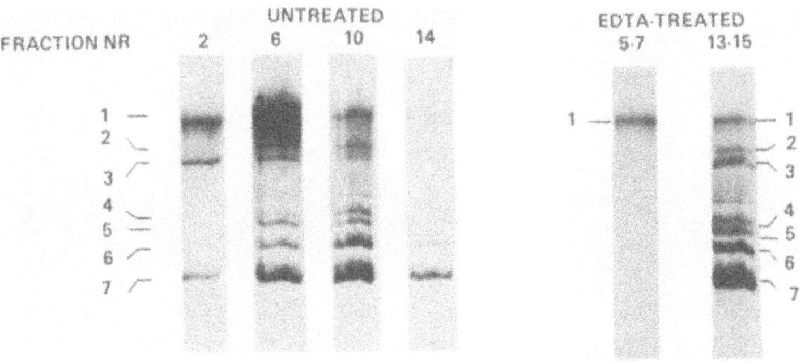

Fig.4. Agarose gel electrophoresis of RNA extracted from polyribosome gradients. Virus-specific mRNAs were labeled and polyribosomes from MHV-A59 infected cells were analyzed as shown in Fig. 3. RNA was extracted, denatured and analyzed by agarose gel electrophoresis. The left part of the figure gives the results for every fourth fraction of the gradient shown in Fig. 3. The numbers 1 to 7 indicate the position of the seven virus-specific poly(A)-containing RNAs isolated from infected cells (Fig. 2) which were run as markers in the same gel. The right hand portion represents an analysis of the RNAs present in the two peaks found after the addition of EDTA to the cell lysate. The fraction numbers refer to the gradients shown in Fig. 3. Equal amounts of radioactivity were loaded on the gel but the lane containing the EDTA-resistant material was only exposed for 12 h, compared to 96 h for the RNAs present in the EDTA-sensitive peak. Other details are given in ref.24 .

2 min at 65°C. For this reason RNA is easily recovered from such gels.

To purify MHV-A59 specific intracellular RNAs for the injection into Xenopus oocytes, RNA was isolated from MHV-A59 infected Sac(-) cells by phenol extraction and ethanol precipitation. A poly(A)-containing fraction was prepared by oligo(dT)-cellulose chromatography. All RNA species were present in this preparation (data not shown). A ^{32}P-labeled poly(A)$^{+}$RNA fraction, isolated from MHV-A59 infected Sac(-) cells grown in the presence of actinomycin D and ^{32}P-phosphate, was added as a marker and the sample was electrophoresed in an agarose-urea gel. Virus-specific RNAs were localized by autoradiography of the wet gel. Bands corresponding with the RNAs 1, 2, 3, 4 + 5, 6 and 7 were excised and the RNAs recovered by phenol extraction and ethanol precipitation. To check the validity of this procedure, small samples of the RNA-preparations were reanalyzed by agarose gel electrophoresis after glyoxal-dimethylsulfoxide denaturation. As shown in Fig.5B pure preparations both of RNA3 and RNA7 were obtained, whereas RNA6 still contained some contamination

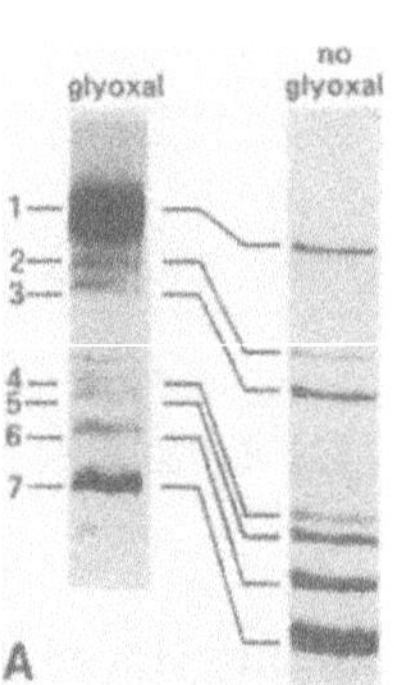

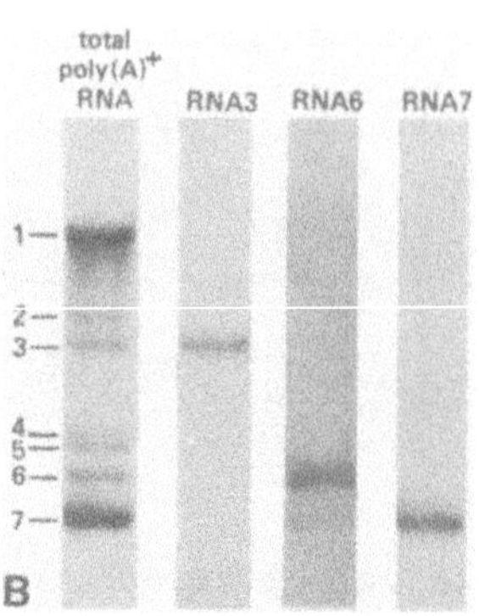

Fig.5. (A): Effect of glyoxal-dimethylsulfoxide denaturation on the electrophoretic separation of MHV-A59 specific intracellular RNAs in a 1% agarose-6M urea gel. Virus-specific RNAs were isolated by phenol extraction and ethanol precipitation from MHV-A59-infected Sac(-) cells labeled with ^{3}H-uridine in the presence of actinomycin D. One sample was denatured with glyoxal in 50% DMSO, another was heated and rapidly cooled in a sample buffer containing 0.25% SDS as described in ref.18. (B): Purification of MHV-A59-specific intracellular RNAs. Cultures of Sac(-) cells were infected with MHV-A59 and incubated in the presence of actinomycin D and ^{3}H-uridine. Cells were harvested at 9 h p.i.; RNA was isolated from the cell lysate by phenol extraction and the polyadenylated fraction was isolated by oligo(dT)-cellulose chromatography. A sample of RNA extracted from MHV-A59-infected Sac(-) cells also grown in the presence of actinomycin D but labeled with $^{32}PO_4$ was added as a marker and the preparation was electrophoresed in a 1% agarose-6M urea gel. RNA bands were visualized by autoradiography of the wet gel. Bands corresponding to RNAs 3, 6 and 7 were excised, melted and phenol-extracted. RNAs recovered after ethanol precipitation were analyzed in a 1% agarose slab gel after glyoxal-dimethylsulfoxide denaturation. A sample of ^{32}P-labeled unfractionated poly(A)$^+$ RNA from infected cells was run as a marker in an adjacent lane of the gel. Other details are given in ref.18.

of RNA7. Similarly, RNA1 and RNA2 were obtained pure, but in the preparation of the RNAs 4 and 5, which were excised from the urea gel and processed together, a significant amount of RNA7 was also detectable, probably due to aggregation (results not shown).

Translation of the RNAs in oocytes of Xenopus laevis

The RNAs thus obtained were microinjected into *Xenopus* oocytes which were subsequently incubated in the presence of ^{35}S-methionine.

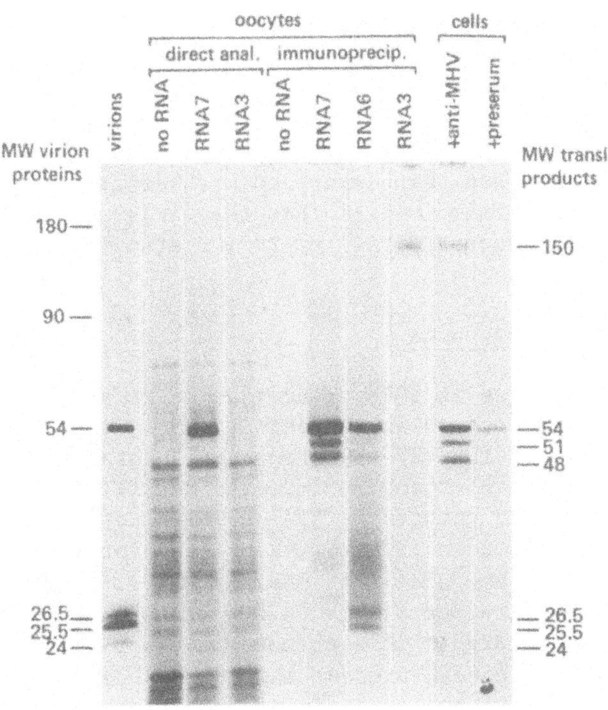

Figure 6. Electrophoretic analysis of the translation products of MHV-A59 specific RNAs 3,6 and 7. Oocytes were injected with RNA or with injection medium only, labeled with ^{35}S-methionine, and subsequently homogenized. Samples of the homogenates were taken for direct analysis in a 12.5% polyacrylamide gel. Other samples were used to prepare immunoprecipitates. These were run in the same gel. Proteins of MHV-A59-infected Sac(-) cells precipitable with the same antiserum, using mouse preimmune serum as a control, as well as ^{3}H-labeled purified virion proteins were run for comparison. The molecular weights are indicated in thousands. For other details see ref. 18.

The oocytes were homogenized and samples of the homogenates were analyzed directly by SDS-polyacrylamide gel electrophoresis. Only in one case when oocytes were injected with RNA7 the synthesis of a novel, presumably viral, polypeptide was observed as shown in Fig.6. Its molecular weight was estimated to be 54,000. In all other cases no such polypeptides were detected above the background of endogenous <u>Xenopus</u> proteins as is illustrated for RNA3 (Fig.6).
We have also done immunoprecipitation on the homogenates of oocytes injected with the virus-specific RNAs. The immune complexes were analyzed by electrophoresis in a SDS-polyacrylamide gel (Fig.6). Injection of oocytes with RNA7 resulted in the detection of three virus-specific polypeptides: one predominant polypeptide of about 54,000 daltons that had already been observed by direct analysis of the homogenate, plus two smaller polypeptides of about 51,000 and 48,000 daltons. The same polypeptides were also produced when oocytes were injected with the preparation of RNA6. Since this preparation contained significant amounts of contaminating RNA7, the appearance of the RNA7-specific polypeptides among the translation products was to be expected. However, three other polypeptides were detected having estimated molecular weights of 24,000, 25,500 and

26,500, the latter two of which were dominant. Injection with RNA3 gave rise to the synthesis of one virus-specific product with an estimated molecular weight of 150,000. No translation products of RNAs 1, 2 and 4+5 were found, except that in the immunoprecipitate of the translation products of RNA 4+5 the products of the contaminating RNA7 appeared. The antiserum used came from mice that had survived MHV-A59-induced hepatitis, but the same results were obtained when the immunoprecipitations were carried out with an antiserum obtained from rabbits that had been immunized with desintegrated purified MHV-A59 virions. This implies that the virus-specific translation products described above are related to the structural proteins of MHV-A59.

Characterization of translation products

The electrophoretic mobilities in SDS-polyacrylamide gels of the polypeptides synthesized in oocytes in response to RNAs 3, 6 and 7 were compared with those of the MHV-A59 structural proteins and with the virus-specific proteins found in infected cells. (Fig. 6.). The 54,000 dalton polypeptide encoded by RNA7 co-electrophoresed with the presumed nucleocapsid protein (27, 28), a phosphoprotein (26), and with a protein of the same size prominent in MHV-A59-infected cells. After immunoprecipitation of the 54,000 translation product two new polypeptides appeared. This phenomenon was also observed with the corresponding protein present in infected cells (Fig.6) and with ^{32}P-labeled virion nucleocapsid protein (data not shown). A similar degradation during immunoprecipitation has been described for the nucleocapsid protein of strain JHM (23).Apparently the nucleocapsid protein is subject to proteolytic degradation even though protease inhibitors were present in the reaction mixture. These data indicate that RNA7 encodes the nucleocapsid protein.

The 24,000, 25,500 and 26,500 molecular weight polypeptides translated from RNA6 comigrated with the lower molecular weight proteins found in purified MHV-A59. Their relative intensities also seemed to correspond. *In vitro* iodination of purified virus using the lactoperoxidase-catalyzed reaction showed all three proteins to be present in the viral envelope (unpublished data). They might be different forms of the same protein differing in their degree of glycosylation.

No counterpart of the 150,000 dalton translation product of RNA3 is present among the virion structural proteins. However, this polypeptide had the same electrophoretic mobility as one of the polypeptides that can be immunoprecipitated from homogenates of infected Sac(-) cells with an antiserum directed against the viral structural proteins. This protein is a glycopeptide containing a protein moiety of about 110,000 daltons.

Even though a more detailed characterization of the translation products described is required, these data together clearly prove that at least three of the seven MHV-A59 subgenomic RNAs are functional messengers. It is not yet clear why no virus-specific translation products were observed upon injection of Xenopus oocytes with RNAs 1, 2 and 4+5. One reason might be that these RNAs do not encode viral structural proteins and that their products therefore were not immunoprecipitated. In addition, the amounts of the RNAs injected into the oocytes, or their efficiencies of translation may have been too low. To overcome these problems we have scaled up the RNA preparation procedure, hoping that injection of saturating quantities of the messengers will allow the detection of products even without immunoprecipitation as was already possible with RNA7.

UV TRANSCRIPTION MAPPING OF THE TARGET SIZES FOR THE MHV-A59 SUBGENOMIC RNAs

UV irradiation of RNA induces uracil dimers (13); UV transcription mapping is based on the assumptions that a) formation of one dimer is a sufficient barrier to stop the transcription of the RNA chain at that point; b) repair is slow or absent; c) the number of hits at a given dose rate will be proportional to the time of irradiation, and to the length of the template (target size). If an RNA is synthesized as a precursor molecule, or if its synthesis is dependent on prior transcription of the other RNAs, a UV target size greater than its physical size will be found. If, on the other hand,

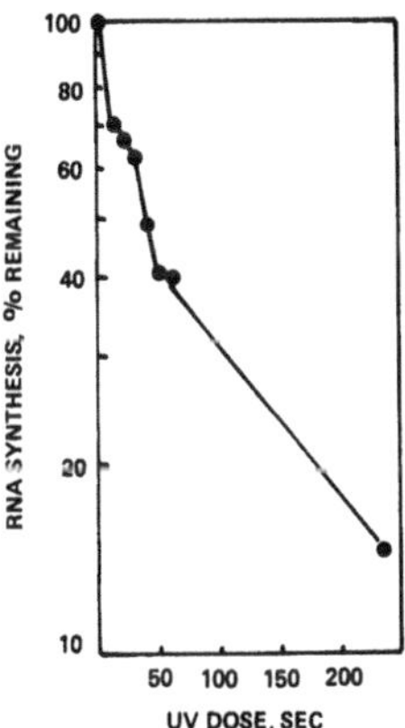

Fig. 7. Effect of UV irradiation on the overall synthesis of virus-specific RNA in MHV-A59 infected Sac(-) cells. Actinomycin D-treated cells were irradiated with UV light (254 nm) at a dose rate of 50 $erg.sec^{-1}.mm^{-2}$ at 6h p.i. and then labeled with 100 μCi/ml ^{3}H-uridine, from 6h 5min to 6h 35min p.i. in the presence of 1 μg/ml actinomycin D. Background incorporation in uninfected cells (6.6 to 7.7% of the incorporation of the unirradiated control) was subtracted to calculate the remaining virus-specific RNA synthesis at the various UV doses. Other details are given in ref. 9a.

the synthesis of a RNA is initiated independently, the physical size will be the same as the UV target size of its template. The efficacy of UV mapping to determine the size of transcription templates for the mRNAs of a number of RNA viruses is well documented (21).

UV inactivation of total MHV-A59-specific RNA synthesis

To determine the target size for the intracellular subgenomic RNAs of MHV-A59, infected cells were UV-irradiated at 6h p.i., the time when virus-specific RNA synthesis starts to increase sharply (see Fig. 3). Almost all RNA synthesized in infected cells between 6 and 8 h p.i. is present in nucleocapsid or polyribosomes (see Fig. 3), and we assume that by this time most of the negative strand templates for the synthesis of viral RNA and mRNAs have been synthesized. Fig.7 shows the effect of increasing UV doses on the synthesis of virus-specific RNA synthesized in the 30 min after irradiation. An average of one hit per RNA template, corresponding to 37% survival, was reached at an UV dose of 3500 $erg.mm^{-2}$. The shape of the dose-response curve indicates a multicomponent character of the template. The same curve was obtained when the labeling was started at 6h 35min p.i., indicating that there was no repair in the first half h after UV irradiation.

Target sizes for the templates of the individual virus-specific RNAs

To determine the effect of UV radiation on the synthesis of the individual RNAs, they were extracted from the cells and separated by agarose gel electrophoresis. The resulting fluorograph

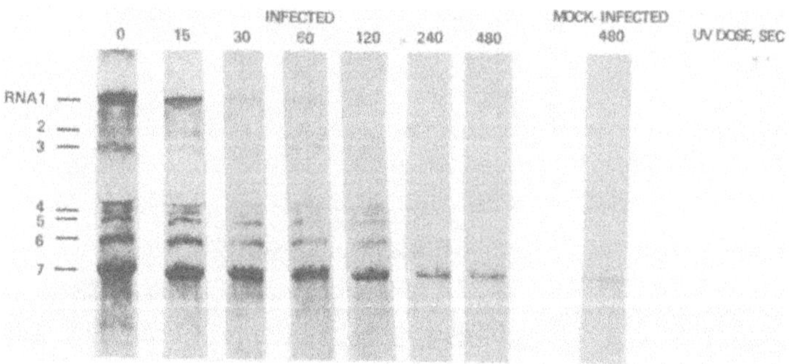

Fig. 8. Agarose gel electrophoresis of the virus-specific RNAs synthesized between 6h 5min and 6h 35min p.i. in MHV-A59 infected cells, exposed to increasing doses of UV irradation. Lanes contain RNA extracted from equal numbers of cells. Denatured nucleic acids were electrophoresed in a urea-containing gel and detected by fluorography. The positions of the seven virus-specific RNAs are indicated.

(Fig.8) indicates that the smaller the RNA, the more resistant its synthesis to UV. The RNA bands were cut from the gel to quantitate the amounts of RNA synthesized. The result of such an experiment is shown in Fig.9.

Using the data from Fig.9 the target sizes were calculated (Table 3). There is an almost perfect agreement between the target size of the template of RNAs 1 to 5 and the physical sizes of these RNAs. This fit is less perfect for RNA 6 and 7, which could be due to a lack of measuring points for the irradiation times between 60 and 240 sec.

The results of these experiments strongly argue that the transcription of RNAs 1 to 7 is initiated independently. They do not, however, allow conclusions concerning the physical size of the template(s), i.e. whether transcription of the subgenomic RNAs occurs on a genome-sized template or on several subgenomic negative-stranded RNAs.

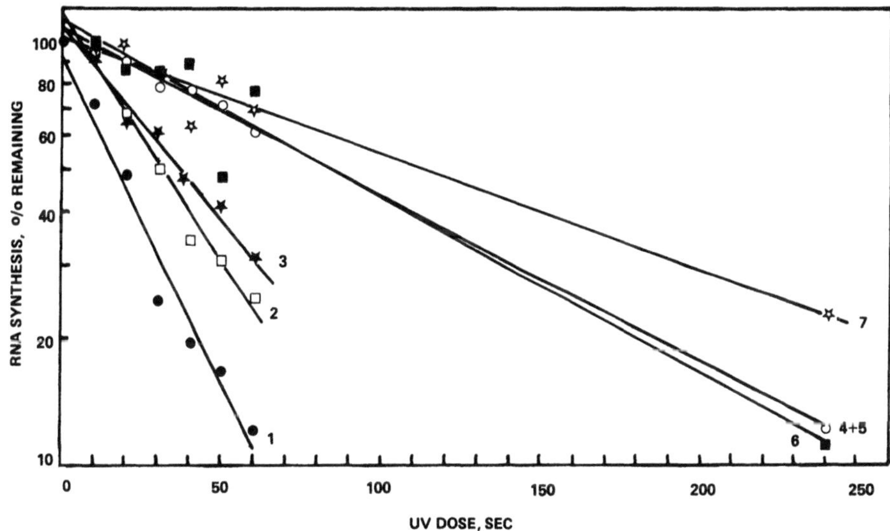

Fig. 9. Effect of increasing doses of UV irradiation on the synthesis of the intracellular RNAs of MHV-A59. Cells were infected, UV irradiated, and labeled as described in the legend of Fig. 7. RNAs were extracted from the cells and separated by electrophoresis (see Fig. 8); RNA bands were cut out of the gel and dissolved by boiling in 0.5 ml of water. RNA4 and 5 were processed together. Liquid scintillation fluid was added and the amount of radioactivity was determined. The graphs were fitted by linear regression analysis. The correlation coefficients (r) varied between 0.97 and 1.00.

Table 3. Comparison of the molecular weights of the MHV-A59 intracellular RNAs and the UV target-sizes of the templates for these RNAs

RNA	K x T [a)]	Target size of template [b)]	RNA size [c)]
	(sec^{-1})	(daltons of RNA x 10^{-6})	
1	3.57×10^{-2}	(5.6)	5.6
2	2.52×10^{-2}	3.9	4.0
3	1.94×10^{-2}	3.0	3.0
4+5	0.90×10^{-2}	1.4	1.2-1.4
6	0.94×10^{-2}	1.5	0.9
7	0.62×10^{-2}	0.97	0.6

a) K x T was calculated from the relationship $\ln(N_t/N_o) = -K \times T \times t$, where N_t is the incorporation of ^{3}H-uridine into RNA after t seconds of UV irradiation; N_o is the RNA synthesis in the unirradiated culture; T is the target size and K is a constant. The calculation was made from the data points illustrated in Fig. 9, using linear regression analysis. The value of K was calculated as 6.38×10^{-9} sec^{-1} by substituting a value of 5.6×10^6 for the target size of RNA1.

b) Using this value of T the target sizes for the other RNAs were calculated.

c) The molecular weights of the denatured virus-specific RNAs were determined by agarose gel electrophoresis (24).

REPLICATION STRATEGY OF MHV-A59

Our data leave little doubt that a hitherto undescribed mechanism is involved in the replication of coronaviruses. In the Baltimore classification system (1) the coronaviruses would belong to a new subdivision of class IV, consisting of positive-stranded, non-segmented, single-stranded RNA viruses inducing multiple subgenomic RNAs in infected cells. Evidence that these RNAs are mRNAs comes from their polyadenylation and the presence in polyribosomes. Moreover three RNAs could be translated in *Xenopus laevis* oocytes.

Since the sum of the molecular weights of the six subgenomic RNAs is 11.1×10^6, almost twice that of the genome, sequence homologies should exist between these RNAs. We have speculated that all subgenomic RNAs and the genome share a homologous region at their 3'-termini.(Fig.10). Direct proof for this assumption is still

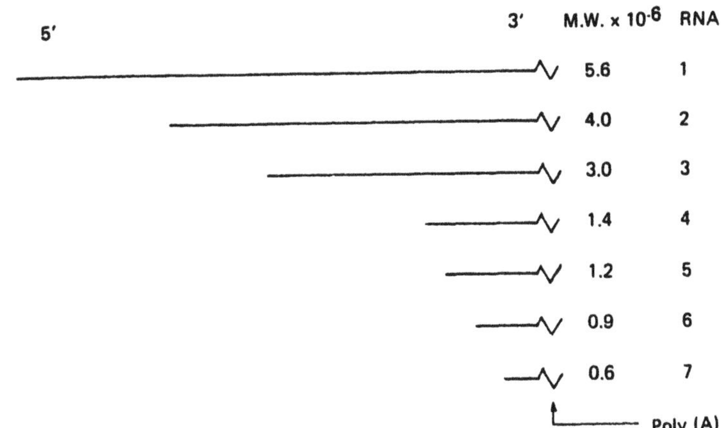

Fig. 10. A model for the sequence homology between mouse hepatitis mRNAs.

lacking. Some corroboration comes from work by Stern and Kennedy on the avian infectious bronchitis virus (25). Six major polyadenylated virus-specified RNAs were found in infected cells. The molecular weights of these RNAs roughly correspond to those found by us for the MHV-A59 mRNAs with the exception that RNA2 was not detected in the avian system. The authors also provide evidence that the sequence of each RNA is contained within the sequences of all larger RNA species and refer to preliminary observations that the subgenomic RNAs share the 3'-end of the genome.

If the model would be correct it could easily explain the size of the translation products of RNAs 3, 6 and 7 by making one further assumption i.e. that only that 5'-terminal part of an RNA not present in the next smaller RNA is translated and that internal initiation of translation does not occur. Thus, only the 1.6×10^6 daltons 5'-terminal region of RNA3 (3.0×10^6 daltons) should be expressed yielding a translation product with a molecular weight of at most about 160,000. Similarly, a polypeptide of up to 30,000 daltons is predicted to be obtained from the 0.3×10^6 daltons 5'-terminal part of RNA6 (0.9×10^6 daltons), and RNA7 (0.6×10^6 daltons) is supposed to act as a monocistronic messenger, coding for a protein with a maximum size of about 60,000 daltons.

Although the Xenopus oocyte translation products should be characterized more thoroughly, they are in good agreement with the data for MHV-JHM of Siddell et al.(23). There seems to be little doubt that RNA6 codes for the smaller glycoprotein and RNA7 for the nucleocapsid protein.

The results of the UV transcription mapping experiments exclude that the subgenomic RNAs are processed or spliced from a common precursor. The data are consistent with the independently initiated transcription of a genome-sized negative-stranded template or a number of smaller templates. A further characterization of the negative-stranded template(s) will discriminate between these two models.

ACKNOWLEDGEMENTS

We thank Dr. A.D.M.E. Osterhaus for his help in the preparation of mouse antiserum against MHV-A59, Dr. R. Huber for her hospitality, help and advice in oocyte experiments, Mrs. Nancy Bleumink-Pluym and Mrs. M. van Kleef-Koopmans for technical assistance and Mrs. Elizabeth Alvarez for the preparation of this manuscript.

REFERENCES

1. Asselbergs, F.A.M. (1979). Ph.D. thesis, University of Nijmegen, The Netherlands.
2. Baltimore, D. (1971). Bacteriol. Rev. 35, 235-241.
3. Cheever, F.S., Daniels, J.B., Pappenheimer, A.M. and Bailey, O.T. (1949). J. Exp. Med. 90, 181-194.
4. Dick, G.W.A., Niven, J.S.F. and Gledhill, A.W. (1956). Brit.J. Expt. Path. 37, 90-98.
5. Gledhill, A.W. and Andrewes, C.H. (1951). Brit. J. Exp. Pathol. 22, 559-568.
6. Haspel, M.V., Lampert, P.W. and Oldstone, M.B.A. (1978). Proc. Natl. Acad. Sci. USA 75, 4033-4036.
7. Herndon, R.M., Griffon, D.E., McCormick, U. and Weiner, L.P. (1975). Arch. Neurol. 32, 32-35.
8. Herndon, R.M., Price, P.L. and Weiner, L.P. (1977). Science (Wash. D.C.) 195, 693-694.
9. Hierholzer, J.C., Broderson, J.R. and Murphy, F.A. (1979).Infect. Immun. 24, 508-522.
9a. Jacobs, L., Spaan, W.J.M., Horzinek, M.C. and Van der Zeijst, B.A.M. (1980). Submitted for publication.
10. Kääriäinen, L. and Söderlund, H. (1978).Curr. Top. Microbiol. Immunol. 81, 15-69.
11. Lampert, P.W., Sims, J.K. and Kniazeff, A.J. (1973). Acta Neuropath. 24, 76-85.
12. Manaker, R.A., Piczak, C.V., Miller, A.A. and Stanton, M.F. (1961). J. Nat. Cancer Inst. 27, 29-45.
13. Miller, R.L. and Plagemann, P.G.W. (1974). J.Virol. 13, 729-739.
14. Nagashima, K., Wege, H. and Ter Meulen, V. (1978). Adv. Exp. Med. Biol. 100, 395-409.
15. Nagashima, K., Wege, H., Meyermann, R. and Ter Meulen, V. (1979). Acta Neuropath. 45, 205-213.
16. Nelson, J.B.(1952). J.Exp. Med. 96, 293-302.
17. Robb, J.A., Bond, C.W. and Leibowitz, J.L. (1979). Virology 94, 385-399.

18. Rottier, P.J.M., Spaan, W.J.M., Horzinek, M.C. and Van der Zeijst, B.A.M. (1980). J. Virol., in press.
19. Rowe, W.P., Hartley, J.W., and Capps, W.I. (1963). Proc. Soc. Exp. Biol. Med. 112, 161-165.
20. Sabesin, S.M. (1972). Am.J. Gastroenterol. 58, 259-274.
21. Sauerbier, W. and Hercules, K. (1978). Ann. Rev. Genet. 12, 329-363.
22. Shatkin, A.J., Banerjee, A.K. and Both, G.W. (1977). Comprehensive Virology, vol. 10. Plenum Press, New York.
23. Siddell, S.G., Wege, H., Barthel, A. and Ter Meulen V. (1980). J. Virol. 33, 10-17.
24. Spaan, W.J.M., Rottier, P.J.M., Horzinek, M.C. and Van der Zeijst, B.A.M. (1981). Virology 107, in press.
25. Stern, D.F. and Kennedy S.I.T. (1980). J. Virol. 34, 665-674.
26. Stohlman, S.A. and Lai, M.C.M. (1979). J. Virol 32, 672-675.
27. Sturman,L.S. (1977). Virology 77, 637-649.
28. Sturman, L.S., Holmes, K.V. and Behnke, J. (1980). J. Virol. 33, 449-462.
29. Virelizier, J.L., Dayan, A.D. and Allison A.C.(1975). Infect. Immun. 12, 1127-1140.
30. Wege, H. and Ter Meulen, V. (1978). J.Gen. Virol. 41, 217-227.
31. Weiland, E., Mussgay, M. and Weiland, F. (1978). J. Exp.Med. 148, 408-423.
32. Weiner L.P. (1973). Arch. Neurol. 28, 298-303.

MURINE CORONAVIRUS RNA

Julian L. Leibowitz* and Susan R. Weiss[§]

*Department of Pathology, University of California, San Diego, School of Medicine, La Jolla, CA 92093 and [§]Department of Microbiology, University of California, San Francisco, School of Medicine (currently at Department of Microbiology, University of Pennsylvania, Philadelphia, PA 19104)

INTRODUCTION

Coronaviruses are ubiquitous in nature and cause several diseases in infected hosts (Robb and Bond, 1979a). The genomic RNA of coronaviruses has been extensively studied in recent years (Lomneczi and Kennedy, 1977; Yogo et al., 1977; Lai and Stohlman, 1978; Wege et al., 1978; Macnaughton and Madge, 1978; Guy and Brian, 1979). These studies have shown that the coronavirus genome is a large, single stranded RNA which is polyadenylated and of positive polarity.

In contrast to the data obtained on virion RNA, there is a paucity of published data on intracellular coronavirus specific RNA. Robb and Bond (1979b) have studied mouse hepatitis virus (MHV) infected cells and found that RNA isolated from virus specific polysomes was heterogeneous in size (10-28S). Recently, Siddell et al. (1980) have shown that RNA of this size codes for two MHV structural proteins. Stern and Kennedy (1980) have identified six virus specific RNAs synthesized in cells infected with avian infectious bronchitis virus (IBV). These IBV specific RNAs have been fingerprinted and form a nested set.

We have been investigating the virus specific RNAs synthesized in cells infected with either MHV-A59 (A59V) or MHV-JHM (JHMV). JHMV is a highly neurotropic strain of MHV and produces a demyelinating encephalomyelitis in infected mice. A59V is weakly neurotropic. Both of these strains of MHV are able to initiate persistent infections in cell culture and in vivo. We have been investigating the replication of these viruses in the hope of eventually understanding how these viruses persist in infected mice.

MATERIALS AND METHODS

Cells

The origin and growth of the murine cell line 17CL-1 has been described previously (Sturman and Takemoto, 1972; Bond et al., 1979).

Virus

The origin and growth of A59V and JHMV virus stocks has been described (Robb and Bond, 1979b). Cells were infected in suspension and virus adsorption was at 37°C for 30 minutes. Following adsorption the cells were centrifuged, resuspended in Dulbecco's Modified Eagle's Medium with 2% fetal bovine serum (DME-2) prewarmed to 37°C and plated into 35 mm (1.5×10^6 cells/dish), 60 mm (5×10^6 cells/dish), 100 mm (1.5×10^7 cells/dish) or 150 mm ($4\text{-}5 \times 10^7$ cells/dish) plastic culture dishes and further incubated at 37°C. For most experiments utilizing ^{32}P-orthophosphate as label, the cells were resuspended and plated in phosphate free DME-2.

Extraction of Intracellular RNA

Cytoplasmic extracts of infected or mock infected 17CL-1 cells were prepared using NP-40 (Borun et al., 1967). Monolayers were rinsed once with cold phosphate buffered saline (PBS), scraped into cold reticulocyte standard buffer (RSB, 0.01 M Tris, pH 7.4, 0.01 M NaCl, 0.0015 M $MgCl_2$) with a rubber policeman and transferred to a tube containing sufficient NP-40 to give a final concentration of 1%. The cell suspension was vortexed gently, incubated on ice for 5 minutes, vortexed again and the nuclei removed by centrifugation at 1,500 g for 2 minutes. The cytoplasmic extract was adjusted to 1% SDS, 0.4 M NaCl, 0.01 M EDTA, and 1.0 mg/ml proteinase K and incubated at 50°C for five minutes and at room temperature for an additional 25 minutes. The RNA was then extracted with phenol chloroform and precipitated with 3 volumes of ethanol.

Preparation of MHV Virion RNA

17CL-1 cells were infected with A59V or JHMV in phosphate free DME-2 as described above. Following virus adsorption the cells were plated in 100 or 150 mm culture dishes and incubated at 33°C. At 4 hours post infection (h.p.i.) ^{32}P-orthophosphate was added to a concentration of 100-1,000 μci/ml. At 16-18 h.p.i. the cell associated virus was released by two cycles of freeze thawing and the resulting lysate clarifeid by centrifugation at 10,000 g for 30 minutes at 4°C. Virus was concentrated by centrifugation for 60 minutes at 35,000 rpm in the SW40 rotor through a 0.5 ml pad of 15% (w/w) potassium tartrate in MSE buffer (0.01 M morpholinopropane sulfonic acid, 0.15 M NaCl, 0.001 M EDTA, pH 6.8). The virus pellets were resuspended by sonciation in 0.5 ml of MSE buffer, layered onto a 12 ml gradient of 5-25% (w/w) potassium tartrate in MSE buffer and centrifuged at 35,000 rpm for 45 minutes in the SW40 rotor. The gradient was fractionated and the virion peak located by counting aliquots of each fraction. For the preparation of highly purified virus, this material was diluted with MSE, layered on a 9 ml 10-40% (w/w) potassium tartrate gradient and centrifuged in the SW40 rotor at 37,000 rpm for 4 hours. The gradient was fractionated, aliquots were counted and the peak of radiolabeled virus collected. This material had a buoyant density between 1.19 and 1.17 g/cc. The virus was diluted with MSE buffer, pelleted at 45,000 rpm for 30 minutes in the SW50.1 rotor and resuspended by sonication in 1 ml of MSE buffer. Virion RNA was extracted in a similar manner to intracellular RNA and precipitated with ethanol after the addition of 50 μg of carrier tRNA.

Virion RNA for fingerprinting was prepared by a slightly different procedure. Virus was concentrated and banded on a 5-25% potassium tartrate gradient and this partially purified virus was diluted with MSE buffer, pelleted in the SW50.1 rotor and the RNA was extracted and precipitated with ethanol as described above. The RNA was collected by centrifugation, dried under a stream of nitrogen and dissolved in 0.1 ml of SDS buffer (0.01 M Tris, 0.01 M NaCl, 0.001 M EDTA, 0.1% SDS, pH 7.4). It was then overlaid on a 5 ml 10-30% (w/w) sucrose in SDS buffer gradient and centrifuged at 46,000 rpm for 107 minutes at 20°C in the SW50.1 rotor. The gradient was fractionated and the peak of virion RNA located by counting aliquots of each fraction. These fractions were pooled, adjusted to 0.4 M NaCl and precipitated with ethanol in the presence of 100 μg of tRNA carrier. This material was used for fingerprinting studies and was homogeneous upon analytical electrophoresis.

Isolation of Poly(A) Containing RNA

Intracellular RNA was extracted and precipitated with ethanol as described. The polyadenylated RNA species were isolated by affinity chromatography over poly(U) Sepharose as described by Wilt (1977).

Agarose Gel Electrophoresis

Analytical electrophoresis. Agarose gel electrophoresis following glyoxal denaturation was essentially as previously described (McMaster and Carmichael, 1977). Samples were electrophoresed at 100 V for 4 hours in horizontal slab gels containing 0.7, 0.8 or 1.0% agarose, 0.01 M phosphate buffer, pH 7.0, 0.002 M EDTA.

Preparative electrophoresis. Labeled intracellular RNA was extracted from 1.2 x 10^8 to 2.0 x 10^8 cells and the poly(A) containing RNA species selected by affinity chromatography. The RNA was denatured with 10 mM methyl mercuric hydroxide and electrophoresed in agarose gels containing 5 mM methyl mercuric hydroxide (Bailey and Davidson, 1976). Electrophoresis was at 100 volts for 6 hours in a horizontal gel containing either 0.8% agarose or 1% low melting agarose, depending on the method used to elute the RNA from the gel (See below.). Following electrophoresis, the majority of the methyl mercury was removed from the gel by soaking in two changes of 750 ml sterile 0.5 M ammonium acetate (Bailey and Davidson, 1976).

RNA Elution

RNA species were located by autoradiography of the wet gels wrapped in Saran. Agarose strips corresponding to the bands seen in the autoradiographs were cut from the gel wit a flamed scalpel. For T_1 fingerprint studies low melting point agarose gels were used and RNA was recovered from gels by melting the agarose at 70°C for 5 minutes in the presence of Tris acetate buffer (10 mM Tris, 20 mM sodium acetate, 5 mM EDTA), 1% 2-mercaptoethanol. Five ml of a hydroxylapatite (HA) slurry, prewarmed to 37°C, was added and the HA was collected by centrifugation and washed twice with Tris acetate buffer (pH 7.3) in a 37°C warm room to remove the liquified agarose. The HA was resuspended in 5 ml of Tris acetate buffer and transferred to disposable columns. The RNA was eluted from HA columns by two washes of 1.0 ml of 0.4 M sodium phosphate, 1 mM EDTA (pH 7.0) which were forced from the columns by centrifugation at 1,000 g for 10 minutes. The phosphate eluates were pooled and the RNA was precipitated with CTAB as described by Stern and Kennedy (1980). The CTAB precipitates were dissolved in 0.2 ml of 50 mM Tris, pH 7.4, containing 1M NaCl and 1 mM EDTA and the RNA was precipitated with ethanol.

RNA to be used in translation studies was electrophoresed in 0.8% standard melting point agarose gels. The RNA species were located as above, agarose strips were excised from the gel with a scalpel and ground up in a tissue homogenizer containing a high salt buffer (10 mM Tris, 0.5 M NaCl, 1 mM EDTA, 1% SDS, 1% 2-mercapto-ethanol). This material was extracted overnight at 4°C on a rocker platform with an equal volume of phenol. The phases were separated by centrifugation, the aqueous phase was re-extracted and the RNA precipitated with ethanol in the presence of rabbit liver tRNA.

Ribonuclease T_1 Fingerprinting

The RNA was digested with 10 µl of ribonuclease T_1 (1 mg/ml) in 10 mM Tris, pH 7.6, at 37°C for 30 minutes. Ten µl of a solution containing 5 M urea, 50% sucrose, 0.1% bromphenol blue and 0.1% xylene cyanol FF was added to the digestion products. The RNAse T_1

resistant oligonucleotides were separated by two dimensional polyacrylamide gel electrophoresis as described by Stern and Kennedy (1980) with the following modification. After electrophoresis in the first dimension, the gel strips were washed for 25 minutes with two changes of 100 mM Tris borate buffer containing 2.5 mM EDTA, pH 8.3, prior to pouring the second dimension gel (Lee et al., 1979).

Following electrophoresis the gels were wrapped with polyethylene sheets and exposed with intensifying screens (Laskey and Mills, 1977).

In Vitro Translation

A rabbit reticulocyte lysate system treated with micrococcal nuclease (Pelham and Jackson, 1976) was used with ^{35}S-methionine as the label.

Polyacrylamide Gel Electrophoresis

Polyacrylamide gel electrophoresis was performed as described by Laemmli (1970).

Tryptic Peptide Map Studies

Tryptic peptide map studies were performed as described previously (Gibson, 1974).

RESULTS

Identification of MHV Specific Polyadenylated RNA species

17CL-1 cells were infected with A59V, JHMV or mock infected and labeled with ^{32}P-orthophosphate from 4-8 h.p.i. in the presence of actinomycin D. The cytoplasmic RNA was extracted and separated into polyadenylated (poly(A)$^{+}$) and non-polyadenylated (poly(A)$^{-}$) classes by chromatography over poly(U) Sepharose. These RNAs were denatured with glyoxal and then analyzed by agarose gel electrophoresis. Seven MHV specific poly(A)$^{+}$ RNAs were reproducibly present in infected cells (Fig. 1). These RNAs have been designated RNAs 1-7, in decreasing order of size. In addition, we have occasionally observed two additional RNA species migrating faster than RNA 7 and minor RNA species migrating between RNAs 1 and 2 and RNAs 3 and 4. These minor species have not been studied extensively as yet.

The largest MHV specific RNA, RNA 1, comigrates with virion RNA and represents the intracellular form of the genome. In contrast to the differences observed between A59V and JHMV specific proteins (Bond et al., 1979), A59V and JHMV specific RNAs co-electrophorese in agarose gels.

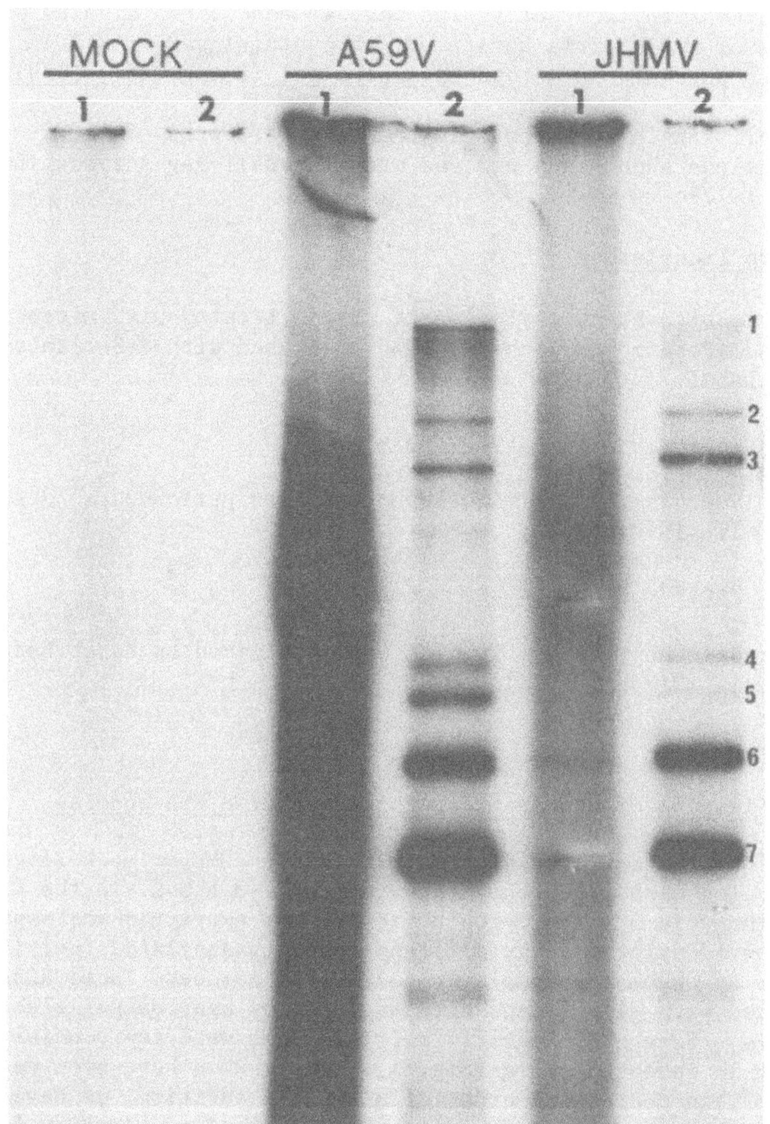

Fig. 1. The identification of MHV specific poly(A)+ RNA species. 17CL-1 cells were infected with A59V, JHMV or mock infected, and labeled with ^{32}P-orthophosphate in the presence of 5 μg/ml actinomycin D from 4-8 hours post infection. Cytoplasmic nucleic acids were extracted, precipitated and chromatographed over poly(U) Sepharose as described by Wilt (1977). The poly(A)$^-$ RNA(1) and poly(A)$^+$ RNA (2) species were glyoxylated and electrophoresed on a 0.8% agarose gel.

The poly(A)$^-$ MHV specific RNA is a heterogeneous mixture. Discrete bands which comigrate with poly(A)$^+$ MHV specific RNA are superimposed on a smear of heterogeneous material.

The sizes of MHV specific RNAs 1-7 were determined by agarose gel electrophoresis with appropriate molecular weight markers (Table 1). A linear-log relationship was obtained over a molecular weight range of 5.5×10^5 to 1.15×10^7 daltons.

Ribonuclease T_1 Oligonucleotide Fingerprint Studies

The sum of the molecular weights of the six subgenomic RNA species exceeds the molecular weight of the genome by approximately 50 percent. To further investigate this observation, the 7 major MHV specific RNAs were purified and compared to each other and to virion RNA using the technique of ribonuclease T_1 fingerprinting.

The individual RNA species and virion RNA were purified from cells labeled with ^{32}P-orthophosphate, digested with ribonuclease T_1 and the resulting oligonucleotides were separated by two dimensional gel electrophoresis. The results are shown in Figures 2 and 3. Poly(A) tracts are seen as streaks in the upper left hand corner of the fingerprints of A59V and JHMV virion RNAs. This confirms the findings of others (Yogo et al., 1977; Lai and Stohlman, 1978; Wege et al., 1978) that the MHV genome is polyadenylated. The seven major A59V and JHMV specific intracellular RNAs are also polyadenylated.

Table 1. The Molecular Weights of MHV Specific RNA

RNA Species	Mol. wt.[a]
Virion RNA	6.1×10^6
RNA 1	6.1×10^6
RNA 2	3.4×10^6
RNA 3	2.6×10^6
RNA 4	1.2×10^6
RNA 5	1.08×10^6
RNA 6	8.5×10^5
RNA 7	6.3×10^5

[a]Molecular weights were determined by electrophoresis after glyoxal denaturation in parallel to the following markers. E. coli rRNA, 17CL-1 cell rRNA, mengovirus RNA, VSV RNA, adenovirus type 2 DNA.

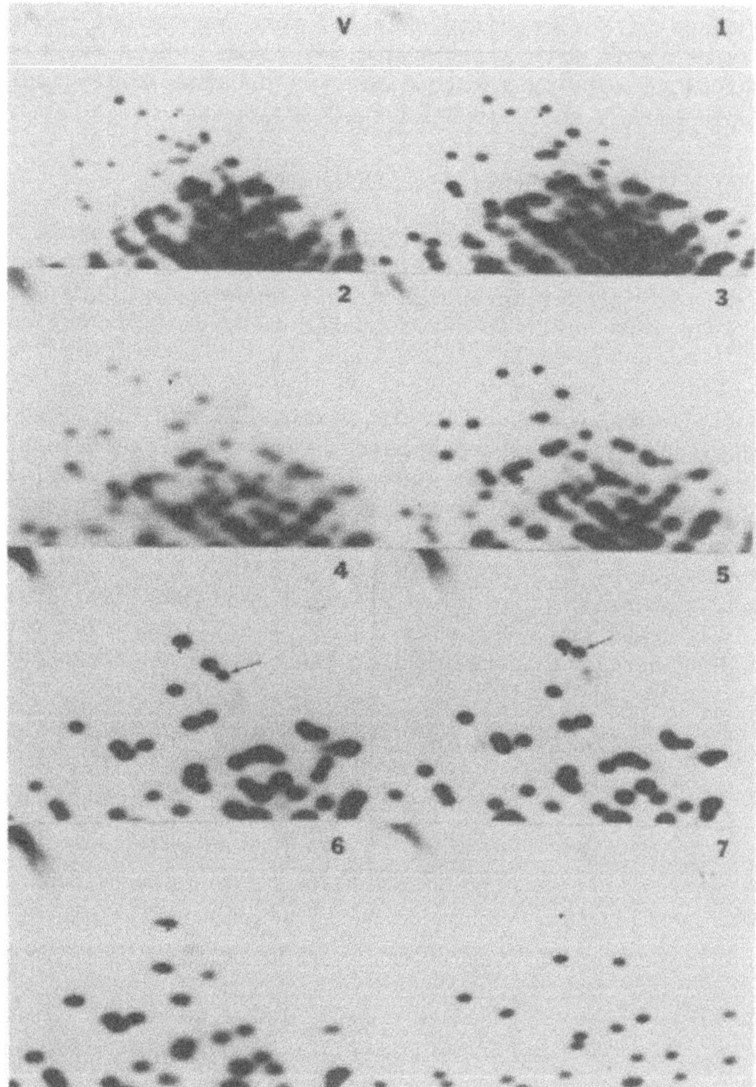

Fig. 2. Oligonucleotide fingerprints of A59V specific RNA. A59V virion (panel V) and intracellular RNAs (panels 1-7) were purified, digested with RNase T_1 and the resulting oligonucleotides separated as described in Materials and Methods. Only the portion of the autoradiographs which contains oligonucleotides migrating more slowly than the bromphenol blue dye markers are shown. The positions of the xylene cyanol dye markers are indicated by asterisks. Unique spots are indicated by arrows.

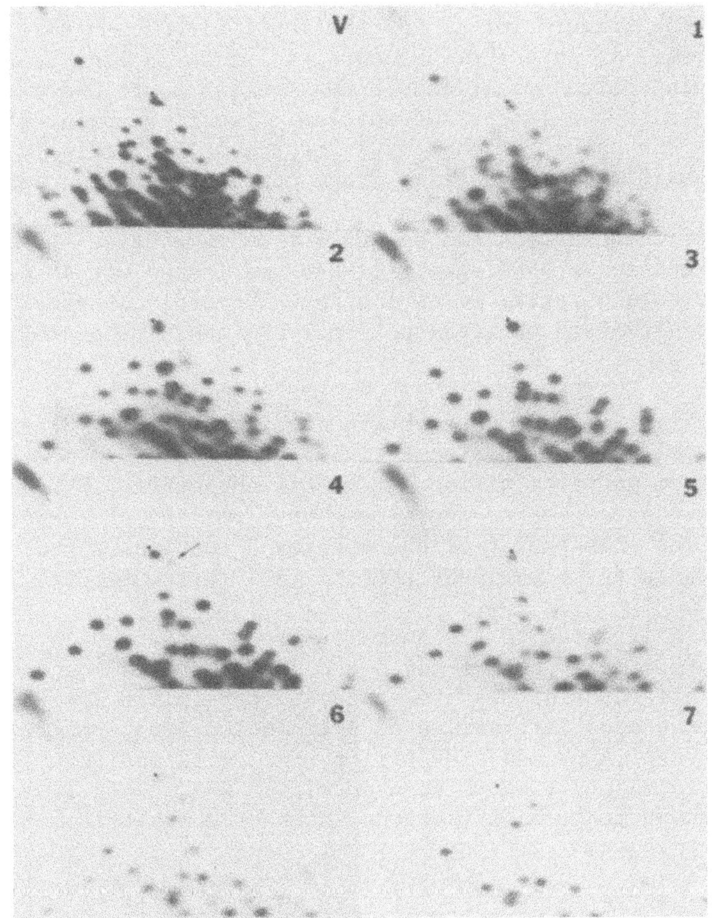

Fig. 3. Oligonucleotide fingerprints of JHMV specific RNA. JHMV virion (panel V) and intracellular RNAs (panels 1-7) were purified and oligonucleotide fingerprints prepared as in Fig. 2. The positions of the xylene cyanol dye marker are shown by asterisks. Unique spots are indicated by arrows.

A comparison of the fingerprints of the seven A59V specific intracellular RNAs with each other and with A59V virion RNA (Fig. 2) reveals several things. The fingerprint of the largest intracellular RNA, species 1, is essentially identical to that of virion RNA. All the oligonucleotides contained in RNA species 2 are present in RNA species 1 and are a subset of these oligonucleotides. Similarly, the fingerprint of RNA species 3 is a subset of the fingerprint of RNA species 2. An examination of the fingerprint of RNA species 4 reveals a new spot which is not present in any of the other A59V specific RNAs (arrow in Fig. 2, panel 4). The remaining oligonucleotides observed in RNA species 4 are a subset of the larger RNA species. The fingerprint of RNA species 5 also contains a spot which is not present in any other RNA species (arrow in Fig. 2, panel 5). The remaining oligonucleotides in RNA species 5 are contained in the fingerprints of the larger RNA species. The fingerprint of RNA species 6 is a subset of that of RNA species 5. Similarly, all the oligonucleotides of RNA species 7 are contained in RNA species 6.

Several conclusions can be drawn from this data. Firstly, the seven intracellular A59V specific RNAs are indeed virus specific and are of the same polarity as virion RNA. Secondly, these RNAs form a nested set with each succeeding larger RNA containing additional sequences.

An analysis of the data obtained with JHMV (Fig. 3) reveals similar results. RNA 1 is essentially identical to genomic RNA isolated from purified virions. The six subgenomic JHMV specific RNAs form a nested set as described above for the A59V specific RNA species. The fingerprint of RNA species 4 contains a spot which is not present in any other JHMV specific RNA (arrow in Fig. 3, panel 4).

The significance of the anomalous spots observed in the fingerprints of A59V RNAs 4 and 5 and JHMV RNA 4 is unknown. If these new oligonucleotides are at the 5' termini of RNAs 4 and 5 they could be truncated derivatives of oligonucleotides present in the fingerprints of A59V and JHMV virion RNA. Alternatively, these new spots are adjacent to spots seen in virion RNA and it is possible that they represent minor modifications, such as methylation, of these oligonucleotides.

In Vitro Translation of Intracellular A59V Specific RNA

The seven subgenomic poly(A)$^+$ RNAs were purified from A59V infected cells by agarose gel electrophoresis as described in Materials and Methods. These RNAs were added to the nuclease treated reticulocyte lysate *in vitro* translation system described by Pelham and Jackson (1976). The products of these translation experiments were analyzed by polyacrylamide gel electrophoresis. The results of one of these experiments are shown in Figure 4. *In vitro* translation of RNA 7 results in the synthesis of two virus specific polypeptides; a minor product which co-electrophoreses with nucleocapsid protein and a major product which migrates slightly faster than the nucleocapsid protein. Analysis of tryptic digests of these two polypeptides and the intracellular nucleocapsid protein by 2-dimensional chromatography and electrophoresis shows that they have identical methionine containing tryptic peptides (Fig. 5). Translation of RNA 6 results in the synthesis of two polypeptides. The larger of these polypeptides comigrates with the major translation product of RNA 7 and has

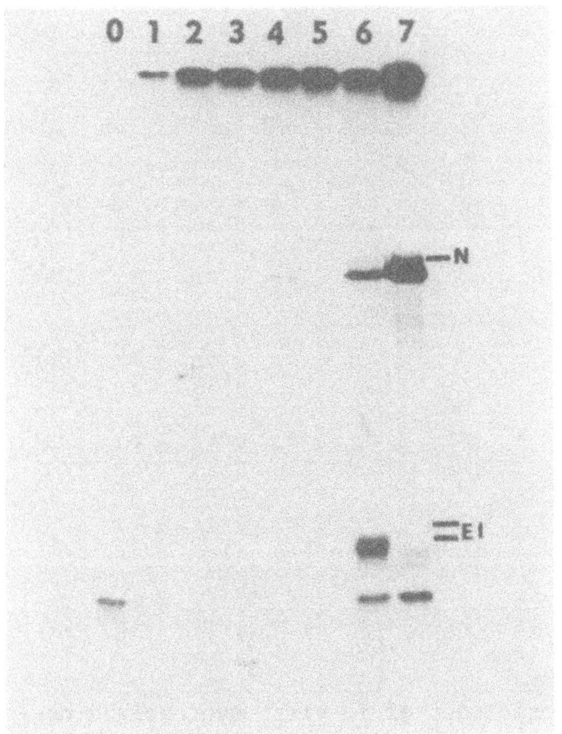

Fig. 4. The translation of A59V specific RNAs. Intracellular RNAs were purified and translated as described in Materials and Methods. The products of the translation were analyzed by polyacrylamide gel electrophoresis on a 10% gel. Lane 0 is the analysis of a translation of a lysate with no added RNA. Lanes 1-7 are the analyses of translations of purified A59V specific RNAs 1-7 respectively. The positions of A59 nucleocapsid (N) and E1 proteins are indicated.

an identical ^{35}S-methionine tryptic peptide map (Fig. 5). The smaller translation product of RNA 6 co-electrophoreses with the lower molecular weight form of the E1 protein. The ^{35}S-methionine tryptic peptide map of this protein and the A59V E1 protein are identical (Fig. 6). Translation of the larger, less abundant RNAs demonstrated one additional product. A longer exposure of the gel shown in Figure 4 demonstrates a minor band with a molecular weight of approximately 35 000 daltons in the translations of RNAs 4, 3 and 2 (date not shown). This material is currently being analyzed further to determine if it corresponds to the previously described non-structural A59V protein of the same molecular weight (Bond et al., 1979).

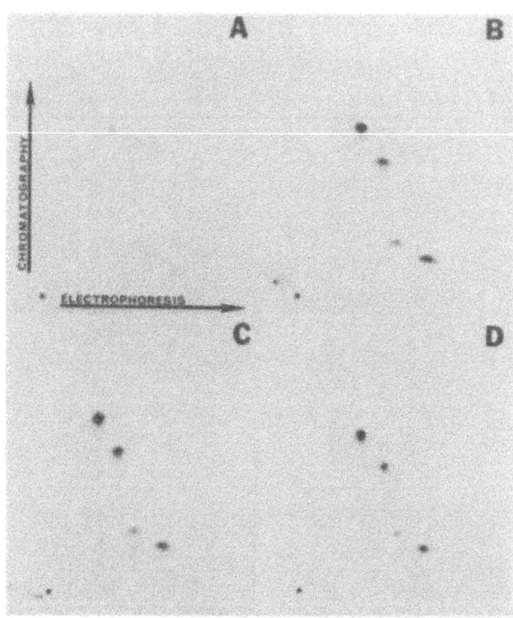

Fig. 5. The tryptic maps of in vitro synthesized nucleocapsid protein. The ^{35}S-methionine labeled in vitro translation products of RNA 7 were purified by polyacrylamide gel electrophoresis, digested with trypsin and analyzed as described by Gibson (1974). The tryptic maps of the major and minor translation products (See text.) are shown in panels B and A, respectively. The translation product of RNA 6 which co-electrophoresed with the major translation product of RNA 7 (see text) was similarly analyzed (panel C), as was ^{35}S-methionine labeled A59V nucleocapsid protein purified from infected cells (panel D). The origins are indicated by asterisks.

Translation of Virion RNA

Following virus purification, intact A59V and JHMV virion RNA was further purified by sedimentation on sucrose gradients. This RNA was translated in the reticulocyte lysate system and the products were analyzed by gel electrophoresis. As shown in Figure 7, the translation of four different preparations of virion RNA resulted in three polypeptides of over 200,000 daltons molecular weight. These polypeptides do not co-electrophorese with any known MHV specific proteins. Experiments to demonstrate these polypeptides in infected cells have been unsuccessful to date. Analysis of these three polypeptides by the limited proteolysis method of Cleveland et al.

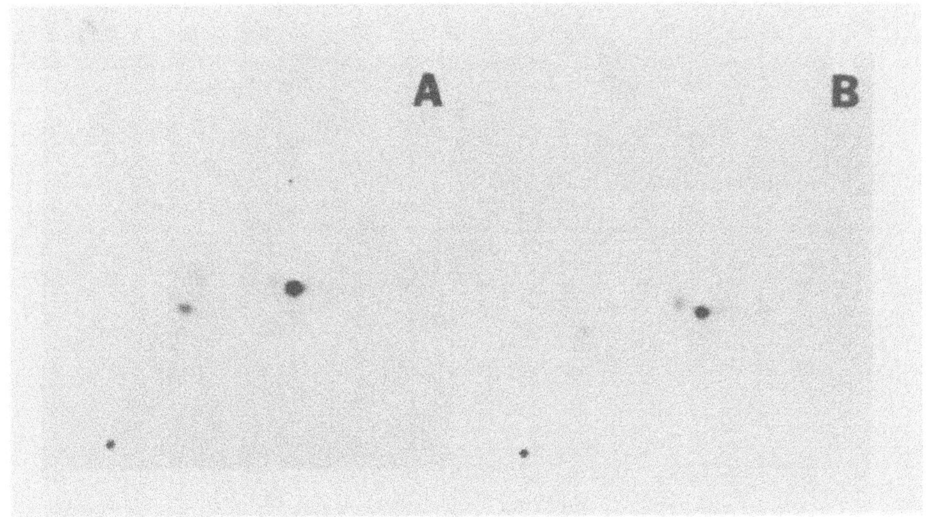

Fig. 6. The tryptic map of in vitro synthesized E1 protein. The translation product of RNA 6 which co-electrophoreses with E1 protein (panel A) and E1 protein prepared from purified A59V (panel B) were analyzed as described in Figure 5.

(1977) shows them to be structurally related to each other (Data not shown.).

DISCUSSION

The data presented above indicate that MHV infected cells synthesize at least seven virus specific RNAs. The largest of these RNAs, RNA 1, is identical to virion RNA as judged by oligonucleotide fingerprinting. The oligonucleotides of the six subgenomic RNAs, RNA 2-6, are contained in the virion RNA. They are therefore of the same polarity as the virion RNA. Oligonucleotide fingerprints of these RNAs show them to make up a nested set in which any RNA contains the sequences present in any other smaller RNA plus additional sequences consistent with its larger size. Similar data have been obtained with another coronavirus, IBV (Stern and Kennedy, 1980). A "Northern blot" analysis using representative and short 3' specific c-DNA probes indicates that the six subgenomic RNA's share sequences at their 3' ends (Weiss and Leibowitz, this symposium). Furthermore, Stern and Kennedy (this symposium) have established a 5' to 3' oligonucleotide spot order for the IBV genome. Their data show that the IBV subgenomic RNAs form a nested set with common 3' ends. Taken together, these data suggest that the MHV specific subgenomic RNAs map from the 3' end of the genome in a similar manner to IBV. A possible model of this arrangement is shown in Figure 8.

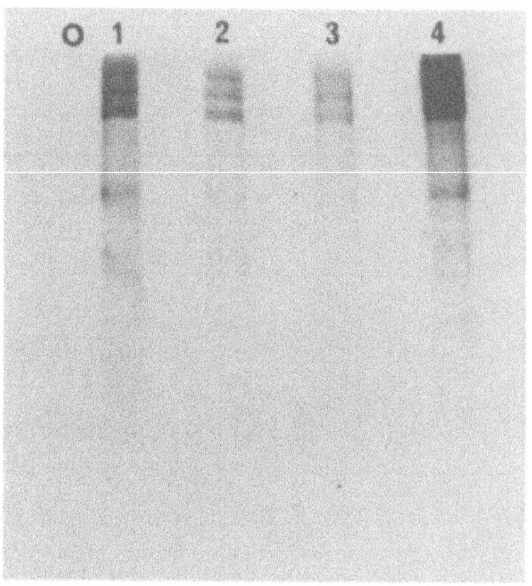

Fig. 7. In vitro translation of virion RNA. Virion RNA was purified and translated in vitro as described in Materials and Methods. The translation products were analyzed by polyacrylamide gel electrophoresis. Lane 0 is the analysis of a translation with no added RNA; lanes 1, 3 and 4, with three different preparations of A59V RNA; lane 2 with JHMV RNA.

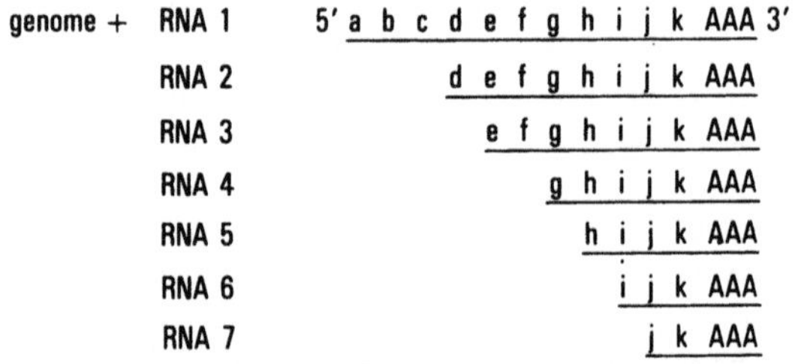

genome +	RNA 1	5' a b c d e f g h i j k AAA 3'
	RNA 2	d e f g h i j k AAA
	RNA 3	e f g h i j k AAA
	RNA 4	g h i j k AAA
	RNA 5	h i j k AAA
	RNA 6	i j k AAA
	RNA 7	j k AAA

Fig. 8. A possible model of the sequence arrangement of MHV specific RNAs.

It is unlikely that any of the six subgenomic RNAs are defective interfering RNAs. The stock virus used in these experiments was 3 passages (A59V) or 4 passages (JHMV) removed from cloning by limiting dilution (Robb and Bond, 1979b). The low M.O.I. used to grow virus stocks (10^{-4} PFU/cell) and to initiate infections in these experiments (0.1 to 0.15 PFU/cell) select against the generation of defective interfering particles. Furthermore, after ten serial undiluted passages of A59V and JHMV in 17CL-1 cells, the RNA gel pattern observed is unchanged from early passage virus (Leibowitz, unpublished data).

At least two, and probably all six, subgenomic RNAs are mRNAs. They are polyadenylated, as expected of mRNAs, and Robb and Bond (1979b) have shown that multiple MHV specific RNA species spanning the size range of the subgenomic RNAs 2-7 are present on polysomes of infected cells. The data presented in this paper demonstrate that RNA 7 codes for the nucleocapsid protein. The small difference in migration of the major in vitro translation product of this RNA and the in vivo nucleocapsid protein could perhaps be due to phosphorylation, as the virion nucleocapsid had been shown to be phosphorylated (Stohlman and Lai, 1979). Translation of RNA 6 results in two products, the E1 protein and the nucleocapsid protein. This result is consistent with the proposed physical arrangement of the genome shown in Figure 8. The E1 protein is encoded in the sequences at the 5' end of RNA 6 (designated j and k) coding for the nucleocapsid. The data we have obtained does not distinguish between the synthesis of the nucleocapsid protein from RNA 6 being due to internal initiation of protein synthesis or degradation of the RNA during the translation resulting in the exposure of an internal initiation site.

Translation of purified virion RNA results in the synthesis of three structurally related polypeptides greater than 200,000 daltons molecular weight. The coding capacity of the 5' end of the genome which is not present in the subgenomic mRNAs (sequences a, b and c in Figure 8) is approximately 270,000 daltons and will accommodate these polypeptides. These polypeptides are likely to function as the intracellular MHV specific RNA polymerase by analogy to other positive stranded RNA viruses. Further work is needed to demonstrate these polypeptides in infected cells or in an in vitro MHV specific RNA polymerase system.

ACKNOWLEDGEMENTS

This work was supported in part by NIH grants NS 07078, NS 13898 and NS 15211 from the National Institute of Neurological and Communicative Disorders and Stroke, and a grant from the National Multiple Sclerosis Society. Dr. Leibowitz is the recipient of Teacher/Investigator Award NS 00418.

REFERENCES

Bailey, J. M., and Davidson, N., 1976, Methylmercury as a reversible denaturing agent for agarose gel electrophoresis, Anal. Biochem., 70:75.

Bond, C. W., Leibowitz, J. L, and Robb, J. A., 1979, Pathogenic murine coronaviruses. II. Characterization of virus-specific proteins of murine coronaviruses JHMV and A59V, Virology, 94:371.

Borun, T. W., Scharff, M. D., and Robbin, E., 1967, Preparation of mammalian polyribosomes with the detergent Nonidat P-40, Biochim. Biophys. Acta, 149:302.

Cleveland, D. W., Fischer, S. G., Kirschner, M. W., and Laemmli, U.K., 1977, Peptide mapping by limited proteolysis in sodium dodecyl sulfate and analysis by gel electrophoresis, J. Biol. Chem., 252:1102.

Gibson, W., 1974, Polyoma virion proteins: a description of the structural proteins of the virion based on polyacrylamide gel electrophoresis and peptide analysis, Virology, 62:319.

Guy, J. S., and Brian, D. A., 1979, Bovine coronavirus genome, J. Virol., 29:293.

Laemmli, U. K., 1970, Cleavage of structural proteins during the assembly of the head of bacteriophage T4, Nature, 227:680.

Lai, M. M. C., and Stohlman, S. A., 1978, RNA of mouse hepatitis virus, J. Virol., 26:236.

Laskey, R. A., and Mills, A. D., 1977, Enhanced autoradiographic detection of ^{32}P and ^{125}I using intensifying screens and hypersensitized film. FEBS Letters, 82:314.

Lee, Y. F., Kitamura, N., Nomoto, A., and Wimmer. E., 1979, Sequence studies of poliovirus type 1, type 2, and two type 1 defective interfering particles RNAs1 and fingerprint of the poliovirus type 3 genome, J. Gen. Virol., 44:311.

Lomniczi, B., and Kennedy, I., 1977, Genome of infectious bronchitis virus, J. Virol., 24:99.

Macnaughton, M. R., and Madge, M. H., 1978, The genome of human coronavirus strain 229E, J. Gen. Virol., 39:497.

McMaster, G. K., and Carmichael, G. C., 1977, Analysis of single- and double-stranded nucleic acids on polyacrylamide and agarose gels by using glyoxal and acridine orange, Proc. Natl. Acad. Sci. U.S.A., 75:4835.

Pelham, H. R. B., and Jackson, R. J., 1976, An efficient mRNA-dependent translation system from reticulocyte lysates. Eur. J. Biochem., 67:247.

Robb, J. A., and Bond, C. W., 1979a, Coronaviridae, in: "Comprehensive Virology," vol. 14, H. Fraenkel-Conrat and R. R. Wagner, eds., Plenum Publishing Corp., New York.

Robb, J. A., and Bond, C. W., 1979b, Pathogenic murine coronaviruses. I. Characterization of biological behavior in vitro and virus specific intracellular RNA of strongly neutotropic JHMV and weakly neurotropic A59V viruses, Virology, 94:352.

Siddell, S. G., Wege, H., Barthel, A., and terMeulen, V., 1980, Coronavirus JHM:Cell-free synthesis of structural protein p60, J. Virol., 33:10.

Stern, D. F., and Kennedy, S. I. T., 1980, Coronavirus multiplication strategy. I. Identification and characterization of virus-specified RNA, J. Virol., 34:665.
Stohlman, S. A., and Lai, M. M. C., 1979, Phosphoproteins of murine hepatitis viruses, Virology, 32:672.
Sturman, L. S., and Takemoto, K. K., 1972, Enhanced growth of a murine coronavirus in transformed mouse cells. Infection & Immunity, 6:501.
Wege, H., Müller, A., and terMeulen, V., 1978, Genomic RNA of the murine coronavirus JHM, J. Gen. Virol., 41:217.
Wilt, F. H., 1977, The dynamics of maternal poly(A)-containing mRNA in fertilized sea urchin eggs, Cell, 11:673.
Yogo, Y., Hirano, N., Hino, S., Shibuta, H., and Matumoto, M., 1977, Polyadenylate in the virion RNA of mouse hepatitis virus, J. Biochem., 82:1103.

COMPARISON OF THE RNAs OF MURINE AND HUMAN CORONAVIRUSES

Susan R. Weiss[1] and Julian L. Leibowitz[2]

[1]Department of Microbiology
University of California
San Francisco, CA
(present address: Department of Microbiology
University of Pennsylvania Medical School
Philadelphia, PA 19104)
[2]Department of Pathology
University of California, San Diego
Medical School
La Jolla, CA 92093

INTRODUCTION

Coronaviruses cause acute and/or persistent disease in many species of animals. One factor that determines target organ and lethality of coronavirus infection is the strain of virus (McIntosh, 1972; Robb et al., 1980). For example most strains of mouse hepatitis virus (MHV), such as A59 and MHV3, were isolated from the livers of infected mice and are primarily hepatotropic (McIntosh, 1974). In contrast the JHM strain of MHV is primarily neurotropic (McIntosh 1974: Bailey et al., 1949). Most MHV strains are closely related serologically (McIntosh, 1974).

Human coronaviruses (HCV), such as the 229E strain, are primarily respiratory viruses (Hamre and Procknow, 1966; McIntosh, 1974). Recently, however, there has been a report of the recovery of putative human coronaviruses from the brain tissue of two multiple sclerosis patients (Burks et al., 1980). At least some human coronavirus strains cross react immunologically with neurotropic murine and porcine coronaviruses (McIntosh, 1974).

Biochemical studies to date have shown that various murine and human coronavirus strains, although biologically distinct, have similar size genome RNAs and structural proteins (Bond et al, 1979;

Robb and Bond, 1979, Hierholzer, 1976, McNaughton and Madge, (1978). We have used molecular hybridization, oligonucleotide fingerprinting, and agarose gel electrophoresis to further compare the genome and intracellular RNAs of MHV strains A59, MHV3 and JHM and HCV strain 229E.

MATERIALS AND METHODS

Cells and Viruses

MHV strains A59 (Sturman and Takemoto, 1972), MHV3 (Dick et al 1956) and JHM (Bailey et al., 1949) were grown in DBT or 17CL-1 mouse cell lines (Sturman and Takemoto, 1972). Human coronavirus strain 229E (Hamre and Procknow, 1966) was grown in human embryonic lung cell line, L-132 (Davis and Bolin, 1960). All viruses were plaque purified twice and stocks grown at a multiplicity of infection (m.o.i.) of approximately 10^{-4} plaque units (pfu) per cell.

RNA Preparation

Preparation of genome RNA. Cells were infected at m.o.i. of 0.1 to 1 to pfu/cell and in some experiments were labeled with ^{32}P-inorganic phosphate or ^{3}H-uridine. MHV was grown at 37°C and harvested at 18-20 hours post infection. 229E was grown at 32°C and harvested at 40 hours post infection. In most experiments, virus was purified from the medium as previously described (Kennedy and Johnson-Lussenberg, 1975-76; Robb et al 1979). RNA was extracted from virions by proteinase K treatment in the presence of 1%SDS, followed by phenol extraction (Weiss et al., 1977) and further purified by sedimentation on a sucrose gradient. Genome RNA sedimented as a uniform peak at about 57S. In some experiments RNA for hybridization was extracted from virus pelleted from the medium, and used without further purification.

Preparation of intracellular RNA. Infected cells were labeled with ^{3}H-uridine in the presence of Actinomycin D (Act D) from 4-9 hours post infection for MHV or 16-24 hours post infection for 229E. Cells were lysed by pipeting in the presence of 1% NP40 in RSB (0.01MTris, pH7.4;0.01M NaCl; 0.005M $MgCl_2$), the nuclei pelleted and RNA extracted from the cytoplasm as described above for virion RNA. In most experiments poly(A)-containing RNA was selected by chromatography on oligo (dT)-cellulose columns (Aviv and Leder, 1972).

RNA Analysis

Oligonucleotide fingerprinting. High specific activity ^{32}P-labeled purified genome RNA was digested with T1 ribonuclease and the resulting olignoculeotides analyzed by two dimensional polyacrylamide gel electrophoresis as previously described (Stern and Kennedy, 1980; Lee et al 1979).

Agarose gel electrophoresis. ^{3}H-uridine labeled RNA was subjected to electrophoresis in 1% agarose gels containing methyl mercury hydroxide as denaturant (Bailey and Davidson, 1976) and gels were flourographed (Chamberlain 1979). Unlabeled RNA was electrophoresed in these gels and then used in RNA blots as described below.

Probe Synthesis

Preparation and characterization of cDNA rep. Purified A59 genome RNA was used as a template to synthesize high specific activity ^{32}P- or ^{3}H-labeled cDNA using avian myeloblastosis virus polymerase and oligomers of calf thymus DNA as primer. Since the calf thymus DNA hybridizes and primes DNA synthesis at random places along the genome RNA, this DNA should be equally representative of the entire genome and thus is designated $cDNA_{rep}$ (Taylor et al., 1976). For liquid hybridization experiments where a single stranded cDNA probe is desirable, $cDNA_{rep}$ was chromatographed on an hydroxylapatite column to remove double stranded DNA (Leong et al., 1972). $cDNA_{rep}$ synthesized by this technique is both specific for viral nucleotide sequences and equally representative of the majority of the genome (see Results section).

Preparation of $cDNA_{3'}$. High specific activity ^{32}P-labeled cDNA was synthesized as above only using oligo$(dT)_{12-18}$ as primer (Tal et al 1977). The oligo(dT) hybridizes to poly(A) at the 3' end of the genome RNA and thus primes DNA synthesis only at the 3' end of the gemome. This cDNA was hybridized to poly(A) and subsequently passed through an oligo(dT) cellulose column to eliminate DNA not covalently linked to oligo(dT). Since this cDNA was not greater than 1000 nucleotides in length (data not shown) it should represent not more than 5% of the 3' end of the genome and thus is designated $cDNA_{3'}$.

Molecular Hybridization

Hybridization in solution was carried out at 68°C in 0.6M NaCl and analyzed by S1 nuclease digestion (Leong et al., 1972).

RNA Blots. RNA was electrophoresed in agarose gels as above, blotted to diazobenzyloxymethyl (DBM) cellulose, and then hybridized with ^{32}P-labeled cDNA and autoradiographed (Alwine et al, 1977).

RESULTS

Homology among the Genomes of A59, MHV3, JHM and 229E

Molecular hybridization. All three MHV strains and 229E contain plus stranded, polyadenylated RNA genomes of about 6 x 10^6 daltons (MacNaughton, 1978). We have used molecular hybridization as a measure of nucleotide sequence homologies among these genomes. For this purpose we synthesized a virus-specific complementary DNA (cDNA) probe, $cDNA_{rep}$, containing sequences homologous to most or all of the A59 genome (see Materials and Methods for details in preparation). To validate the specificity of $cDNA_{rep}$ we measured the rates of hybridization of ^{32}P-labeled $cDNA_{rep}$ with cytoplasmic RNA extracted from A59-infected and uninfected cells (Fig.1). In this Crt analysis (Leong et al., 1972) $cDNA_{rep}$ did not hybridize with uninfected cell RNA even at very high Crt values where hybridization went to completion with infected cell RNA. Thus $cDNA_{rep}$ is sufficiently free of host sequences to serve as probe for virus-specific RNA. Furthermore, $cDNA_{rep}$ contains sequences equally representative of at least 65% of the A59 genome (data not shown).

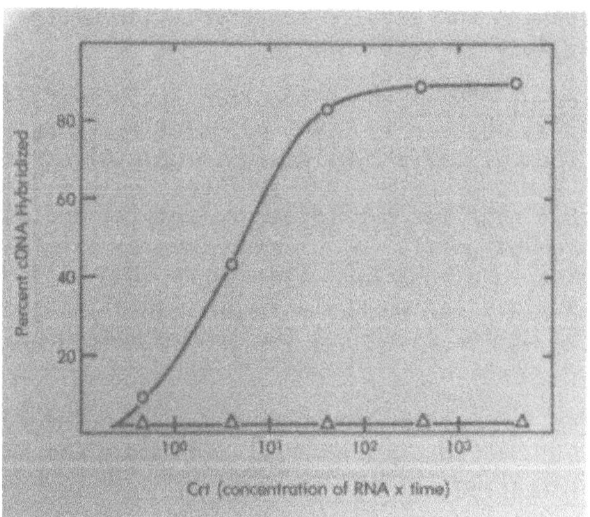

Figure 1. Kinetics of hybridization of $cDNA_{rep}$ with cytoplasmic RNA from A59-infected and uninfected cells. Various amounts (80μg to 8 ng) of RNA were hybridized with 4000 cpm (0.5 ng) of ^{32}P-labeled $cDNA_{rep}$ to the indicated Crt values. Hybridization was assayed by digestion with S1 nuclease. (0) infected cell RNA (Δ) uninfected cell RNA.

The A59 $cDNA_{rep}$ was hybridized to completion with RNA in vast excess, to genome RNA and intracellular RNAs of all four viruses. These hybridizations were done in solution, under stringent conditions and assayed by S1 nuclease digestion (see Materials and Methods for details). The results are summarized in Table 1. All three MHV genomes contain extensive sequence homology. The A59 and MHV3 genomes contain more homology than the A59 and JHM genomes. We could detect no sequence homology between A59 $cDNA_{rep}$ and the 229E genome under these hybridization conditions. Under the less stringent hybridization conditions used for RNA blotting there is some cross reactivity between 229E RNA and A59 $cDNA_{rep}$ (see below).

Oligonucleotide fingerprints. Genome RNAs were also compared by oligonucleotide fingerprinting analysis. Figure 2 shows the results of two dimensional gel electrophoresis of T1 ribonuclease digests of ^{32}P-labeled genome RNAs. The oligonucleotides that are large enough to be significant in the comparison of the RNAs are found in the top third of the fingerprints. In agreement with the hybridization results, oligonucleotide fingerprinting suggests that all three MHV genomes are related. The most closely related are the A59 and MHV3 genomes having most of the significant oligonucleotides in common. The JHM and MHV3 genomes are the next most closely related pair and the JHM and A59 genomes are more distantly related. By this technique, the 229E genome shows little if any homology with the MHV genomes.

Comparison of Murine and Human Coronavirus Intracellular RNAs

Agarose gel electrophoresis. Murine and avian coronaviruses generate multiple subgenomic polyadenylated intracellular putative mRNAs of the same polarity as genome RNA (Stern and Kennedy, 1980; Leibowitz et al, manuscript in preparation). We have found that human coronavirus 229E generates a similar set of intracellular subgenomic RNAs. RNA was extracted from the cytoplasm of coronavirus infected cells that had been labeled with ^{3}H-uridine for several hours, late in infection, in the presence of Act D to inhibit host cell RNA synthesis. Poly(A)- containing RNA was selected and electrophoresed in agarose gels as shown in Figure 3. Lane a shows the position of purified A59 genome RNA on these gels. Each MHV strain generates six subgenomic RNAs ranging in molecular weight from 0.62 to 3.6 x 10^{6} daltons (Figure 3, Table 2). This is in basic agreement with Leibowitz et al., (manuscript in preparation) and the RNAs have been numbered as in that paper. For all three strains, the RNAs are of the same sizes and present in approximately equal relative proportions with the possible exception that in the case of JHM, RNAs 4 and 5 may be less abundant relative to the other RNAs. The extra band between RNAs 2 and 3 observed in MHV3 RNA, as well as other extra bands are occasionally observed. We do not know the significance of these bands. Lanes f and g show a

Table 1. Homology Among the A59, MHV3, JHM, and 229E Coronavirus Genomes

Source of RNA	Percent Hybridization of A59 $cDNA_{rep}$ [a]
A59	100
MHV3	87
JHM	74
229E	0

a. A59 $cDNA_{rep}$ was hybridized to completion with a vast excess of RNA from virions or infected cells. These values are averages of 2-3 experiments and have been normalized to 100% hybridization of A59 $cDNA_{rep}$ with its homologous A59 RNA. The actual values for hybridization of A59 $cDNA_{rep}$ with A59 RNA ranged from 85-100%.

comparison of the human and murine coronavirus subgenomic RNAs. Again in the case of 229E, there are six size classes of RNAs (numbered in analogy to the MHV RNAs) but each is of lower molecular weight than its MHV counterpart (Figure 3, Table 2). There is little genome sized RNA detected in the infected cell with any of these viruses.

RNA Blots

Blotting with $cDNA_{rep}$. We also used molecular hybridization to study coronavirus intracellular RNAs. Hybridization with cDNA probes is a very sensitive technique that may be used to detect small amounts of virus-specific intracellular RNA in the presence of a vast excess of cellular RNA, without the use of Act D. This technique of "RNA blotting" is illustrated in Figures 4 and 5. RNA extracted from A59-infected DBT cells late in infection, RNA extracted from uninfected DBT cells, and A59 virion RNA were electrophoresed in an agarose gel, blotted onto DBM paper and hybridized with $cDNA_{rep}$ (Alwine et al., 1977). As shown in Figures 4 and 5, there is no hybridization detected with RNA from uninfected cells. As expected virion RNA contains one major species of about 6×10^6 daltons. All six subgenomic RNAs are detected in RNA from infected

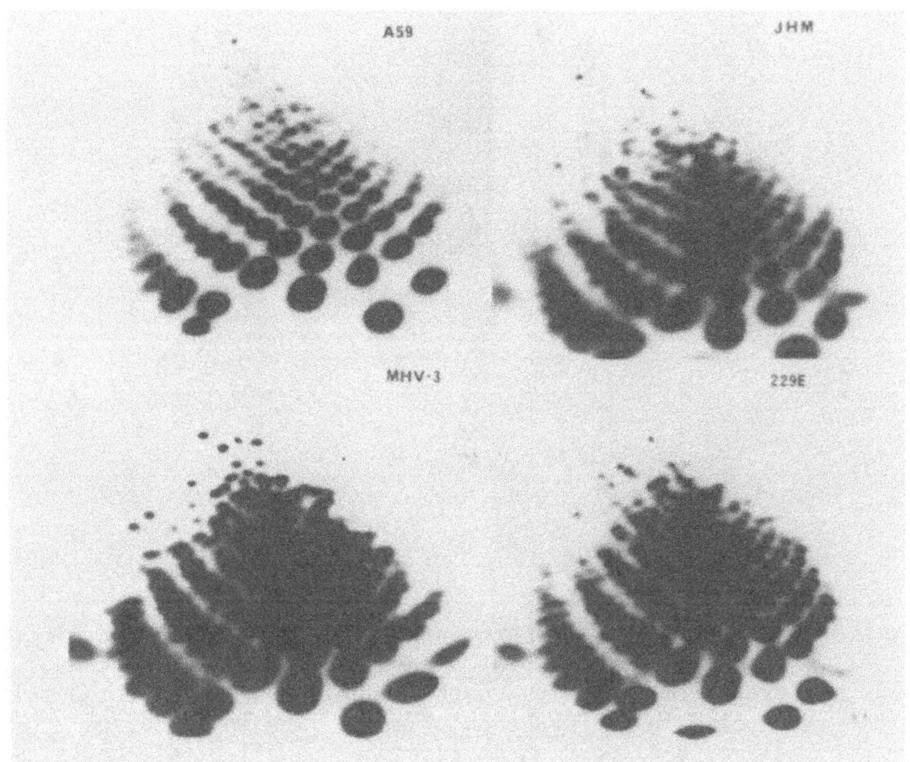

Figure 2. Olignoculeotide fingerprints of coronavirus genomes. High specific activity ^{32}P-labeled purified coronavirus genome RNAs were incubated with T1 ribonuclease and analyzed by two dimensional polyacrylamide gel electrophoresis. The asterisk shows the positon of the xylene cyanol blue dye marker.

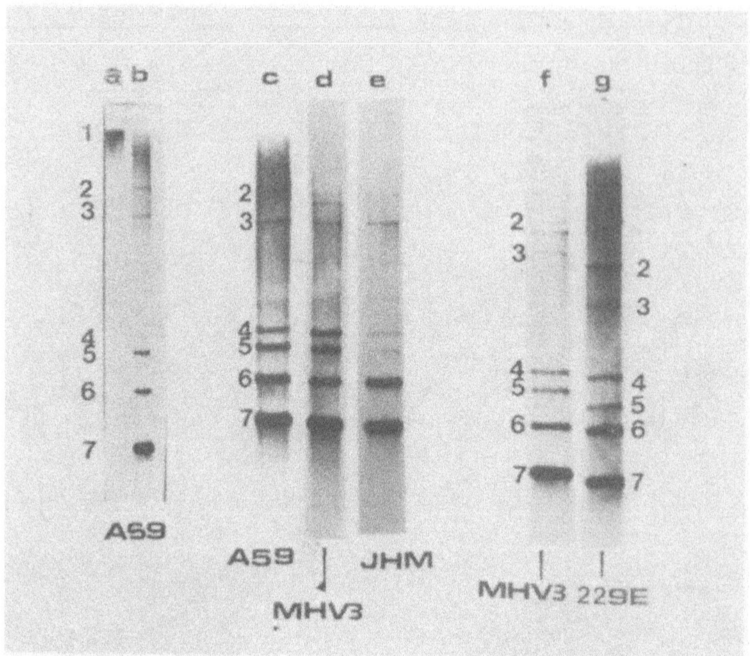

Figure 3. Agarose gel electrophoresis of ^{3}H-uridine labeled virus-specific intracellular RNA. ^{3}H-uridine labeled RNAs, extracted from virus particles (lane a) or infected cells labeled in the presence of Act D late in infection (lanes b-g) were chromotographed on oligo (dT)-cellulose columns and electrophoresed in 1% agarose gels containing 10 mM methyl mercury hydroxide.

lane a. A59 genome RNA
b. A59-infected cell cytoplasmic RNA
c. A59-infected cell cytoplasmic RNA
d. MHV3-infected cell cytoplasmic RNA
e. JHM-infected cell cytoplasmic RNA
f. MHV3-infected cell cytoplasmic RNA
g. 229E-infected cell cytoplasmic RNA

Table 2. Molecular Weights of Coronavirus Subgenomic RNAs

RNA	Molecular Weight (X 10^{-6} Daltons)[a]	
	Murine	Human
1 (GENOME)	6.0	(6.0)[b]
2	3.6	2.8
3	3.0	2.1
4	1.3	1.25
5	1.2	1.0
6	0.90	0.84
7	0.62	0.60

a. The murine coronavirus RNAs were coelectrophoresed with murine ribosomal 45S, 32S, 28S and 18S RNA standards. A plot of logarithm of the molecular weights of these RNAs vs. distance migrated formed a straight line. The sizes of the viral RNAs were determined from this calibration curve. The size of the human RNAs were determined by coelectrophoresis with the murine coronavirus RNAs.

b. We did not analyze the 229E genome by gel electrophoresis. However, MacNaughton (1978), by gel electrophoresis, and we, by sucrose velocity sedimentation, have found the 229E and MHV genomes to be the same size.

cells, although RNAs 2 and 3 are difficult to see over background. The same pattern is obtained with RNA that was synthesized in the presence or absence of Act D (Figure 5A). All six RNAs are detected with A59 $cDNA_{rep}$ when either MHV3 or JHM intracellular RNAs are analyzed (data not shown). As with directly labeled RNA, there is little if any genome sized RNA detected in the infected cell.

Preliminary blotting experiments suggest that A59 $cDNA_{rep}$ can be used to detect 229E intracellular RNA in a blot, but only when RNA is present at a level ten fold higher than that needed to detect MHV RNA. Hybridization conditions used in a blot (41°C, 50% formamide) are less stringent than those for solution hybridization (as described above) and thus would be expected to allow the detection of more poorly matched hybrids, not detected by solution hybridization (see Discussion).

The 3' ends of virus-specific intracellular RNAs. cDNA probes, specific for certain regions of the viral genome can be used to analyze the genetic content of virus-specific intracellular RNAs. The subgenomic RNAs of an avian coronavirus, infectious bronchitis

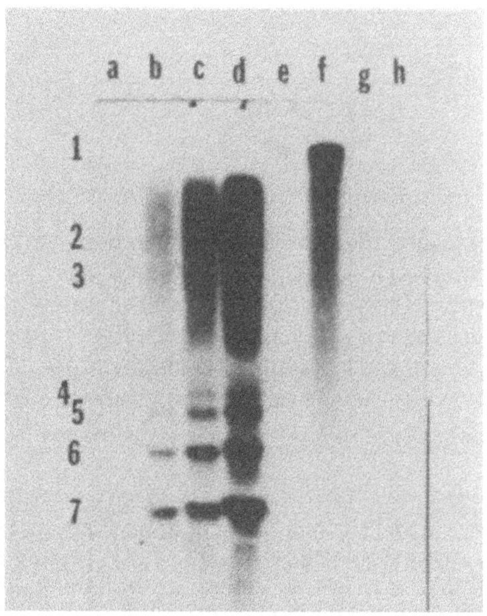

Figure 4. Hybridization of virus-specific RNA in gels. Unlabeled RNAs were electrophoresed as in Figure 3, transferred to DBM paper and hybridized with approximately 2 x 10^6 cpm of ^{32}P-labeled $cDNA_{rep}$.

lane a. 2μg A59-infected cell cytoplasmic RNA
b. 6μg A59-infected cell cytoplasmic RNA
c. 20μg A59-infected cell cytoplasmic RNA
d. 60μg A59-infected cell cytoplasmic RNA
e. 2ng A59 genome RNA
f. 20ng A59 genome RNA
g. 6μg uninfected cell cytoplasmic RNA
h. 60 μg uninfected cell cytoplasmic RNA

virus (IBV) and MHV strains A59 and JHM form nested sets. That is, all the RNAs overlap in sequence so that each RNA contains all the sequences of the next smaller one and in addition extra sequences

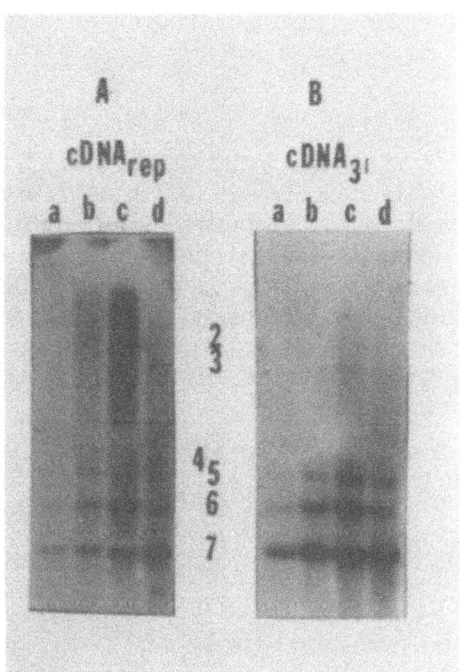

Figure 5. Hybridization of infected cell RNAs with $cDNA_{rep}$ and $cDNA_{3'}$. RNAs were electrophoresed in agarose gels, transferred to DBM paper and hybridized with $cDNA_{rep}$ (panel A). The probe was removed and the blot hybridized with $cDNA_{3'}$ (Panel B).

lane a. 2μg A59-infected cell cytoplasmic RNA
b. 6μg A59-infected cell cytoplasmic RNA
c. 20μg A59-infected cell cytoplasmic RNA
d. 6μg A59-infected cell cytoplasmic RNA, synthesized in the presence of Act D.

(Stern and Kennedy, 1980; Leibowitz et al., manuscript in preparation). In the case of IBV, all subgenomic RNAs contain sequences homologous to the 3' end of genome RNA and extend various distances toward the 5' end (Stern and Kennedy, personal communication). To test this for MHV, we synthesized $cDNA_{3'}$, a probe complementary to the 3' end of A59 genome RNA (see Materials and Methods for details). This probe was hybridized to MHV intracellular RNA in a blot (Figure 5). As with $cDNA_{rep}$, RNAs 2-6 are detected with $cDNA_{3'}$, suggesting that all RNAs contain sequences homologous to the 3' end of genome RNA. The larger RNAs (2 and 3) are more difficult to detect with $cDNA_{3'}$ than with $cDNA_{rep}$. This is probably because, as suggested by the direct labeling experiment above (Figure 3), RNAs 2 and 3 are less abundant than RNAs 4-7 and hybridization with $cDNA_{3'}$ should be a measure of the number of RNA molecules in each band rather than the total amount of RNA in each band.

DISCUSSION

The A59 and MHV3 strains of MHV are primarily hepatropic while the JHM strain is highly neurotropic (McIntosh 1974). We have shown here by oligonucleotide fingerprinting and by molecular hybridization that JHM has diverged from the other two strains in its nucleotide sequence as well as in its biology. The oligonucleotide fingerprints revealed less homology among the three MHV strains than the hybridization experiments. This would be expected because the former technique is more likely to reflect small change, even one base, in RNA sequence.

All three strains of MHV generate six subgenomic intracellular putative mRNAs. It is unlikely that any of these are defective viral genomes as all virus was plaque purified and stocks were grown at low m.o.i. There are no obvious strain dependent differences in the subgenomic RNAs that could reflect the different tropism of JHM.

We have found no homology between A59 $cDNA_{rep}$ and 229E RNA when measured by a stringent solution hybridization assay. However, when hybridization criteria are lowered as in an RNA blot, a low level of homology is detected. Thus human and murine coronaviruses are probably related, but quite diverged from each other. Recently a similar phenomenon has been observed for murine and simian papova virus genomes (Hawley et al, 1980). Homology among these genomes may be demonstrated only under relaxed hybridization conditions.

229E is an unusual strain of HCV in that it is tissue culture adapted and does not grow in mouse brains. Most other strains of HCV, exemplified by OC43, do not grow in tissue culture and must be propagated in human tracheal organ culture or in suckling mouse brains (McIntosh, 1974). The putative human coronaviruses isolated from multiple sclerosis brain tissue are more closely related to

OC43 than 229E (Burks et al 1980). We plan to analyze OC43 RNA for possible sequence homology with MHV and 229E.

Both avian and murine coronavirus putative mRNAs have been shown to overlap in sequence and to contain the same 3' sequences (Stern and Kennedy, 1980, personal communication; Liebowitz et al. manuscript in preparation). This is the case for several other classes of animal viruses (Cancedda et al 1975; Oppermann et al 1977; Deininger et al., 1979). In most cases each subgenomic RNA serves as mRNA for the its 5' gene. We and others (Leibowitz and Weiss, this volume; Sidell et al., 1980) have started to analyze the mRNA capacities of the MHV intracellular RNAs. In cell-free translation experiments RNAs 6 and 7 have been shown to code for the 25,000 dalton virion glycoprotein and nucleocapsid structural proteins respectively.

We have synthesized and characterized MHV-specific cDNA probes. The use of high specific activity labeled probes either in solution hybridization or in RNA blots is sensitive enough to detect < 1 copy/cell of virus-specific genome RNA (Parker and Stark, 1979; Spector et al., 1978). These probes will be especially useful in the analysis of virus-specific RNA in situations where viral RNA may be present in very small quantities such as during persistent infection in cultured cells or in animals. Furthermore, cDNAs representing specific portions of ghe genome will be useful in analyzing the genetic content of virus-specific RNAs.

Acknowledgements. Susan R. Weiss would like to thank Dr. J. Michael Bishop, in whose lab some of this work was carried out.

REFERENCES

Alwine, J.C., Kemp, D.J. and Stark, G.R. 1977, Method for detection of specific RNAs in agarose gels by transfer to diazobenzyloxymethyl paper and hybridization with DNA probes. Proc. Nat. Acad. Sci 74: 5350-5354.

Aviv, H. and Leder, P. 1972, Purification of biologically active globin messenger RNA by chromatography on oligothymidylic acid cellulose. Proc. Nat. Acad. Sci. 69: 1408-1412.

Bailey, O.T., Pappenheimer, A.M., Sergent, F., Cheever, M.D., and Daniels, J.B. 1949, A murine virus (JHM) causing disseminated encephalomyelitis with extensive destruction of myelin. J. Expt. Med. 90: 195-212.

Bailey, J. and Davidson, N. 1976, Methyl mercury as a reversible denaturing agent for agarose-gel electrophoresis. Analyt. Biochem. 70: 75-85.

Bond, C.W., Leibowitz, J.L., and Robb, J.A. 1979, Pathogenic murine coronaviruses, II. Characterization of virus-specific proteins

of murine coronavirus. Virology 94: 371-384
Burks, J., DeVald, B.L., Jankovsky, L.D. Gerdes, J.C. 1980, Two coronaviruses isolated from central nervous system tissue of two multiple sclerosis patients. Science 209: 933-934.
Cancedda, R., Villa-Kamaroff, L., Lodish, H.F., and Schlesinger, M. 1974, Initiation sites for translation of sindbis virus 42S and 26S messenger RNAs. Cell 6: 215-222
Chamberlain, J.P. 1979, Fluorographic detection of radioactivity in polyacrylamide gels with the water soluble fluor, sodium salicylate. Analyt. Biochem. 48: 132-135.
Deininger, P., Esty, A., LaPorte, P., and Friedman, T. 1979, Nucleotide sequence and genetic organization of the polyoma late region: features common to the polyoma early region and SV40. Cell 18: 771-779.
Dick, G.W.A., Niven, J.S.F., Gledhill, A.W. 1956, A virus related to that causing hepatitis in mice (MHV). Brit. J. Expt. Path. 37: 90.
Hamre, D. and Procknow, J.J. 1966, A new virus isolated from the human respiratory track. Proc. Soc. Expt. Biol. Med. 121: 190-193.
Hierholzer, J.C. 1976, Purification and biophysical properties of of human coronavirus 229E. Virology 75: 155-165.
Howley, P.M., Israel, M.A., Law, M.F., Martin, M.A. 1980, Proc. Nat. Acad. Sci. 254: 4876-4883.
Kennedy, D.A. and Johnson-Lussenberg, C.M. 1975-1976. Isolation and morphology of the internal component of human coronavirus; 229E. Intervirology 6: 197-206.
Lee, Y.F., Kitamura, N., Nomato, A. and Wimmer, E. 1979, Sequence studies of poliovirus type 1, type 2, and two type 1 defective interfering particles RNAs. J. Gen. Virol. 44: 311-322.
Leong, J.A., Garapin, A.C., Jackson, N., Fanshier, L., Levinson, W., and Bishop, J.M. 1972, Virus-specific ribonucleic acid in cells. producing Rous sarcoma virus: Detection and characterization. J. Virol. 9: 891-902.
McNaughton, M.R, 1978, The genomes of three coronaviruses. FEBS Letters 94: 191: 194.
McNaughton, M.R. and Madge, M.H. 1978, The genome of human coronavirus 229E. J. Gen. Virol. 39: 497-504.
McIntosh, K. 1974, Coronaviruses: A comparative review. Current Topics in Microbiology and Immunology. 63: 85-129
Opperman, H., Bishop, J.M., Varmus, H.E. and Levintow, L. 1977, A joint product of the genes gag and pol of avian sarcoma virus: a possible precursor of reverse transcriptase. Cell 12: 993-1005.
Parker, B. and Stark, G. 1979. Regulation of simian virus 40 transcription: Sensitive analysis of the RNA species present early in infection by virus or viral DNA. J. Virol. 31: 360-369.
Robb, J.A. and Bond, C.W. 1980. Coronaviridae. Comprehensive Virology 14: 193-245.

Robb, J.A., Bond, C.W. and Leibowitz, J.L. 1979, Pathogenic murine coronaviruses. I. Characterization of biological behavior in vitro and virus specific intracellular RNA of strongly neurotropic JHMV and weakly neurotropic A59V viruses. Virology 94: 385-399,

Siddell, S.G., Wege, H., Barthel, A. and ter Meulen V. 1980. Cell-free synthesis of structural protein pp60.

Spector, D.H., Smith, K., Padgett, T., McCombe, P., Roulland-Dussoix, D., Moscovici, C., Varmus, H.E., and Bishop, J.M. 1978. Uninfected cells contain RNA related to the transforming gene of avion sarcoma viruses. Cell 13: 371-379.

Stern, D. and Kennedy, S.I.T. 1980, The coronavirus multiplication strategy. I. Identification and characterization of virus specific RNA. J. Virol. 34: 665-674.

Sturman, L.S. and Takemoto, K.K. 1972, Enhanced growth of a murine coronavirus in transformed mouse cells. Infection and Immunity 6: 501-507.

Tal, J., Kung, H.J., Varmus, H.E. and Bishop, JM 1977. Characterization of DNA complementary to nucleotide sequences adjacent to poly(A) at the 3' terminus of the avian sarcoma virus genome. Virology 78: 183-197.

Taylor, J.M., Illmensee, R., and Sommers, S. 1976, Efficient transcription of RNA into DNA by avian sarcoma virus polymerase. Biochim. Biophys. Acta. 442: 324-330.

Weiss, S.R., Varmus, H.E. and Bishop, J.M. 1977, The size and genetic composition of virus-specific RNAs in the cytoplasm of cells producing avian sarcoma-leukosis viruses. Cell 12: 983-992.

BIOCHEMISTRY OF CORONAVIRUSES 1980

Brian W.J. Mahy

Division of Virology, Department of Pathology,

University of Cambridge, England

INTRODUCTION

The coronavirus is something of a wolf in sheep's clothing. Originally identified as a large pleomorphic enveloped RNA virus with unique external morphological features and a helical internal nucleocapsid (Tyrrell et al., 1975), the close parallels with negative strand RNA viruses prompted many investigators to search for a coronavirion transcriptase. It soon became clear however, that, despite their morphological appearance, the coronaviruses possess an infectious genome RNA which must, by definition, be of positive polarity.

Considerable advances in our knowledge of coronavirus biochemistry have been made during the past two years, most of which are described in this volume, but still there are enormous gaps, particularly in understanding the mechanism by which these viruses multiply in the infected host cells.

THE GENOME

Several laboratories have determined the size of coronavirus genome RNA by gel electrophoresis in comparison with marker RNAs of known size. Table 1 summarises some of the values reported in this volume, and indicates an average genome molecular weight for a variety of different coronaviruses of 6 to 7 x 10^6. Thus coronavirus genome RNA is larger than that of any other known single-stranded RNA virus, and might be expected to code for as many as twelve average sized (50K) polypeptides.

A major question regarding coronavirus RNA is whether or not it consists of non-covalently bound subunits. Despite reports that the RNA of porcine (Garwes et al., 1975) or human (Hierholzer et al., this volume) coronaviruses dissociates on heating or in the presence of chaotropic agents, the weight of evidence suggests that this is a technical artifact. There is clear published data that avian (Lomniczi and Kennedy, 1977; Schochetman et al., 1977), murine (Lai and Stohlman, 1978; Wege et al., 1978) as well as porcine (Brian et al., 1980) and human (MacNaughton and Madge, 1978) RNAs do not dissociate into a subunit form as does oncornavirus RNA. Furthermore, complexity measurements of the avian coronavirus genome indicate that it is haploid (Lomniczi and Kennedy, 1977).

The presence of poly (A) within the genome RNA has been reported by several laboratories, though curiously most found that only 30 % of the genome RNA molecules were polyadenylated. The possibility that some genome RNA molecules do not contain poly (A), as with certain picornavirus RNAs (Frisby et al., 1976) cannot be ruled out. But since all the evidence derives from selection of the coronavirus genome RNA by binding to oligo-dT columns, the most likely explanation for only 30 % binding is that the poly (A) stretch is quite short so that some molecules do not bind sufficiently strongly.

Indeed, by binding to poly(U) sepharose after ribonuclease A digestion, a 2s poly (A) fraction was obtained from human coronavirus OC43, which is consistent with a poly(A) length of only 19 adenylate residues (Hierholzer et al., this volume). So far it has not been unequivocally established that the poly (A) is 3'-terminal, though this is presumed to be the case (MacNaughton and Madge, 1978).

Both Lai and Stohlman (this volume), for murine hepatitis virus, and Stern et al. (this volume) for avian IBV have found that the 5'-terminus of the genome RNA contains a methylated cap structure, which in the latter case is apparently of the form m^7GpppA (Kennedy, personal communication). This further emphasizes the positive strand nature of the coronavirus genome, which

Table 1. Comparative Sizes of Coronavirus-Specific RNAs Molecular Weights (X 10^{-6}) from Gel Electrophoresis

VIRUS	GENOME RNA	SUBGENOMIC RNAs						SOURCE
	1	2	3	4	5	6	7	(THIS VOLUME)
AVIAN IBV	6.9	-	2.6	1.5	1.3	0.9	0.8	STERN ET AL.
HUMAN 229 E	6.5	NOT REPORTED						HIERHOLZER ET AL.
HUMAN 229 E	6.0	2.8	2.1	1.3	1.0	0.8	0.6	WEISS AND LEIBOWITZ
HUMAN OC43	6.1	NOT REPORTED						HIERHOLZER ET AL.
MURINE A59	6.1	3.4	2.6	1.2	1.1	0.9	0.6	LEIBOWITZ AND WEISS
MURINE A59	5.6	4.0	3.0	1.4	1.2	0.9	0.6	VAN DER ZEIJST ET AL.
MURINE JHM	6.7	3.4	2.8	1.4	1.2	0.9	0.6	WEGE ET AL.
MURINE JHM	6.0	3.6	3.0	1.3	1.2	0.9	0.6	WEISS AND LEIBOWITZ
PORCINE TGEV	6.8	3.2	(1.6)*	1.4	(1.1)*	0.9	0.7	DENNIS AND BRIAN

*MINOR RNA SPECIES FOUND

must function directly as mRNA in the infected cell. Evidence that the isolated genome RNA is infectious has been obtained for murine (Wege et al., 1978), avian (Schochetman et al., 1977; Lomniczi, 1977) and porcine (Norman et al., 1968; Brian et al., 1980) coronaviruses.

INTRACELLULAR VIRUS-SPECIFIC RNAs

When coronavirus-infected cells are radioactively labelled with ^{3}H-uridine in the presence of sufficient actinomycin D to inhibit host cell mRNA synthesis, seven virus-specific polyadenylated RNAs can normally be detected. In this respect coronavirus genome expression differs from that of picornaviruses (where only genome-sized RNA functions as mRNA) or caliciviruses and togaviruses (where two mRNA species are found) but has some similarity to that of the other major group of positive strand viruses, the oncornaviruses.

It is clear from Table 1 that there is good agreement between various investigators on the sizes of the intracellular RNAs. In each case, RNA of genome size can be detected in infected cells in addition to six subgenomic RNA species, with the exception of IBV, where only five subgenomic RNAs are reported (Stern and Kennedy, 1980).

The sum of the molecular weights of the six subgenomic RNAs is considerably greater than that of the genome RNA; this reflects the fact that the intracellular RNAs share common sequences. Both Weiss and Leibowitz, and Stern et al. (this volume), have shown that all the virus-specific RNAs share a common 3'-terminal sequence. T_1 ribonuclease mapping studies indicate that all RNAs can be arranged as a 'nested set', with the sequence of each RNA being contained within the sequences of all larger RNAs, extending inward from the 3'-terminus of genome RNA (Leibowitz and Weiss, Stern et al., this volume).

In vitro translation of the subgenomic RNAs in micrococcal nuclease-treated rabbit reticulocyte or L cell lysates (Siddell et al this volume; Leibowitz and Weiss this volume) or in Xenopus oocytes (van der Zeijst et al. this volume) indicates that the size of any particular translation product corresponds to the difference in coding capacity between any one RNA and the next smallest RNA. For example, RNA 7 encodes the 60 K nucleocapsid protein, and RNA 6 a 23K precursor to the envelope protein gp25. Similarly, the largest molecular weight difference is found between RNAs 3 and 4 (about 1.2 x 10^6) and this allows RNA 3 to encode the major high molecular weight envelope protein. Thus only the 5'-terminal portion of each subgenomic RNA is translated, and presumably there must exist a termination signal to prevent further read-through. It is still not clear how the genome RNA normally acts as a mRNA; the in vitro translation products which have been observed are of high molecular weight and do not correspond to any intracellular virus-specific proteins so far observed (Leibowitz and Weiss this volume). However, since the virion RNA is infectious, it is likely to encode one or more non-structural proteins required for its own replication.

The mechanism by which the virus-specific RNAs are synthesised is as yet unknown. Since they have the same polarity as genome RNA they must be transcribed from a complementary (negative strand) RNA template. No such template, or double-stranded replicative intermediate molecule, has yet been identified. Assuming that it exists, there are two likely mechanisms for subgenomic RNA synthesis: transcription of a full length plus strand copy of the template followed by processing into six smaller mRNAs, or independent initiation of the synthesis of each mRNA on the template molecule. Evidence that the latter scheme may be correct has been obtained by van der Zeijst et al (this volume), who determined the UV target sizes of the subgenomic RNA species induced in murine A59 virus-infected cells. Complete agreement was found between the physical sizes of RNAs 1 to 5 as determined by agarose gel electrophoresis and the calculated UV dose required to block their synthesis. These data appear to rule out the possibility that coronavirus RNAs are processed from a large precursor molecule. The existence of a short 5'-terminal sequence common to all the RNAs and derived by a splicing or polymerase jumping mechanism cannot, however, be excluded.

The nature of the virus-specific RNA polymerase complex is unknown, although Dennis and Brian (this volume) have found a cytoplasmic membrane-associated RNA-dependent RNA polymerase activity in cells infected with porcine coronavirus. On the other hand, Evans and Simpson (1980) have presented evidence that avian coronavirus replication requires participation of the host cell nucleus and is sensitive to inhibition of host cell DNA-dependent RNA polymerase form II by a-amanitin.

Since avian coronavirus multiplication is quite insensitive to 1 ug/ml actinomycin D in the growth medium (Kennedy, personal communication) and enucleated cells will apparently support the growth of murine coronavirus (Bond, personal communication) it is difficult to reconcile these findings until further experimental work has been carried out.

VIRUS-SPECIFIC PROTEINS

Many investigators have studied the number and sizes of the virion structural proteins, and a summary of results reported in this volume for a variety of coronaviruses is presented in Table 2. In all viruses studied so far, three major virion proteins can be detected. The most prominent of these is a 50 - 60 K protein which in association with RNA forms the helical nucleocapsid. As might be predicted from studies of negative strand virus nucleocapsid proteins, the coronavirus protein is found to be phosphorylated, presumably to facilitate interaction with the genome RNA. Siddell et al. (1981) have described a virion protein kinase activity but it is not clear whether this is a virus-specific enzyme or in which virion-associated proteins the kinase activity resides. Phosphorylation occurs on serine, but not threonine residues (Stohlman and Lai, 1979; Siddell et al., 1981).

The other two well-defined virion proteins are envelope glycoproteins. The largest forms the petal-like structure (peplomers) of the 'crown' and apparently has a conventional mode of synthesis and glycosylation similar to the glycoprotein of other enveloped viruses. This glycoprotein, which some investigators refer to as envelope 2 protein, is found in some viruses in related forms, with molecular weights of 90 K and about 180 K. The processing events which give rise to these two forms are at present unclear. The tryptic peptide patterns of the 90 K species and 180 K species are apparently identical (Sturman and Holmes, 1977). The high molecular weight form is trypsin sensitive, as are the spike glycoproteins of myxoviruses (Klenk and Rott, 1980) and is converted by trypsin treatment into the 90 K form(s) (Sturman and Holmes, 1977). As a consequence the relative amount of gp 90 to gp 180 may vary depending on the proteolytic activity in the host cell in which the virus is grown. This in turn reflects virus infectivity, since cleavage of gp 180 -gp 90 is probably required for infectivity (Storz et al., this volume). An interesting model for the structure of this large envelope glyco-

Table 2. Comparison of Coronavirus Structural Proteins

VIRUS	NUCLEOCAPSID	MEMBRANE	ENVELOPE	OTHER	SOURCE
					(THIS VOLUME)
AVIAN IBV	PP 51	gp 31	gp 90	gp 84 P 14	STERN ET AL.
BOVINE BECV	P 50	gp 23	gp 90/180	gp 65	STORZ ET AL.
BOVINE BECV	50	28	125	65 50 45 36	LAPORTE AND BOBULESCO
CANINE CCV	P 50	gp 32	gp 204	gp 22	GARWES
HUMAN 229 E	P 50	gp 24	gp 105	gp 160 P 22	MACNAUGHTON
HUMAN 229 E	P 47	gp 17	gp 105/gp 196	gp 165 gp 66 gp 31	HIERHOLZER ET AL
HUMAN OC43	P 47	gp 15	gp 104/gp 191	gp 165 gp 60 P 30	HIERHOLZER ET AL
MURINE A59	P 50	gp 23	gp 90/180		STURMAN
MURINE A59	60	25	170		BOND ET AL.
MURINE JHM	63	25	170		BOND ET AL.
MURINE JHM	PP 60	gp 25	gp 98/170	gp 65 P 23	SIDDELL ET AL.
PORCINE TGEV	P 50	gp 30	gp 200		GARWES

protein, containing a single trypsin-sensitive site and disulphide bonds necessary for the conformation of the molecule is presented by Sturman (this volume), and based on studies with murine coronavirus A 59.

There is general agreement that the smaller envelope glycoprotein (gp 25) fulfils a similar role in virion structure to that of the matrix protein of negative strand viruses, though in contrast the corona-virion protein is glycosylated. Some investigators refer to it as envelope I, but 'membrane protein' would probably be a more easily recognized designation. This protein is embedded in the lipid bilayer, and is largely unaltered by incubation of the virion with bromelain, which removes the peplomers, although the carbohydrate moiety is lost by such treatment (Sturman, 1977).

Glycosylation of this membrane protein is unusual in that it is insensitive to tunicamycin, in contrast to all other virus glycoproteins studied so far (including the 90 K coronavirus glycoprotein), (Holmes et al., Niemann and Klenk, this volume). This indicates that dolichol-linked N-acetylglucosamine plays no part in its synthesis, and it is probably that the carbohydrate linkages are of the o-glycosidic type as found in mucin (Niemann and Klenk, this volume). These results strongly suggest a novel mode of synthesis for the 25 K glycoprotein, involving a different cellular compartment to that involved in 90 K glycoprotein synthesis. In agreement, with this idea, it is found that neither mannose nor fucose can be incorporated into this protein (Storz et al, this volume). When coronavirus infects cells in the presence of tunicamycin, synthesis of the 90 K peplomer protein is inhibited, but 'bald' particles still bud out from the cells, and contain only the nucleocapsid and 25 K membrane protein: the particles are non-infectious, however (Holmes et al; Sturman, this volume).

Table 2 shows that in addition to the three well-defined virion proteins, several investigators report an additional glycoprotein of about 65 K and an additional 30 K protein has been reported for human coronavirus. Definition of the role and location of these additional proteins in the virion must await further investigation.

Currently there is no concensus of opinion regarding the virus-induced non-structural proteins found in coronavirus-infected cells. Comparison of results from different laboratories lead to no useful conclusions, but now that well defined virus-cell systems are under investigation, particularly with the murine and porcine viruses, a great deal will be learnt in this area over the next few years. Such studies are necessary to provide a firm basis for investigation of the wide range of persistently-infected cells now available. Unravelling the molecular basis of this persistence both in vitro and ultimately in vivo, is a major goal for future research.

REFERENCES

Brian, D.A., Dennis, D.E. and Guy, J.S. (1980). Genome of porcine transmissible gastroenteritits virus. J. Virol. 34: 410-415.

Evans, M.R. and Simpson, R.W. (1980). The coronavirus avian infectious bronchitis virus requires the cell nucleus and host transcritpional factors.

Frisby, D., Smith, J., Jeffers, V. and Porter, A. (1976). Size and location of poly (A) in encephalomyocarditis virus RNA. Nucleic Acids Res. 3, 2789-2809.

Garwes, D.J., Pocock, D.H. and Wijaszka, T.M. (1975). Identification of heat-dissociable RNA complexes in two porcine coronaviruses. Nature, London 257, 508-510.

Klenk, H.D., and Rott, R. (1980). Cotranslational and post-translational processing of viral glycoproteins. Current Topics in Microbiol. and Immunol., 90, 19-48.

Lai, M.M.C. and Stohlman, S.A. (1978). RNA of mouse hepatitis virus. J. Virol. 26, 236-242.

Lomniczi, B. (1977). Biological properties of avian coronavirus RNA. J. gen. Virol. 36, 531-533.

Lomniczi, B. and Kennedy, I. (1977). Genome of infectious bronchitis virus. J. Virol. 24, 99-107.

Macnaughton, M.R. and Madge, M.H., (1978). The genome of human coronavirus strain 229E. J. gen. Virol. 39, 497-504.

Norman, J.O., and McClurkin, A.W. (1968). Infectious nucleic acid from a transmissible agent causing gastroenteritis in pigs. J. Comp. Pathol. 78, 227-235.

Schochetman, G., Stevens, R.H. and Simpson, R.W. (1977). Presence of infectious polyadenylated RNA in the coronavirus avian bronchitis virus. Virology 77, 772-782.

Siddell, S.G., Barthel, A. and ter Meulen, V. (1981). Coronavirus JHM. A virion-associated protein kinase. J. gen. Virol. 52, in press.

Stern, D.F. and Kennedy, S.I.T., (1980). Coronavirus multiplication strategy. II. Mapping the avian infectious bronchitis virus intracellular RNA species to the genome. J. Virol. 36, 440-449.

Stohlman, S.A. and Lai, M.M.C. (1979). Phosphoproteins of murine hepatitis viruses. J. Virol. 32, 672-675.

Sturman, L.S. (1977). Characterization of a coronavirus I. Structural proteins: effects of preparative conditions on the migration of protein in polyacrylamide gels. Virology 77, 637-649.

Sturman, L.S. and Holmes, K.V. (1977). Characterization of a coronavirus. II. Glycoproteins of the viral envelope: tryptic peptide analysis. Virology 77, 650-660.

Tyrrell, D.A.J., Almeida, J.D., Cunningham, C.H., Dowdle, W.R., Hofstad, M.S., McIntosh, K., Tajima, M., Zakstelskaya, L.Y., Easterday, B.C., Kapikian, A. and Bingham, R.W. (1975). Coronaviridae. Intervirology 5, 76-82.

Wege, H., Müller, A., and ter Meulen, V. (1978). Genomic RNA of the murine coronavirus JHM. J. gen. Virol. 41, 217-227.

IN VIVO AND IN VITRO MODELS OF DEMYELINATING DISEASES

Ole Sorensen, Marion Coulter-Mackie, Dean Percy and
Samuel Dales

Cytobiology Group, Department of Microbiology and
Immunology, University of Western Ontario, London
N6A 5C1 Canada.

INTRODUCTION

One feature characterizing chronic viral infections of the nervous system (NS) associated with progressive degenerative disease is the capacity of the viral agent to maintain itself in a persistent, and/or latent state for prolonged periods. Ability of DNA viruses of the herpes or papova type to remain covert intermittently or for indefinite periods within nuclei of neurons, particularly in peripheral nerve ganglia, has been clearly documented (1-4). RNA viruses of the retrotype such as Visna and C-type of wild mice which, via a provirus intermediate, can become integrated into the host's genome, likewise possess the potential for maintaining persistent or latent infections in the NS (5, 6). It is, however, puzzling how neurotropic RNA agents, among them coronaviruses with +RNA genomes and paramyxoviruses with -RNA genomes, may be perpetuated in the same manner as the viruses mentioned above. As part of our continuing programme of investigations of mechanisms by which NS diseases are produced by some RNA viruses we have studied on the one hand the pathological process in the central nervous system (CNS) of rodents and on the other cell-virus interactions in selected lines of rodent cells of neural and other derivation.

I CENTRAL NERVOUS SYSTEM DISEASE IN THE RAT PRODUCED BY MURINE CORONAVIRUS

A neurotropic strain of mouse hepatitis virus (MHV) was isolated over 30 years ago and designated as JHM (7). This isolate was shown to produce encephalomyelitis and demyelination in mice of various strains (8). Furthermore intracerebral (ic) inoculation of JHMV into white rats produced either fatal or transient neurologic disease, with evidence of demyelinating foci. Demonstration that JHMV could establish persistent or latent infections in a rat cell line of Schwann cell derivation (9) prompted us to study the slowly progressing rat CNS disease caused by JHMV.

(a) Influence of Age and Genetic Constitution of the Host on the Disease Process

Initial experiments by us showed that neurologic disease of rats could be reproducibly initiated by intracerebral (ic) inoculation of JHMV, employing a standard dose of 5×10^4 plaque forming units (pfu). Fewer pfus per inoculum failed to elicit reproducibly either the clinical or histopathological symptoms of disease. By comparison very few pfus are required to initiate disease in mice (8). Intraperitoneal (ip) injection of JHMV or a related viscerotropic MHV_3 at concentrations up to 5×10^5 pfu did not produce any evident disease, nor did the ic injection of MHV_3. Therefore potential host cells in the rat CNS appear to discriminate between the neurotropic and viscerotropic strains of MHV, while those of the mouse do not (10).

When outbred Wistar, Long-Evans or Sprague-Dawley rats are inoculated at two days of age neurologic disease becomes manifested within seven days post inoculation (pi). The symptoms observed include ataxia, tremors and posterior paresis. Deaths in these strains occur during the first 14 days pi and about 3 days after onset of clinical symptoms (Table 1). If animals are injected at 5 days of age, disease is observed later at 15-26 days pi (Table 1). In the latter group posterior paresis or paralysis occurs without apparent effect on forelimb movement. It is highly noteworthy that occasional remissions occur in animals surviving to weaning. Some rats which did not die of acute encephalitic disease by the time of weaning exhibited delayed paralysis and upon autopsy had discrete foci of CNS demyelination. However, some of these rats survived with remissions of neurologic signs and were apparently free of demyelinative lesions.

Inoculation of inbred Wistar-Lewis and Fischer 344 rats caused clinical symptoms which appeared later and the proportion of animals with fatal disease was lower than among the outbred strains (Table 1). By comparison ic inoculation of JHMV into 2 or 5 day old Wistar-Furth rats revealed that this strain is unusually susceptible to rapid encephalitis and death. Paralysis becomes evident only when 10 day old animals are injected (Table 1).

In the resistant strains tested, the longest latent period

Table 1. The Susceptibility of Various Strains of Rat to Paralysis and Death Following JHMV Innoculation

Rat Strain	Age at Inoculation	Number of rats paralysed at death/number of deaths — Time (days pi)				Number deaths**	Number Inoculated
		1-7	8-14	15-21	> 21		
Wistar	2	0/4	1/12	0	0	16	30
	5	0	0	1/2	7/7	9	29
	10	0	0	0	0	0	12
	15	0	0	0	0	0	10
	30	0	0	0	0	0	6
Long-Evans	2	0/1	1/5	3/2	1/2	10	16
Sprague-Dawley	2	0/8	2/9	4/4	2/2	23	33
Fischer 3-1/4	2	0	0/2	2/2	0	4	12
	5	0	0	0	3/3	3	6
Wistar-Lewis	2	0	0	0/1	2/3	4	15
	5	0	0	0	1/1	1	10
Wistar-Furth	2	0/19	0/9	0	0	28	30
	5	0/5	0/8	0	0	13	14
	10	0	6/8	9/9	5/5	22	24

* each animal was inoculated ic with 5 x 10^4 pfu JHMV.
** rats died or were killed *in extremis*.
(Data from reference (11)).

recorded was 99 days pi in a rat manifesting posterior paresis. In this particular animal recovery of hind limbs coordination returned within 40 days.

To ascertain the genetic control of sensitivity of rats to JHMV an F_1 cross between Wistar-Lewis and Wistar-Furth was bred and animals inoculated ic at 10 days of age. As shown in Table 2, none of the animals became paralysed within 21 days pi and the mortality rate was approximately as low as that of the resistant Wistar-Lewis strain. Thus high survival rate to JHM appears to be genetically dominant.

Table 2

Rate of paralysis and mortality in the F_1 Wistar-Lewis x Wistar-Furth*

Days after inoculation				No. of deaths	No. inoculated
1-7	8-14	15-21	21		
0	0/5**	0	0/1	6	47

* 10 day old animals were inoculated ic with 5 x 10^4 pfu JHMV

** ratio animals paralysed/dead

(b) Histopathological Findings

A survey among rats of different strains revealed that the location of histological lesions, identified by means of standard procedures for light and electron microscopy (11), is altered with time elapsing after inoculation (latency period) and the distribution of gray and white matter lesions is also altered (Figure 1). When deaths occur within 1 week pi cerebral gray and white matter lesions are prominent, with those in the gray matter predominating. There was evidence of necrotizing meningioencephalitis with destruction of both gray and white matter, proliferation of endothelial cells and minor infiltration of polymorphonucelar and mononuclear cells into the CNS parenchyma. There was a high incidence of necrotic foci in the cerebral cortex and hippocampal gyrus.

First signs of spiral cord involvement were detected in animals killed or dying 2 weeks pi. These foci were predominantly in the white matter. Animals examined 3 weeks pi exhibited prominent white matter lesions in the rhombencephalon and the cord (Figure 1).

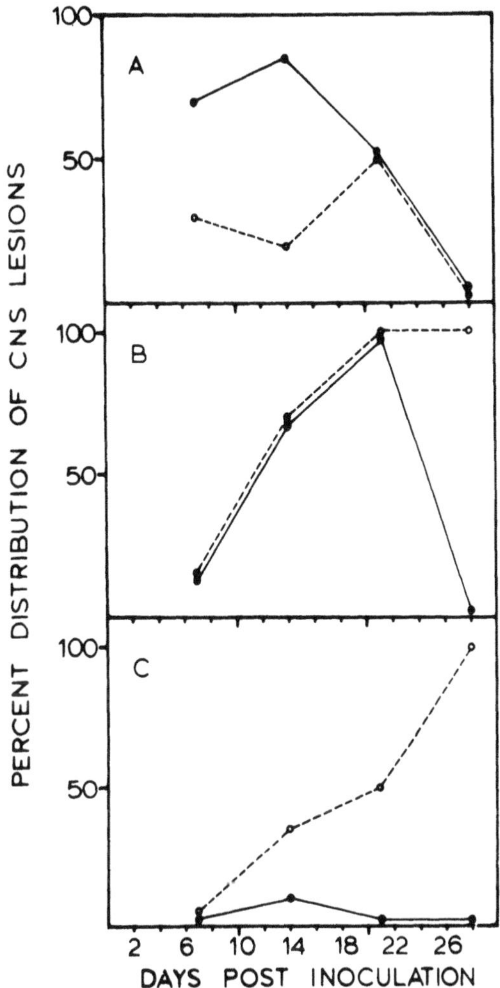

Fig. 1 - Cumulative data on frequency and distribution of white and gray matter lesions in CNS of all rats that died or were killed in extremis after intracerebral inoculation of JHM virus at 2 days of age (A, cerebrum; B, rhombencephalon; C, spinal cord; closed circles, gray matter; and open circles, white matter). (Data from reference (11)).

Specific involvement of the white matter was more evident in rats killed eight days pi or later. Some gray matter destruction was also evident in rats dying eight to 21 days pi (Figure 1). In the CNS of rats in which clinical symptoms developed 15 or more days pi, white matter lesions were more common and more extensive than those in the gray matter. Pathologic changes in the white matter involved various areas of the cerebrospinal axis but were most prominent in the pons, cerebellar folia, myelencephalon, spinal cord, and optic nerve. Characteristically, there was vacuolation of white matter coupled with disruption of normal architecture, absence or scarcity of myelin, and minimal perivascular cuffing with mononuclear cells. Frequently, macrophages with numerous cytoplasmic vacuoles were evident in areas of myelinoclasis implying that breakdown of myelin was followed by phagocytosis of this material. Multinucleated cells, interpreted to be gemistocytic astrocytes, were occasionally observed in demyelinated areas of spinal cord.

It is noteworthy that up to the time of weaning some rats, which did not die of acute encephalitic disease manifested delayed paralytic symptoms and discrete foci of demyelination in the CNS. Some of these paralyzed rats survived with remission of neurologic signs, and were also devoid of lesions on histological and electron microscopic examination, implying that remyelination after paralysis may occur. Similar findings have been reported recently by others (12, 13). Generally, demyelinating foci were absent from rats without clinical signs. To date, exacerbations have not been encountered.

(c) Optic Neuritis

Optic neuritis was prominent in seven of 15 inoculated rats that died or were killed 12 to 25 days pi. Whenever optic nerve involvement was found in a particular rat, there were concurrent lesions in the brain and spinal cord. In optic nerves from rats examined as early as 12 days pi, the lesions were characterized by fragmentation of myelin sheaths, disruption of the normal architecture, and noticeable infiltration by mononuclear cells. In material taken 21 to 25 days pi, areas of demyelination in optic nerves resembled closely demyelinating lesions observed elsewhere in the cerebrospinal axis, including thinning, fragmentation, and dispersal of the myelin covering around individual axons, and infiltration by phagocytic cells.

In view of the tropism of JHMV for oligodendrocytes throughout the CNS, the observed demyelination in the optic nerve might have been due to killing of this cell type. The extent of the lesions observed might reflect the nature of CNS myelination where segments of many axons may be myelinated by a single oligodendrocyte (14).

The optic nerve lesions, when identified, occurred only in those rats that also had lesions elsewhere in the CNS, suggesting great susceptibility of oligodendrocytes in this region to JHMV. Conversely, lesions were not observed in the cerebrospinal axis of rats with optic nerves devoid of lesions. In this context, it is intriguing to note that in man, optic neuritis is frequently associated with multiple sclerosis, and it has been suggested that optic neuritis may be a manifestation of the same disease (15, 16).

(d) JHMV Replication in the Central Nervous System

To assay for the presence of infectious virus, inoculation ic of brain homogenates from JHMV-infected Sprague-Dawley rats was made into suckling mice. Inoculated mice that died displayed typical JHMV histopathologic findings. The data obtained demonstrated the presence of infectious virus in rats during the first 20 days pi. All rats tested both with clinical symptoms, and some without, proved to be positive for JHMV. After injection ic of 3×10^5 LD_{50} JHMV/rat, rats without symptoms killed five or ten days pi yielded in some cases about 3×10^4 LD_{50} JHMV/g of brain. JHMV was also isolated from animals displaying typical symptoms 15 and 20 days pi.

Systematic electron microscopic examination of lesions of the optic nerve, spinal cord, rhombencephalon, or cerebrum, where extensive demyelination and tissue damage occurred failed to provide evidence for the presence of coronavirus. Intracellular viral replication was observed infrequently and only after extensive searching. Invariably the coronavirus particles were confined to oligodendrocytes of the optic nerve and spinal cord of animals sacrificed 12-24 days pi. The appearance of assembling or mature JHMV is indistinguishable from that previously described in rodents and cultured cells as illustrated in our companion article. The process is characterized by virus budding into cytoplasmic vacuoles and the accumulation of intracytoplasmic nucleocapsid material.

(e) Concluding Remarks

Applicability of the rat model for investigating virus-induced progressive demyelinating diseases possesses certain attractive features that deserve further attention. Of particular interest is, first, the delayed onset of neurologic disease with apparent remission after prolonged paralysis; second, the progressive changes in the location and frequency of demyelinating foci in relation to increased length of the latent period; and third, the appearance of demyelinating lesions in the optic nerve.

II INTERACTION OF CORONAVIRUSES IN VITRO WITH CELLS OF NEURAL AND OTHER DERIVATION

(a) Cell Lines

Capability of JHMV and MHV_3 to initiate in rodents chronic and perhaps latent CNS infections raises fundamental questions about the nature of cell-virus interrelationships involving specific neural cell types. With this in mind we undertook a series of studies to examine the infectious process in the less complex in vitro setting and employed established lines of glial, neuronal, and non-nervous system derivation. For comparative purposes interactions with the subsclerosing panencephalitis Hallé and Edmonston vaccine strains of measles, another virus type with neurotropic potential, were examined in parallel with those conducted on the coronaviruses (9, 17). The cell lines employed and their presumed derivation are listed in Table 3. Among them the L-2 murine fibroblasts are fully permissive for JHMV and MHV3 and Vero monkey cells for both the measles isolates. These lines served not only as the prototype permissive host but were also used for propagating virus stocks and plaque assays.

Table 3. Cell Lines

Designation	Species	Type	Cerebroside sulfate (determined by [^{35}S]sulfate incorporated)[a] (dpm/mg of protein)
RN2-2	Rat	Schwannoma	5650
C6	Rat	Astrocytoma	<300
HTC	Rat	Hepatoma	3800
L6	Rat	Myoblast/myocyte	ND[b]
L-2	Murine	Connective tissue fibroblastic	<300
C1300	Murine	Neuroblastoma "axonal"	<300
G26-20	Murine	Oligodendroglioma	ND[b]
G26-24	Murine	Oligodendroglioma	8400
Vero	Monkey	Kidney epithelial	4200

[a] Determined as described in Materials and Methods.
[b] Not done.

(Data from reference (17))

The rat RN2-2 Schwannoma was selected for the most detailed investigations because it ① can be persistently infected by both JHMV and the measles isolates and ② may have the same stem cell origin as oligodendrocytes in the CNS. In this regard it should be remembered that JHMV exhibits rather specific tropism for oligodendrocytes of the rat CNS when a chronic disease occurs, as described above (11).

(b) Persistence and Latency

When RN-2 cells are infected with JHMV with a low multiplicity (moi) of 0.1 at 33° persistence is established immediately (9). Cytopathic effects (CPE) in the form of syncytia formation and cell killing are limited to discrete foci and never involve the entire culture. Coincidentally virus is continually shed for indefinite periods into the medium in amounts fluctuating cyclically (Figure 2). Among all cell lines examined the ability of RN-2 cells to discriminate between the neurotropic and viscerotropic subtypes of coronavirus appears to be a unique property of this Schwannoma line. It remains to be shown whether the results obtained in vitro are in some manner, related to suppression of MHV_3 infection in the CNS of the rat, described above.

Concerning the viral and/or cellular regulation of persistence it may be highly significant that measles viruses undergo replication patterns in RN2-2 cells at 33° essentially identical to those recorded for the coronaviruses, without, however, eliciting any overt cytopathology in the host (17).

Upon temperature shift up from 33° to 40° production of JHMV and measles viruses from persistently infected RN2-2 cells ceases rapidly (17). Since, however, the progeny virions assembled at 33° are not themselves thermolabile the thermosensitivity of replication is most probably controlled by host function(s). A comparative analysis with respect to data on infection of RN2-2 cells by JHMV, MHV_3, SSPE-Hallé and Edmonston measles strains was extended to a variety of other rat and mouse lines (17). The data, summarized in table 4, show that at 33° JHMV and MHV_3 were also produced in cyclical waves of the type evident in the Schwannoma cultures (Figure 2), in rat L6 myoblasts, HTC hepatoma cells and murine G26-20 or G26-24 oligodendroglioina lines. However, the coronaviruses failed to replicate in the C6 astrocytoma line (table 4). Murine C1300 neuroblastoma is permissive for the corona (table 4), and measles (18) agents.

A very striking correlation was observed between capacity of these viruses to establish persistence at 33° and become restricted, usually in a complete manner when cultures are kept at 40° (table 4). Intermediate degrees of suppression of virus production occur at 37°. These findings imply that a host function(s) which interferes with the productive virus cycle is activated or enhanced in activity after elevation of the temperatures from 33° to 37° or 40°.

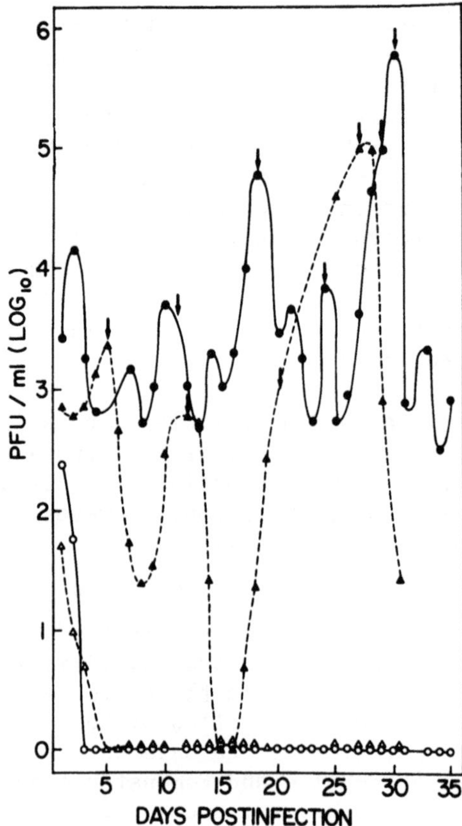

Infection of Rat Glial Cells with Murine Hepatitis Virus

Fig. 2 - Monolayers of RN2-2 cells were infected as described in the text. Virus present in the medium was assayed using the plaque assay on L-2 cells as described in Experimental Procedures. Circles, solid line-experiment 1; triangles, dashed line-experiment 2. Open symbols-MHV_3 infection; closed symbols-JHM infection. Arrows indicate when the cells were subcultured.
(Data from reference (9)).

The relative quantities of cell-associated cerebroside sulfate, a glycolipid species characteristically found in myelin membranes, were ascertained to determine whether persistence and/or latency are correlated with this glycolipid. It may be significant that RN2-2, HTC and G-26-24 cell lines, in which JHMV persistence can be established have cerebroside sulfate levels at least an order of magnitude greater than those of C6 astrocytoma line (table 3), in which infection is aborted (table 4).

(c) Reversibility of Latency

Arrest of virus production at 40° is reversible within certain time limits. The interval elapsing before latently infected RN2-2 cells resume a state of persistence upon temperature shift down to 33° depends upon the duration that cultures are kept at the restrictive temperature. With JHMV, if latency is maintained for 10 days virus production upon shift down, is resumed after a lag of 2-3 days. If the latent state is prolonged beyond 2 weeks the lag period is likewise extended. In the case of Halle measles virus latently infected RN2-2 cells can be maintained for 8 weeks before losing their capacity to resume a state of persistence at 33° (unpublished).

(d) Replication of Other Agents in RN2-2 Cells

The relative ease with which persistent infections with the coronaviruses and measles strains are established and the associated thermosensitivity of the replication process suggested that infections with many virus types may indiscriminately become persistent. To investigate this possibility monolayers of the various cell types are infected at 33° and 40° with IHD-W vaccinia virus at an m.o.i. of 5 pfu or vesicular stomatitis virus (VSV) at an m.o.i. of 0.01 pfu. After 24 hr of incubation, the concentrations of VSV and vaccinia are determined by plaque titration on L-2 cell monolayers. VSV infection of the RN2-2, C6, HTC, and C1300 produces an extensive CPE and yields high titers of virus at both 33° and 40°. VSV infection of the G26-20 and G26-24 cell lines, however, appears to be persistent at both temperatures, yielding low titers of virus over a period of at least several days, with no evidence of CPE. Vaccinia virus causes extensive CPE at both temperatures in the RN2-2, C6, HTC, and C1300 cell lines, although viral production decreases at 40° by 60% in the C1300 and by 90% in the C6 cells. In the vaccinia-inoculated G26-24 cell line kept at either temperature, the infection is apparently aborted since there is no rise in titer between 2 and 24 hr after inoculation; however, a virus induced CPE occurs. These combined observations indicate that with all the cell lines tested, temperature related persistence and latency of the type associated with corona

Table 4. Summary Data on Persistence and Thermolability of Virus Replication in Various Cell Lines Tested

Cell line	Virus	Outcome of infection			Temperature-sensitive restriction of replication
		Lytic	Abortive	Persistent	
L-2	JHM	+			
	MHV_3	+			
Vero	Edmonston	+			
	Hallé	+			
RN2-2	JHM			+	+
	MHV_3		+		
	Edmonston			+	+
	Hallé			+	+
HTC	JHM			+	(+)[a]
	MHV_3			+	+
	Edmonston			+	+
	Hallé			+	+
C6	JHM		+		
	MHV_3		+		
	Edmonston			+	+
	Hallé			+	+
L6	JHM			+	(+)[a]
	MHV_3			+	+
	Edmonston			+	(+)[a]
	Hallé			+	+
G26-20	JHM			+	+
	MHV_3			+	+
	Edmonston		+		
	Hallé		+		
G26-24	JHM			+	(+)[a]
	MHV_3			+	+
	Edmonston		+		
	Hallé		+		
C1300	JHM			(+)[b]	
	MHV_3			(+)[b]	(+)[c]
	Edmonston	ND[d]		ND[d]	
	Hallé	ND[d]		ND[d]	

[a] Restriction partial.
[b] In equilibrium between lytic and persistent.
[c] Virus progeny partially thermolabile.
[d] Not done.

(Data from reference (17)).

and measles viruses does not occur after infection with VSV or vaccinia.

(e) Heterologous Virus Challenge

To determine whether the JHM persistently infected RN2-2 cultures are resistant to superinfection by an unrelated virus, VSV was inoculated onto either uninfected or persistently infected RN2-2 cells (passage 5 or 6) at an m.o.i. of 0.1. Following incubation for 24 hr at 33° the yield of pfu of VSV in the supernatant of each culture was assayed on monolayers of both L-2 and RN2-2 cells. In two separate experiments, yields of VSV from the JHMV persistently infected RN2-2 culture, whether determined on L-2 cells or RN2-2 monolayers, are only about 10% of those from uninfected RN2-2 cells (9). RN2-2 cultures kept at 40° latently infected with Hallé-measles when challenged with the heterologous virus produce VSV at a rate only 5% that made in cultures not harboring latent measles (unpublished). After >8 weeks at 40°, when, upon shift down, rescue of measles can no longer be effected, replication of VSV returns to the normal level (unpublished).

Although the molecular events underlying the maintenance of persistence or latency in the systems under study here remain to be elucidated, in other virus carrier states chronic infections have been explained by effects involving defective interfering (DI) particles or by inhibition of virus production due to interferon, sometimes in a cyclical fashion (19), or due to selection of genotypically changed variants of the virus (20).

Involvement of DI particles in the present studies seems to be unlikely because the inoculation was made at low m.o.i. and medium was changed daily, which should have minimized the production or accurmulation of DI particles.

Evidence with the JHM and measles persistent infections of RN2-2 cells for involvement of an interferon-like mechanism comes from the partial resistance to superinfection with VSV (19). It is not possible, however, to transfer interference against VSV to uninfected RN2-2 cells by soluble material in the culture medium taken from persistently infected RN2-2 cultures. Clearly additional work is required to ascertain whether interferon or some other factors function in the chronic infectious process under study by us.

(f) Identification and Rescue of Latent Virus

Attempts have been made to rescue latent virus from RN2-2 cells at 40°. Treatment with low amounts (0.1 μg/ml) of

Actinomycin D to suppress host related transcription or co-cultivation with indicator cells induces appearance of pfus, albeit in low amounts, in the case of measles. Similar attempts are in progress with JHMV.

Fate of the virus in the temperature restricted state is being studied currently using cDNA probes and nucleic acid hybridization. Todate it is evident that a cDNA specific for the measles genome (21), can detect among total RN2-2 cellular extracts genomic RNA in decreasing amounts up to 5-7 days after temperature shift up to 40°. Preliminary observations by immunofluorescence and light microscopy indicate that viral genome RNA can persist beyond the period of active expression into viral antigens. Use of similar probing techniques is being initiated for the coronaviruses.

(g) Concluding Remarks

Taken together, the results described in this report suggest that the host cell has a profound influence in regulating the replication process of agents with neurotropic potential. The relative ease with which persistence and thermosensitivity develop in the cell lines examined provides new systems for inquiries into the molecular events and mechanisms by means of which certain viruses operate as slowly acting pathogens in the nervous system.

ACKNOWLEDGEMENTS

Supported by the Multiple Sclerosis and Medical Research Council of Canada. O. Sorensen is a holder of an MRC studentship. We are grateful to Professor G. Strejan for his advice regarding the use of pure strains of rats.

REFERENCES

1. K. Kristensson, B. Svennerholm, L. Persson, A. Vahlne, and E. Lycke, Latent herpes simplex virus trigeminal ganglionic infection in mice and demyelination in the central nervous system, J. Neurol. Sci. 43:253 (1979).

2. B.L. Padgett, and D.L. Walker, New human papovaviruses, Prog. med. Virol. 22:1 (1976).

3. D.M. Lonsdale, S.M. Brown, J.H. Subak-Sharpe, K.G. Warren, and H. Koprowski, The polypeptide and the DNA restriction enzyme profiles of spontaneous isolates of herpes simplex

virus Type 1 from explants of human trigeminal, superior cervical and vagus ganglia, J. gen. Virol. 43:151 (1979).

4. .J. Townsend, and J.R. Baringer, Central nervous system susceptibility to herpes simplex infection, J. Neuropath. and Exptl. Neurol. 37:255 (1978).

5. M.B. Gardner, V. Klement, R.W. Rougey, P. McConahey, J.D. Estes, and R.J. Heubner, Type C-virus expression in lymphoma-paralysis-prone wild mice, J. Natl. Cancer Inst. 57:585 (1976).

6. J.R. Martin, and N. Nathanson, Animal models of virus-induced demyelination, Progr. Neuropath. 4:27 (1979).

7. T.O. Bailey, A.M. Pappenheimer, F. Cheever, and J.B. Daniels, A murine virus (JHM) causing disseminated encephalomyelitis with extensive destruction of myelin: II. Pathology, J. Exp. Med. 90:195 (1949).

8. S.F. Cheever, J.B. Daniels, A.M. Pappenheimer, and O.T. Bailey, A murine virus (JHM) causing disseminatated encephalomyelitis with extensive destruction of myelin: I. Isolation and biological properties of the virus, J. Exp. Med. 90:181 (1949).

9. A. Lucas, W. Flintoff, R. Anderson, D. Percy, M. Coulter, and S. Dales, In vivo and in vitro models of demyelinating diseases: I. Tropisms of the JHM strain of murine hepatitis virus for cells of glial origin, Cell 12:553 (1977).

10. C. LePrevost, J.L. Virelizier, and J.M. Dupuy, Immunopathology of mouse hepatitis virus type 3 infection: III. Clinical and virologic observation of a persistent viral infection, J. Immunol. 115:640 (1975).

11. O. Sorensen, D. Percy, and S. Dales, In vivo and in vitro models of demyelinating diseases: III. JHM virus infection in rats, Arch. Neurol. 37:478 (1980).

12. K. Nagashima, H. Wege, and V. ter Meulen, Early and late CNS-effects of coronavirus infection in rats, Adv. Exp. Med. Biol. 100:395 (1978).

13. K. Nagashima, H. Wege, R. Meyermann, and V. ter Meulen, Coronavirus induced subacute demyelinating encephalomyelitis in rats: A morphological analysis, Acta Neuropathol. 44:63 (1978).

14. R.P. Bunge, Glial cells and the central myelin sheath, Physiol. Rev. 48:197 (1968).

15. E. Nikoskelainen, and P. Riekkenen, Optic neuritis: A sign of multiple sclerosis or other diseases of the central nervous system, Acta Neurol. Scand. 50:690 (1974).

16. D. Santoli, Z. Wroblewska, E.N. Cremer, S.F. Lief, and N. Schatz, Acute optic neuritis: A virologic study in relation to multiple sclerosis, J. Med. Virol. 1:201 (1977).

17. A. Lucas, M. Coulter, R. Anderson, S. Dales, and W. Flintoff, In vivo and in vitro models of demyelinating diseases: II. Persistence and host regulated thermosensitivity in cells of neural derivation infected with mouse hepatitis and measles viruses, Virol. 88:325 (1978).

18. R. Lunden, A. Vahlne, and E. Lycke, Measles virus infection of mouse neuroblastoma (C1300) cells (40933), Proc. Soc. Exptl. Biol. Med. 165:55 (1980).

19. T.J. Wiktor, and H.F. Clark, Chronic rabies virus infection of cell cultures, Infec. Immun. 6:988 (1972).

20. J.S. Youngner, and D.D. Quagliana, Temperature sensitive mutants isolated from hamster and canine cell lines persistently infected with Newcastle disease virus, J. Virol. 16:1332 (1975).

21. M.B. Coulter-Mackie, W.C. Bradbury, S. Dales, W.F. Flintoff, and V.L. Morris, In vivo and in vitro models of demyelinating diseases: IV. Isolation of Halle measles virus specific RNA from BGMK cells and preparation of complementary DNA, Virology 102:327 (1980).

EVOLUTION OF A CORONAVIRUS DURING PERSISTENT INFECTION *IN VITRO*

Kathryn V. Holmes and James N. Behnke

Pathology Dept., Uniformed Services University of the Health Sciences, 4301 Jones Bridge Road, Bethesda, Maryland 20014

INTRODUCTION

Coronaviruses usually infect epithelial cells of the gastroenteric or respiratory tracts. They frequently cause local infections which may be fatal in young animals, but which are usually mild or asymptomatic in adults. *In vitro*, coronaviruses may induce virulent, cytolytic and cell fusing effects in some host cells but cause a moderate, persistent infection in other cell types. Thus the host or the host cell appears to be of critical importance in determining the outcome of coronavirus infection. This report will focus on the role of the host cell in coronavirus replication and on the mutually dependent changes induced in the host cell and the virus during the establishment of a persistent infection *in vitro*.

Strong selective pressures may act on coronavirus populations *in vitro* and *in vivo*. The local immune response of the host probably selects for strains of virus with altered viral attachment proteins. Indeed, a large number of strains of each of the animal coronaviruses has been isolated. This observation suggests that a variety of mutants of at least one of the viral glycoproteins (probably the peplomeric glycoprotein E2) can be functional.

The host cell appears to be of critical importance for the replication of coronaviruses. Many coronaviruses show stringent species and tissue specificity during primary isolation. During adaptation to tissue culture selection of viruses with altered antigenicity or virulence often occurs. Such selection may operate at several different stages in the intracellular replication of the virus. Three of the many examples of the dependence of coronaviruses on host cell functions will be mentioned here. Sturman and Takemoto

(1972) showed that the yield of infectious mouse hepatitis virus (MHV) was much greater from transformed BALB/c 3T3 cells than from non-transformed cells. Lucas et al (1978) demonstrated that the replication of MHV3 is temperature sensitive in neuronal cells but not in nonneuronal cells. Evans and Simpson (1980) recently observed that a host transcriptional function may be required for replication of infectious bronchitis virus (IBV) in BHK21 cells. Very little is known about the cellular functions which are responsible for such host dependent differences in coronavirus replication.

To analyze the interactions between a coronavirus and its host cell, we have studied the development of persistent coronavirus infection *in vitro* using the well-characterized A59 strain of MHV in the normally permissive 17 clone 1 (17Cl 1) line of spontaneously transformed BALB/c 3T3 cells. A59 virus replicates efficiently in these cells and it produces large plaques in 17Cl 1 cells at both 32°C and 39.5°C. Yields of 10^8 to 10^9 PFU/ml of released infectious virus are obtained within 24 hours, yet a persistent infection can readily be established in this host cell system.

In this report, we will describe the normal maturation of coronaviruses and discuss the establishment and characterization of a persistent infection *in vitro* with MHV. We will analyze the evolution of the virus during the establishment of the persistent infection and suggest one possible mechanism for coronavirus persistence.

MATURATION AND RELEASE OF CORONAVIRUSES

To study the sequence of events in coronavirus maturation, 17 Cl 1 cells infected with A59 were examined by TEM at intervals after virus inoculation. The events shown here for the acute infection were later found to be similar in the cells producing virus in persistently infected cultures. After the latent period virions were seen within the rough endoplasmic reticulum (RER) and the Golgi apparatus (Fig. 1). Virions in the RER were spherical and had electron lucent centers. Helical nucleocapsids could be observed within these "immature" virus forms, and shift to a lower temperature could apparently block virus release from the RER (Fig. 2). As the acute infection at 37°C progressed the virions moved through the Golgi into smooth walled vesicles (SWV). During this process virions became flattened, disc shaped and electron dense. These SWV containing "mature" virus particles migrated to the plasma membrane (PM) and fused with it to release virions into the medium. Released virions frequently readsorbed to the PM, but virions were never observed to bud from the PM. Late in the infectious cycle, large inclusions of viral nucleocapsid were observed in the cytoplasmic matrix.

A schematic drawing of the sequence of events which we believe occurs during coronavirus maturation is shown in Figure 3. Viral

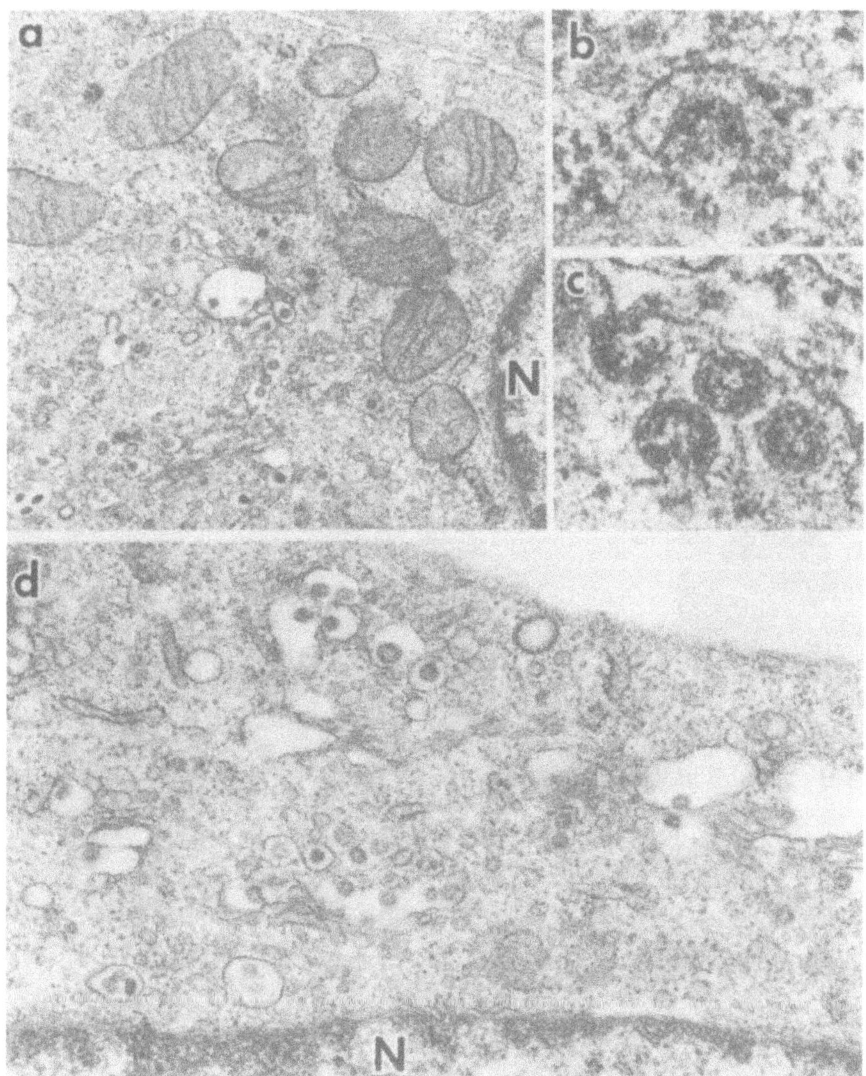

Fig. 1. Maturation of coronaviruses. Virions in the RER and Golgi apparatus 9 hrs. after virus inoculation. Virions budding into the RER are shown in b and c.

glycoproteins as well as virions migrate from RER through the Golgi to the PM where they can be detected by immunoelectronmicroscopy (data not shown). Several host cell functions are required for assembly and release of coronaviruses. We have suggested at this meeting that the glycosylation of the E1 and E2 glycoproteins may utilize two different cellular pathways. Also Doller and Holmes

(1980) showed that these two viral glycoproteins migrate differently within the infected cell, presumeably using different host cell glycoprotein transport systems. To be released from the infected cell, coronaviruses apparently utilize the cellular secretory apparatus. Thus cellular mechanisms for glycosylation, glycoprotein transport and secretion all appear to be required for efficient release of coronaviruses.

ESTABLISHMENT OF PERSISTENTLY INFECTED CULTURES

A persistent infection was established by inoculation of 17 Cl 1 cells with plaque purified MHV at a multiplicity of 3 PFU/cell. Cultures were held at 37°C. Cytopathology (CPE) was extensive during the first 24 hours, but approximately 5% of the cell survived

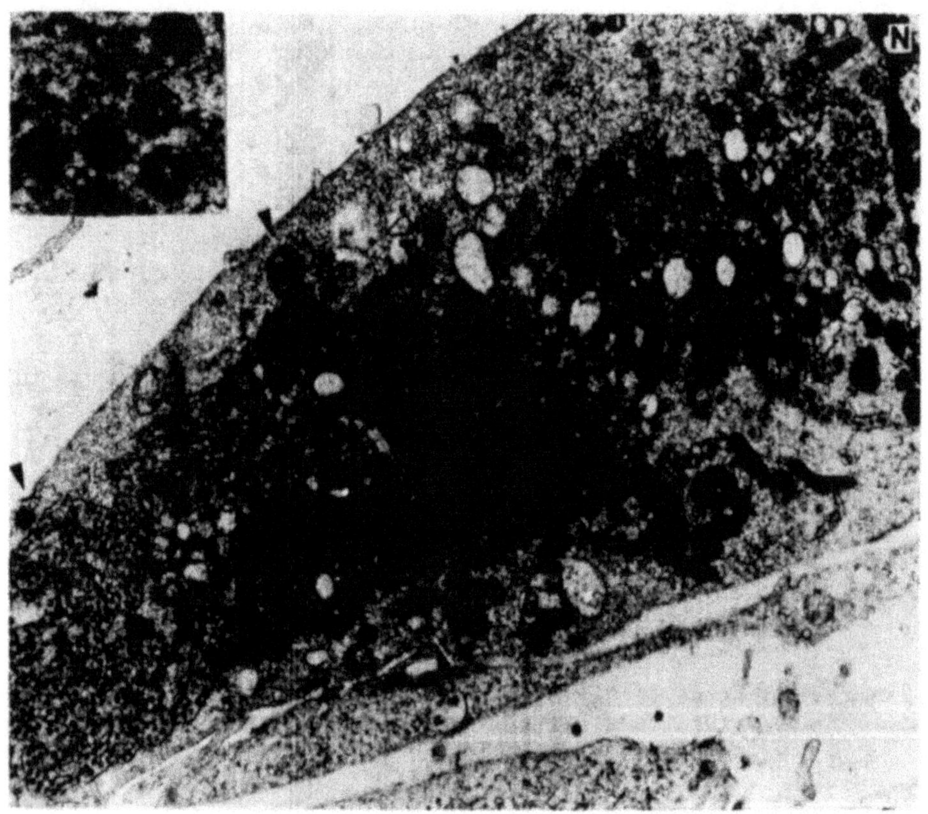

Fig. 2. Effect of temperature shift on virus release. A cell infected with A59 was grown at 37°C for 8 hr then shifted to 32°C for 16 hr. Numerous spherical virions accumulated in the RER and few smooth walled vesicles (arrows) full of mature virions were observed. Inset shows helical nucleocapsids in virions (arrows).

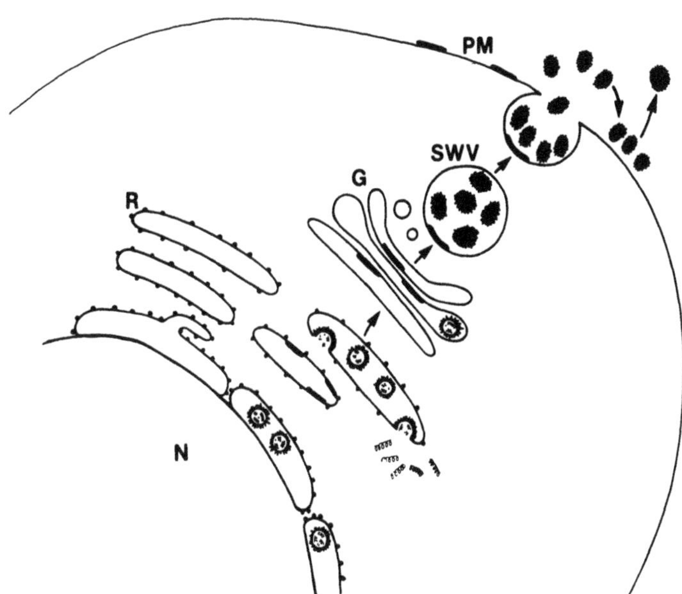

Fig. 3. Sequence of events in coronavirus maturation. The following symbols have been used: N, nucleus; R, rough endoplasmic reticulum; G, Golgi apparatus; SWV, smooth walled vesicles; PM, plasma membrane. Helical nucleocapsid can be seen within spherical "immature" virions in the RER, whereas "mature" virions in SWV and on PM are flattened and electron opaque.

and grew out to form a confluent monolayer. Cultures were passaged twice a week. The supernatant fluid containing released virus was harvested at every passage for plaque assay and a portion of the cells were stored in liquid nitrogen at frequent intervals. Viral structural proteins in the cells were detected by labelling with fluorescent antibody. Cell fusion occurred on the day following trypsinization for about the first six passages, but little or no CPE was observed in later passages. Persistently infected (PI) cultures exhibited a normal growth pattern except for a crisis period at approximately the fourteenth passage when they grew very slowly for several weeks. After recovery, the characteristics of the PI cultures have not changed. The cultures have been maintained for more than 100 passages. The PI cultures showed no CPE (Fig. 4). All of the PI cells were resistant to superinfection with the original wild type (WT) large plaque A59. WT A59 did not grow or induce cytopathic effects in these cultures (Fig. 4), and did not produce plaques on PI cultures. However, unrelated viruses such as VSV or Semliki Forest virus formed plaques on PI cultures as well as on uninfected cells. At every passage 10 to 20% of the cells were positive for MHV viral antigens. TEM showed normal development of virions in 10 to 20% of the cells and no evidence of virus replication in the remaining cells.

CHARACTERIZATION OF VIRUS FROM PI CULTURES

The PI cultures continually shed virus throughout these experiments. In the first two passages the virus produced was predominantly large plaque virus like the WT A59. By the 7th passage however, a wide variety of plaque morphology virus mutants had developed (Fig. 5). Plaque phenotypes including large, medium and small, turbid or clear, ragged or smooth were observed. The proportion of small plaque virus in the population increased irregularly (Fig. 6) until, by the 22nd passage only small plaque virus was detected.

Initially we believe that all of the small plaque viruses from the 22nd passage were temperature sensitive (ts), since no plaques were observed at 39.5°C under conditions in which WT A59 plaqued normally. However, we discovered that supplementation of the medium with additional fetal calf serum permitted detection at 39.5°C of small plaques caused by non-ts mutants which developed more slowly than WT A59. Thus the conditions necessary for plaquing small plaque non-ts mutant virus at 39.5° were different from those used for WT A59. The proportion of small plaque viruses which was temperature sensitive varied during passage of the chronically infected cells (Fig. 7). No regular pattern was evident (Fig. 8) and PI cultures always contained both ts and non-ts small plaque virus.

Several ts mutants have been plaque purified and characterized.

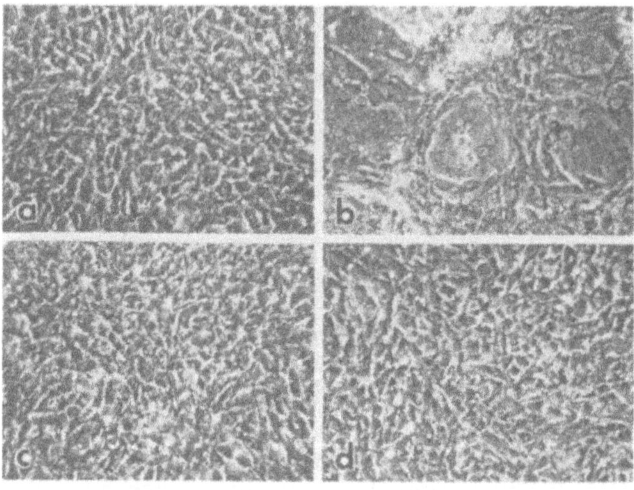

Fig. 4. Effects of A59 infection on normal and persistently infected cells. Normal 17 clone 1 cells (a) showed cell fusion and rounding 24 hr. after infection (b). Persistently infected cultures (c) were indistinguishable from normal cells and showed no CPE 24 hr. after superinfection with A59(d).

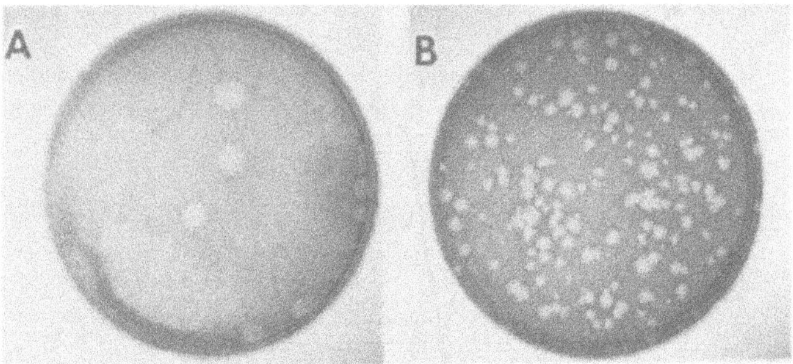

Fig. 5. Development of plaque morphology mutants during persistent infection. Large plaques from WT A59 are shown in A and a variety of plaque morphology mutants from the 7th passage of PI cultures are shown in B.

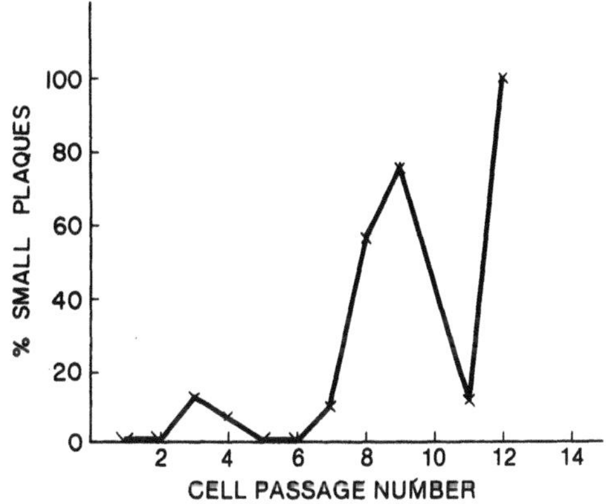

Fig. 6. Selection of small plaque mutants during persistent infection.

One mutant from the 22nd passage called 22B will not replicate at 39.5°C. Growth curves of WT A59 and 22B are shown in Fig. 9. This mutant appears to be a multiple step mutant. At the non-permissive temperature, synthesis of viral specific RNA by 22B was not detectable (Fig. 10; Behnke and Holmes, 1978). Thus 22B appears to have an early defect in viral RNA synthesis. In addition, 22B virions are less stable than WT A59 and SDS PAGE shows altered migration of the E2 glycoprotein.

MECHANISMS OF CORONAVIRUS PERSISTENCE

To study the interactions between ts and non-ts viruses, mixed infections of WT A59 and 22B were done at permissive and non-per-

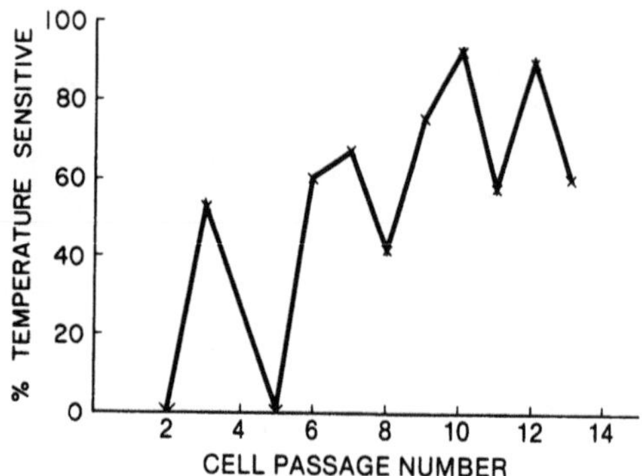

Fig. 7. Development of temperature sensitive virus during persistent infection. % ts virus was calculated using the titer at 32°C as total virus and the titer at 39.5°C as non-ts virus.

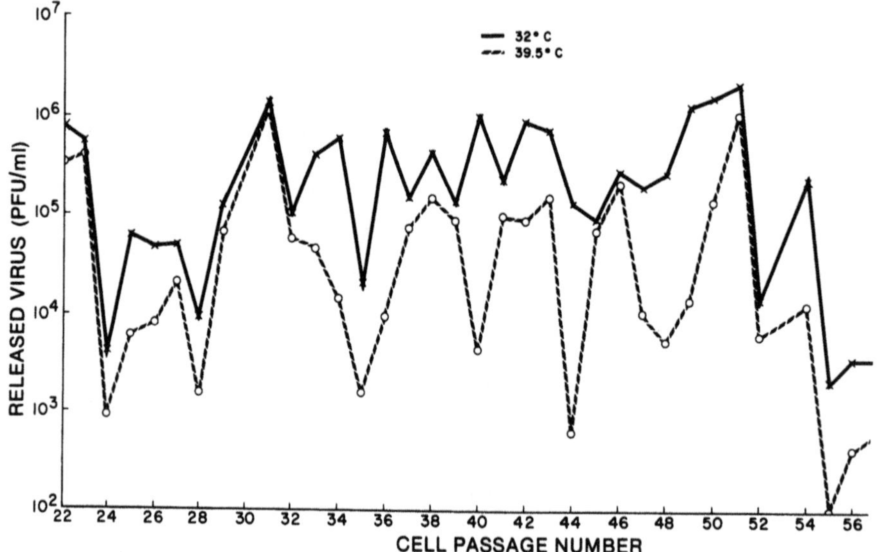

Fig. 8. Yields of released virus from persistently infected cultures. Virus from passages of PI cultures was assayed at 32°C and 39.5°C.

missive temperatures (Table 1). Both viruses replicated after co-infection at 32°, but at the non-permissive temperature the mutant virus could not replicate and interfered with the replication of the wild type virus. This conditional interference with the replication of wild type virus may be an important reason for modulation of viral virulence in persistently infected cell cultures. Studies are continuing on the mechanism of inhibition of virus replication at the non-permissive temperature.

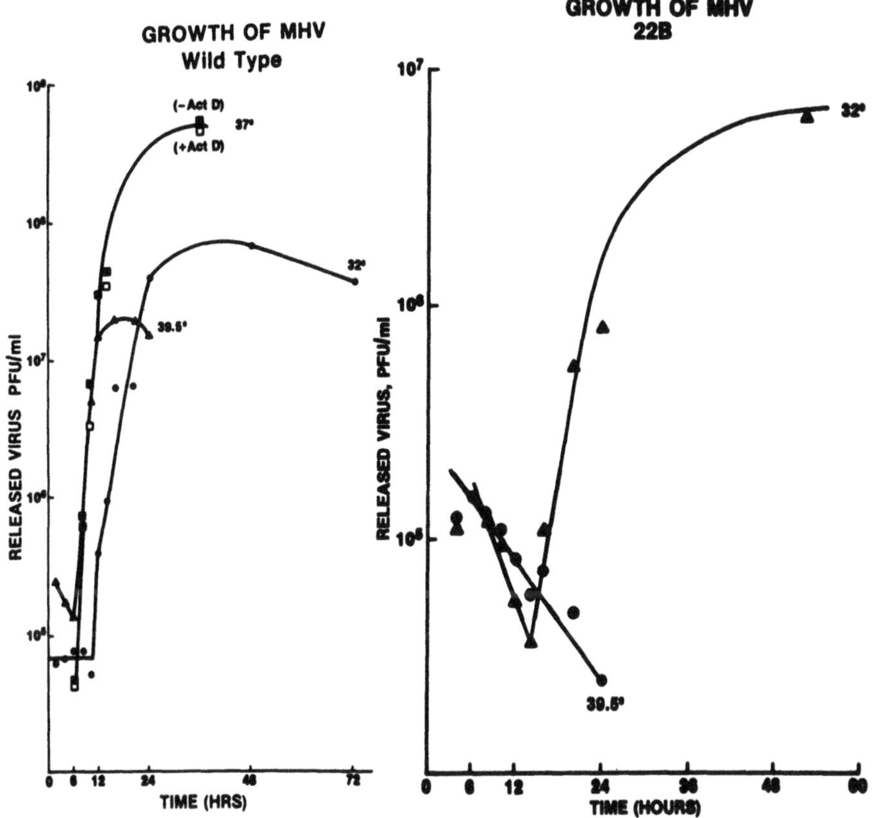

Fig. 9. Growth of WT A59 and the ts mutant 22B at different temperatures. The yield of virus in the supernatent fluid was assayed at 32°. □ yield from cultures treated with 5 μg/ml Actinomycin D; ■ yield without Actinomycin D.

Three mechanisms have been demonstrated for the establishment of persistent infections in a variety of virus-cell systems (Friedman and Ramseur, 1979). The development of ts mutants and their interference with the replication of wild type virus has been shown in rhabdoviruses, togaviruses, and paramyxoviruses. Development of defective interfering particles which interfere with the replication of wild type virus is another factor in persistent infections. Generation of DI virus particles of VSV has been shown to depend upon the host cell (Kang and Allen, 1978). Generation of ts mutants may similarly depend upon a host cell mechanism. The third mechanism for the maintenance of persistent infection *in vitro* is production of interferon (IF). From our persistently infected cell cultures little IF could be detected and VSV could plaque efficiently on the PI cultures. This suggests that IF may not be an important factor in the persistence of A59 virus in these cultures. However,

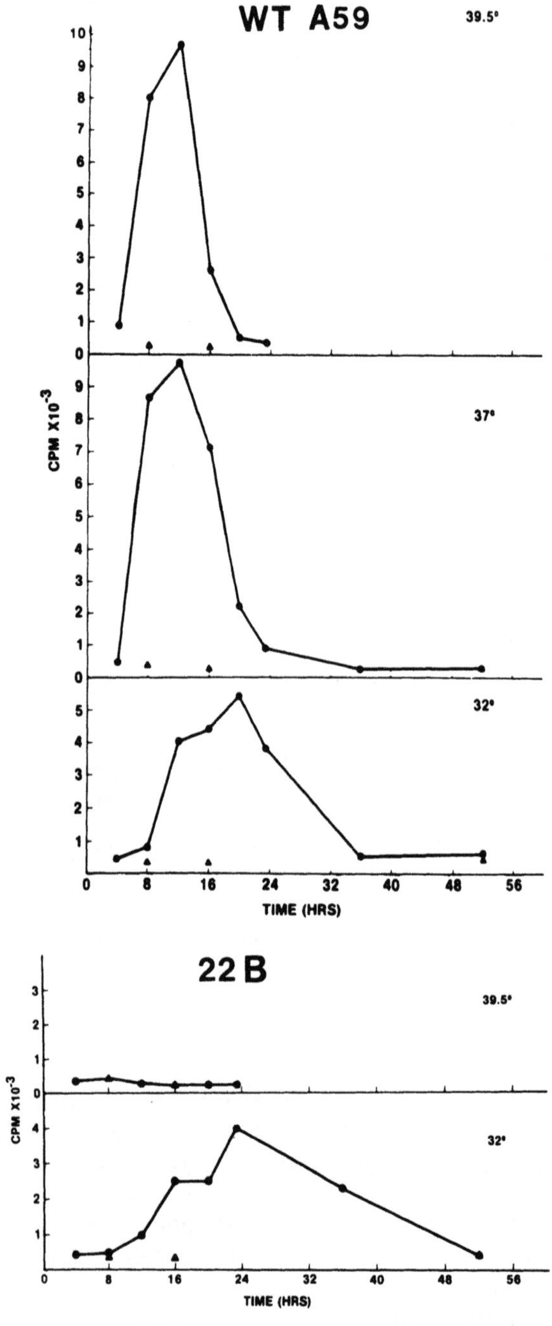

Fig. 10. Synthesis of viral RNA by WT A59 and mutant 22B at different temperatures. ●Incorporation of ^3H uridine into acid insoluble label 4 hr. after the addition of 5 μg/ml Actinomycin D. Cells were labeled for 1 hr. at the times indicated. ▲Incorporation of ^3H uridine into similarly treated uninfected control cells.

Table 1

Inoculum	24 Hour Virus Yield (x 10^4 PFU/ml)* 32°	37°	39.5°
WT A59	8L	105L	73L
ts mutant 22B	56s	2s	0s
Mixed infection (WT A59 - 22B)	6L 43s	1L 1s	1L 0s

*All virus was titered at 32°
L represents large plaque virus
s represents small plaque virus

Table 1. Conditional interference with the replication of wild type A59 by a small plaque, ts mutant derived from a persistently infected culture.

if A59 were sensitive to much lower levels of IF than VSV, IF could still be an important factor in this system. Therefore we cultured PI cells in the presence of anti-IF antibodies and looked for changes in the yield of infectious virus and development of CPE in PI cultures (Sekellick and Marcus, 1979). The persistent infection was not cured by anti-IF antibody and only a modest increase in the yield of infectious virus was detected in anti-IF antibody treated cultures in comparison with those treated with normal rabbit serum. Even passage of the PI culture in the presence of anti-IF antibody did not abrogate the persistent infection nor lead to the development of CPE. Of the three mechanisms for persistent infection shown to operate in other persistent virus infections, we have found only one which may be involved here. That is the development of ts mutants which cause conditional interference with the replication of non-ts virus.

To summarize these experiments, the cells in the PI culture were selected for resistance to viral CPE and became selective for small plaque virus and for ts mutants that could interfere with the growth of non-ts virus. This development of virus resistant cells and coronavirus mutants is like the process of evolution _in vitro_. Similar observations have been made on persistent infections with VSV (Holland et al., 1979). Some unknown factor(s) in the host cell limits replication of wild type virulent virus. This then becomes a selective system for virus variants. Such variants may be preexisting spontaneous mutants or may be the result of host cell action on viral replication. Simultaneously in this process host cells resistant to viral CPE have been selected by the cytolytic effects of virus replication. The virus-cell system has been stabilized to give no apparent CPE and to yield only one plaque morphology of virus. However detailed study has shown that this apparently simple *in vitro* system is very complex.

Similar mechanisms may operate during persistent infections of cells in the respiratory or enteric epithelium *in vivo*, and may in part be responsible for some of the problems associated with the isolation of coronaviruses from persistently infected animals. Additional factors in persistent coronavirus infections *in vivo* are the effects of the host's immune response. Coronaviruses, unlike viruses which bud from the plasma membrane, mature intracellularly before viral antigens are present on the surface of the infected cell. Thus the immune system may not be able to identify and destroy infected cells prior to the maturation of infectious virus. This intracellular maturation, the ability of coronaviruses to replicate in macrophages and the superficial location of virus-infected cells may be additional important mechanisms for coronavirus persistence *in vivo*.

ACKNOWLEDGEMENTS

The authors are grateful for the excellent technical assistance of R. Allen, M. Sharar, K. Clelland, and B. O'Neill. This work was supported by research grant R07403 from the Uniformed Services University of the Health Sciences. The opinions expressed in this report are the private views of the authors and should not be construed as official or as necessarily reflecting the views of the Uniformed Services University of the Department of Defense.

REFERENCES

Behnke, J. N. and Holmes, K. V., 1978, Macromolecular Synthesis of a Temperature Sensitive Mutant of Mouse Hepatitis Virus., *Abstr. Amer. Soc. Microbiol*., p. 251.

Doller, E. W. and Holmes, K. V., 1980, Different Intracellular Transportation of the Envelope Glycoproteins El and E2 of the Coronavirus MHV *Abstr. Amer. Soc. Microbiol*., p. 267.

Evans, M. R. and Simpson, R. W., 1980, The Coronavirus Avian Infectious Bronchitis Virus Requires the Cell Nucleus and Host Transcriptional Factors, *Virol 105*: 582.

Friedman, R. M. and Ramseur, J. M., 1979, Mechanisms of Persistent Infections by Cytopathic Viruses in Tissue Culture. *Arch. Virol*., 60:83.

Holland, J. J., Grabau, E. A., Jones, C. L., and Semler, B. L., 1979, Evolution of Multiple Genome Mutations during Long Term Persistent Infection by Vesicular Stomatitis Virus, *Cell 16*: 495.

Holmes, K. V., 1978, Persistent Infection with a Coronavirus, *IV Internat. Congr. Virol. Abstr*., p. 453.

Kang, C Y. and Allen, R., 1978, Host Function-Dependent Induction of Defective Interfering Particles of Vesicular Stomatitis Virus, *J. Virol*. 25:202

Lucas, A., Coulter, M., Anderson, R. and Dales, S., 1978, In Vivo and In Vitro Models of Demyelinating Diseases. II. Persistence and Host Regulated Thermosensitivity in Cells of Neural Derivation Infected with Mouse Hepatitis and Measles Viruses, Virol. 88: 325.

Sekellick, M. J. and Marcus, P. I., 1979, Persistent Infection II. Interferon-Inducing Temperature-Sensitive Mutants as Mediators of Cell Sparing: Possible Role in Persistent Infection by Vesicular Stomatitis Virus, Virol. 95: 36.

Sturman, L. S. and Takemoto, K. K., 1972, Enhanced Growth of a Murine Coronavirus in Transformed Mouse Cells, Infect. Immun. 6: 501.

PERSISTENT INFECTION WITH MOUSE HEPATITIS VIRUS, JHM STRAIN IN DBT CELL CULTURE

Norio Hirano, Naoaki Goto,* Shinji Makino
and Kosaku Fujiwara*

Department of Veterinary Microbiology, Iwate University
Morioka 020, and *Department of Veterinary Pathology
University of Tokyo, Bunkyo-ku, Tokyo 113, Japan

SUMMARY

After inoculation with JHM strain into DBT cell monolayers, a persistently infected DBT cell culture was established without producing typical cytopathic changes after about 15th passages. By immunofluorescence virus specific antigen was demonstrated in 10 to 15% DBT cells. This persistently infected culture (JHM-CC) was resistant to superinfection with parental JHM, but such resistance was not shown against vesicular stomatitis virus. JHM-CC virus produced small plaques on DBT cell monolayers. Temperature sensitive (TS) mutant, defective interfering (DI) particle or interferon was not detected in the JHM-CC. To intracerebral inoculation with JHM-CC virus, cortisone treated ICR mice survived without showing clinical signs, however, demyelinating lesions were produced in the brain and spinal cord of them.

INTRODUCTION

Mouse hepatitis virus (MHV), a member of coronavirus group, is known to cause hepatitis, encephalitis or enteritis in mice (Robb and Bond, 1978). Among MHV strains, JHM has strong neruotropism characterized by acute and chronic demyelinating encephalitis in mice. Recently, Stohlman and Weiner (1978) reported a persistent infection of JHM in neuroblastoma cells, suggesting that it may provide useful model for studying the mechanism of chronic infection in animal and man.

This study deals with the establishment of carrier culture and some properties of viruses originating from the culture.

MATERIALS AND METHODS

Virus and cell culture : Plaque-purified JHM was propagated in DBT cells and infectivity was assayed by the method as reported previously (Hirano et al, 1974, 1978). DBT cells were grown in Eagle's minimum essential medium (MEM) containing 10% calf serum and 10% tryptose phosphate broth. For virus harvesting and cell maintenance, serum content was reduced to 5%.

Immunofluorescence : Direct immunofluorescence was performed using fluorescein isotyiocyanate-conjugated rabbit IgG against MHV-2 (Hirano et al., 1978). The samples were treated with conjugated antiserum at 37 C for 1 hr.

Interferon assay : Interferon assay was performed by a plaque reduction test using vesicular stomatitis virus (VSV, New Jersy strain) and L cell system as reported previously (Taguchi et al, 1976).

Animal inoculation : Four-week-old male ICR mice were obtained from a breeder colony which was serologically checked for the absence of MHV infection (Fujiwara, 1969). Mice were inoculated intracerebrally (i.c.) with 0.02 ml of virus material, and some mice were injected subcutaneously with 2.5 mg cortisone acetate shortly after virus inoculation.

RESULTS

Establishment and some characterization of a persistently infected DBT cell line : Within 12 hr postinoculation (p.i.) with original JHM, cytopathic effect (CPE) with syncytium formation was evident on DBT cell monolayers and most cells became detached from the glass. However, a few cells still remained and appeared normal in morphology. These remaining cells grew up after changing culture medium and formed a new monolayer. When about 50 to 70% of cell monolayer was established on the glass, passage was done, and syncytium formation was observed in a part of newly established monolayers. After 16th or more passages, syncytium was never formed, and this cell culture was designated as JHM-CC.

By direct immunofluorescence about 10 to 15% cells of the JHM-CC monolayer were found to have virus specific antigen. Especially, strong fluorescence was observed in cells characterized by rounding appearance.

When the culture fluid of JHM-CC was inoculated into a fresh DBT cell monolayer, smaller plaques than those produced by parental JHM were produced in DBT cells. The sizes of plaques formed by JHM-CC virus and JHM were 0.5 to 0.8 and 2 to 4 mm in diameter, respectively (Figure 1). Virus yield was not changed during 80 to 110th passage levels. Figure 2 showed yield of small plaque forming viruses from JHM-CC at the 110 to 130th passage levels.

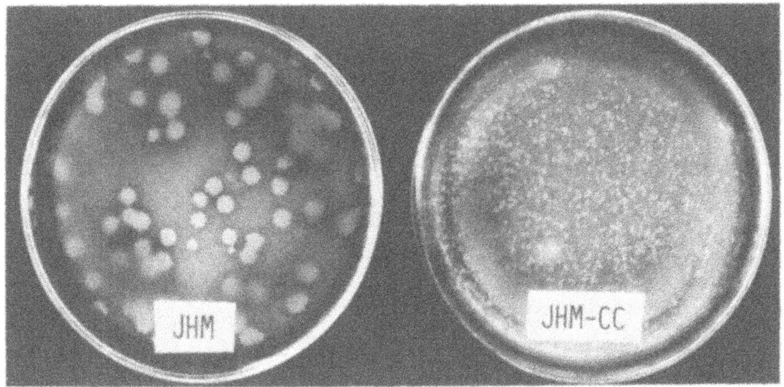

Figure 1. Plaques produced on DBT cell monolayer by JHM and JHM-CC virus at 48 hr p.i.

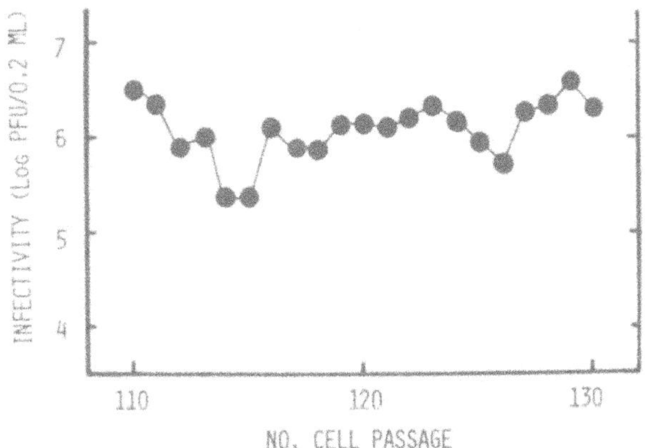

Figure 2. Yield of small plaque forming viruses from the JHM-CC at 110 to 130th passage levels.

JHM-CC monolayers as well as DBT cell monolayers which had been inoculated with JHM (3 PFU/cell) were incubated at different tempertures, 31, 37 and 39 C, and the infectivity of culture fluid was examined at the same temperatures as test incubation at 24 and 72 hr p.i. on DBT cells. As shown in Table 1, there was no difference in virus yield between given temperatures in JHM-CC as well as JHM-infected DBT cells, suggesting that JHM-CC virus is not a temperature sensitive mutant.

From the results obtained, it was evident that JHM-CC virus was less virulent to DBT cells than parent JHM.

To see neurovirulence of JHM-CC virus for mice, 4-week-old ICR

Table 1. Effect of temperatures on virus growth

Virus		Temperature 31	37	39
JHM*	exp.1	6.5**	6.8	6.7
	exp.2	6.5	6.4	6.5
JHM-CC***	exp.1	5.6	5.3	5.5
	exp.2	5.4	5.5	5.3

* JHM harvested at 24 hr p.i. ** Log PFU/0.2 ml
*** JHM-CC harvested at 72 hr p.i.

mice were inoculated i.c. with 10^3 or 10^4 PFU of JHM-CC virus as well as JHM virus. As shown in Table 2, within 3 to 5 days p.i., most of JHM-inoculated mice developed typical central nervous system disorders and died of encephalitis within 10 days. After inoculation with 10^3 to 10^4 PFU of JHM-CC virus, all mice survived for 14 days without any clinical signs even with cortisone treatment. No virus was recovered from the brains of JHM-CC inoculated mice which were sacrificed at 14 days while histopathologically some demyelinating lesions were found in the brain and spinal cord of the survived mice as shown in Figure 3. After inoculation with 10^5 PFU of JHM-CC virus, extensive demyelination was found in the brain stem and cerebellum of the inoculated mice killed at 4 weeks p.i. as shown in Figure 4.

Table 2. Neurovirulence of JHM and JHM-CC virus for 4-week-old mice

Virus	Dose (PFU)	Mortality	Time to death
JHM	10	3/5*	8.3 (7-9)**
	10^2	5/5	8.4 (6-9)
JHM-CC	10^3	0/5	-
	10^4	0/5	-
	10^4 (C)***	0/5	-

* No. dead/tested, 14 days p.i
** Mean time to death in days with range in parenthesis
*** 2.5 mg cortisone administration shortly after virus inoculation.

Resistance of JHM-CC to superinfection : The monolayers of JHM-CC and uninfected DBT cells were inoculated with JHM or other MHV strains (3 PFU/cell). As shown in Table 3, although typical CPE was produced in control DBT cells within 12 hr p.i., no change was detected for 48 hr in the superinfected JHM-CC with JHM or other

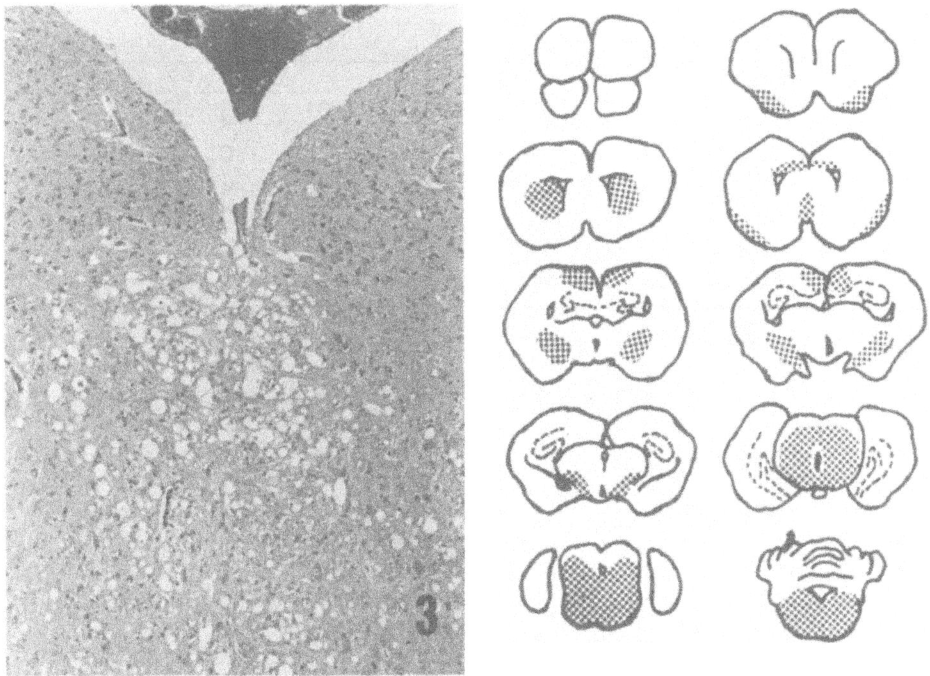

Figure 3. Demyelinating lesions in midbrain of the survived mice after inoculation with 10^4 PFU of JHM-CC virus. Killed at 14 days p.i.

Figure 4. Distribution of demyelinated lesions in the mice inoculated with 10^5 PFU of JHM-CC virus. Killed at 4 weeks p.i.

MHV strains. No progeny of the challenged MHV was recovered from the superinfected JHM-CC, whereas the control DBT cell culture yielded more than 10^6 PFU of MHV after challenge. These findings suggest that JHM-CC interfere with the growth of challeged MHV.

Next, JHM-CC was tested for susceptibility to VSV challenge. JHM-CC and DBT cell monolayers were inoculated with VSV at different doses. After virus inoculation, complete CPE was observed in both JHM-CC and DBT cells, and about 10^7 PFU of VSV were recovered from the both inoculated cultures irrespective of inoculum doses at 24 hr p.i. (Table 4).

Interferon activity was not detected in JHM-CC by assay using VSV and L cell system.

To see the existence of DI particles, DBT cell monolayers were inoculated simultaneously with both JHM virus (3 PFU/cell) and virus from JHM-CC (2 PFU/cell). As control, another group of DBT cell monolayers received a single inoculation with the same dose of JHM. After virus inoculation at 37 C for 1 hr, the inoculated cultures were washed with MEM, given maintenance medium and then incubated

Table 3. Resistance of JHM-CC to superinfection with MHV

Challenge with	CPE		Yield	
	DBT	JHM-CC	DBT	JHM-CC
MHV-1	+	-	6.8*	<1.0
MHV-2	+	-	7.3	<1.0
MHV-3	+	-	6.8	<1.0
JHM	+	-	6.6	<1.0
MHV-A59	+	-	6.8	<1.0

* log PFU/0.2 ml

Table 4. Susceptibility of JHM-CC to superinfection with VSV

VSV (PFU/cell)	Yield	
	DBT	JHM-CC
100	7.5*	6.9
10	7.7	7.0
1	7.7	7.2

* log PFU/0.2 ml

at 37 C for 12 or 24 hr. Within 12 hr p.i. typical syncytium formation was found in the cultures inoculated with two viruses and no difference was seen in yield of JHM virus between single or double infected cultures as shown in Table 5. This suggests that there exists no DI particles in the JHM-CC virus stock.

Table 5. Co-infection of JHM and JHM-CC viruses on DBT cells

Virus (PFU/cell)	Yield	
	12 hr	24 hr p.i
JHM (3)	5.7*	4.1
JHM (3) + JHM-CC (2)	5.8	4.4

* log PFU/0.2 ml

DISCUSSION

The presistent infection seems to result from multiple factors involved in the virus-cell interaction such as the generation of TS mutants (Preble and Younger, 1975), formation of DI particles (Huang and Baltimore, 1970), presence of some virus inhibiting factots (ter Meulen and Martin, 1976) or induction of interferon. However, the persistent infection established with JHM in JHM-CC seems not due to the presence of DI particles, TS mutants or interferon.

Virus specific antigen was found in only 10 to 15% cells of JHM-CC through the experiments. The persistently infected "carrier culture" was divided into three types by Walker (1964), and the persistent case of JHM-CC seems to correspond to that in which the infection is perpetuated in a minority of cells while the most cells are resistant.

JHM-CC virus produced smaller plaques than parent JHM virus in DBT cells and it was less virulent for mice. The correlation between virus plaque size and virulence is well documented with pair of plaque size mutants from a patental stock (Takemoto, 1966). In this case, smaller plaque mutants tend to be less virulent, as shown in this study.

Recently, Stohlman and Weiner (1978) established a persistent infection of JHM in murine neuroblastoma cells and stated that the carried viruses capable causing acute encephalitis were not TS nor plaque mutants. Weiner (1973) described that fatality of JHM infection in mice was dependent upon host age and inoculum dose and that demyelination frequently occurred in non-fatal infection. JHM-CC virus never produced acute encephalitis which is common in parental JHM infection and demyelination occurs in chronic stage of mice that have shown no clinical signs of acute phase.

The persistent infection in JHM-CC in vitro and in vivo system would be helpful in studying the mechanism of chronic and persistent infection with human and animal coronaviruses.

REFERENCES

Fujiwara, K., 1969, Problems in checking inapparent infections in laboratory mouse colonies. An attempt at serological checking by anamnestic response. In : Difining of the laboratory animals. Nat. Acad. Sci. Wash., D.C. 77-97.

Hirano, N., Fujiwara, k., Hino, S., and Matumoto, M., 1974, Replication and plaque formation of mouse hepatitis virus (MHV-2) in mouse cell line DBT culture. Arch. ges. Virusforsch. 44:298-302.

Hirano, N., Murakami, K., Fujiwara, K., and Matumoto, M., 1978, Utility of mouse cell line DBT for propagation and assay of mouse hepatitis virus. Japan. J. Exp. Med. 48:71-75.

Huang, A. S., and Baltimore, D., 1970, Defective viral particles and viral disease prosesses. Nature (London) 226: 325.

Preble, O. T., and Younger, J.S., 1975, Temperature-sensitive viruses and the etiology of chronic and inapparent infection. J. Inf. Dis. 131:467.

Robb, J. A., and Bond, C. W., 1978, Coronaviridae. Comprehensive Virology 14:

Stohlman, S. A., and Weiner, L. P., 1978, Stability of neurotropic mouse hepatitis virus (JHM strain) during chronic infection of neuroblastoma cells. Arch. Virol. 57:53-61.

Taguchi, F., Hirano, N., Kiuchi, Y., and Fujiwara, K., 1976, Difference in response to mouse hepatitis virus among susceptible mouse strain. Japan. J. Microbiol. 20:293-302.

Takemoto, K. K., 1966, Plaque mutants of animal viruses. Prog. Med. Virol. 8:314-348.

ter Meulen, V., and Martin, S. J., 1976, Genesis and maintenance of a persistent infection by canine distemper virus. J. Gen. Virol. 32:431-440.

Walker, D. L., 1964, The viral carrier state in animal cell culture. Prog. Med. Virol. 6:111-148.

Weiner, L. P., 1973, Pathogenesis of demyelination induced by mouse hepatitis virus (JHM strain). Arch. Neurol. 28: 293-303.

CHARACTERISTICS OF A LONG TERM IN VITRO PERSISTENT INFECTION WITH HUMAN CORONAVIRUS 229E

G. Chaloner-Larsson and C.M. Johnson-Lussenburg

Department of Microbiology and Immunology
School of Medicine, University of Ottawa
Ottawa, Ontario, K1N 9A9, CANADA

INTRODUCTION

In October of 1978, we were successful in establishing an in vitro persistent infection of a human cell line (L132) with human coronavirus, strain 229E (229E). These persistently infected cells have been shedding virus since that time (over 300 cell passages) to the same high titer of 10^5-10^6pfu/ml every 48 hours. We have been concerned with studies on both the virus isolated from the cultures (termed VH) and the persistently infected cell cultures per se (termed L132/229E or simply HV). Our preliminary findings have been described at previous meetings and a report has been submitted for publication. A brief summary of these results will be given here to provide the necessary background to our present work.

The persistent VH coronavirus was found to be indistinguishable from our stock 229E strain on the basis of morphology and neutralization by specific antiserum. The L132/229E cultures were resistant to superinfection by 229E virus but supported replication of poliovirus (Sabin). So far, of the treatments tried (short term incubation at 41°C or 33°C, six week incubation at 39°C, overgrowth at room temperature or 37°C and cloning), none have been successful in curing the cells of the persistent virus. Our experimental data have eliminated the involvement of interferon or reverse transcriptase in persistence, and since we could show no interference of replication in mixed infections, we have concluded that defective interfering particles are unlikely to play a role in the maintenance of the persistent state. Evidence has been accumulating which suggests that temperature sensitive (or temperature dependent) step(s) either in host cell metabolism or in virus replication must be involved in this persistent system.

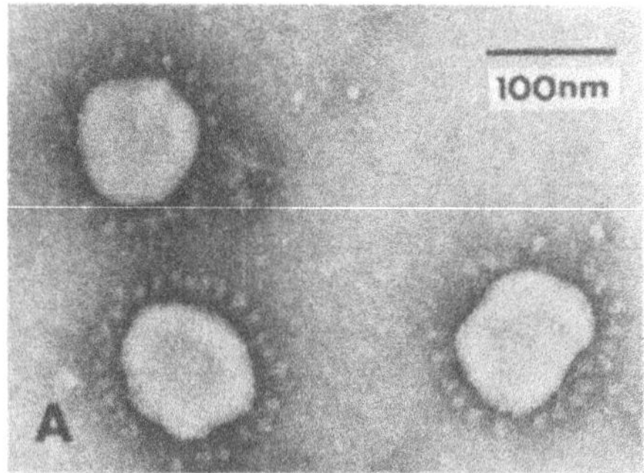

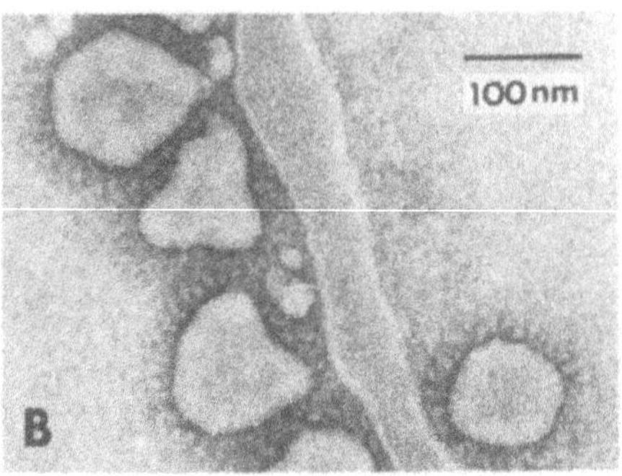

Fig.1. Typical negatively stained virions as found in purified preparations of 229E (A) and supernatant fluids from VH persistently infected cultures (B). Bars represent 100 nm.

In this communication, we will report our recent results which provide further information on the characteristics of both the coronaviruses isolated from the persistent cultures (VH viruses) and the persistently infected cell culture systems (HV cells).

PROPERTIES OF CORONAVIRUS ISOLATED FROM PERSISTENTLY INFECTED CELLS

In several independent attempts, the only successful persistently infected cultures have arisen at 37°C (vide infra) and of these, two, VH1 and VH4 have been studied in detail. The morphology of these viruses was compared with 229E by examining negatively stained preparations of each in the electron microscope. No difference could be seen between the persistently shed virions and the 229E virions as is shown in Figs. 1A and 1B.

Effect of Temperature on Infectivity of VH Viruses

Throughout these studies, temperature has played an unknown but key role in establishing and maintaining the persistently infected cell cultures. To determine whether there was any change in the persistent progeny virus which could be correlated with temperature, the effect of temperature on the stability of the VH and 229E viruses was examined. Suspensions of VH1, VH4 and 229E were incubated at 37°C or 45°C and samples taken at regular intervals were assayed for plaque forming ability on L132 cells. As can be seen in Fig. 2A, there is an almost immediate loss of infectivity of each virus within the first hour at 45°C, while inactivation proceeds more slowly at 37°C being almost complete in 8 hours. There is however, no essential difference in the effect of either temperature on all three viruses.

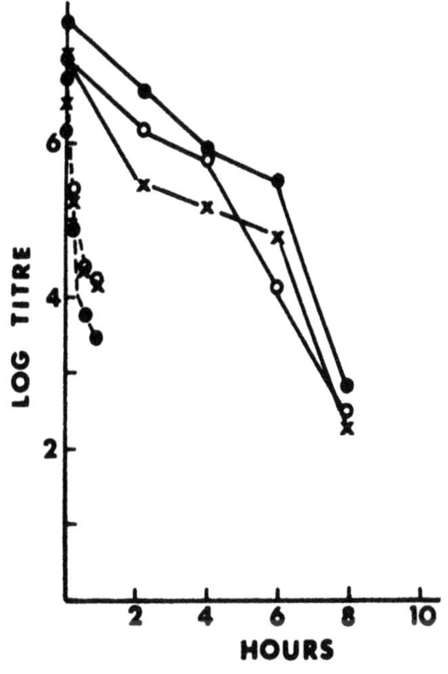

Fig. 2. Effect of temperature on virus infectivity. Clarified infected cell extracts in medium M199 were incubated at 37°C or 45°C. At intervals aliquots were taken and frozen at -20°C. Samples were thawed and titrated by plaque assay[5]. Infectivity is expressed as log pfu/ml. --- 45°C; —— 37°C.

Physical Characteristics of the VH Viruses

The density of the purified VH virions and size of the VH genome was determined. VH virus, labelled in situ with [5-^{3}H]uridine or ^{14}C-amino acids, and VH virus isolated and similarly labelled during an acute infection of L132 cells, were harvested, purified and compared with the standard 229E virus prepared in parallel. The density of the virus as determined by isopycnic sucrose gradient analysis was the same for 229E and VH virus (1.18-1.19 gm/cc; Figs. 3C and 3D). These results also revealed no differences in the VH virus whether harvested directly from the persistent cultures or after propagation in L132 cells at 33°C, the same conditions optimal for growth of our standard virus (data not shown).

RNA isolated from the VH viruses and 229E by treatment with proteinase K/SDS[1] was examined in isokinetic sucrose gradients. As can be seen in Figs. 3A and 3B, the VH and 229E isolated RNA gave the same profile of a single large molecular weight species.

Studies on the Replication of VH Coronaviruses

While an incubation temperature of 37°C is optimal for cell growth and was required for the establishment of persistence, both the iso-

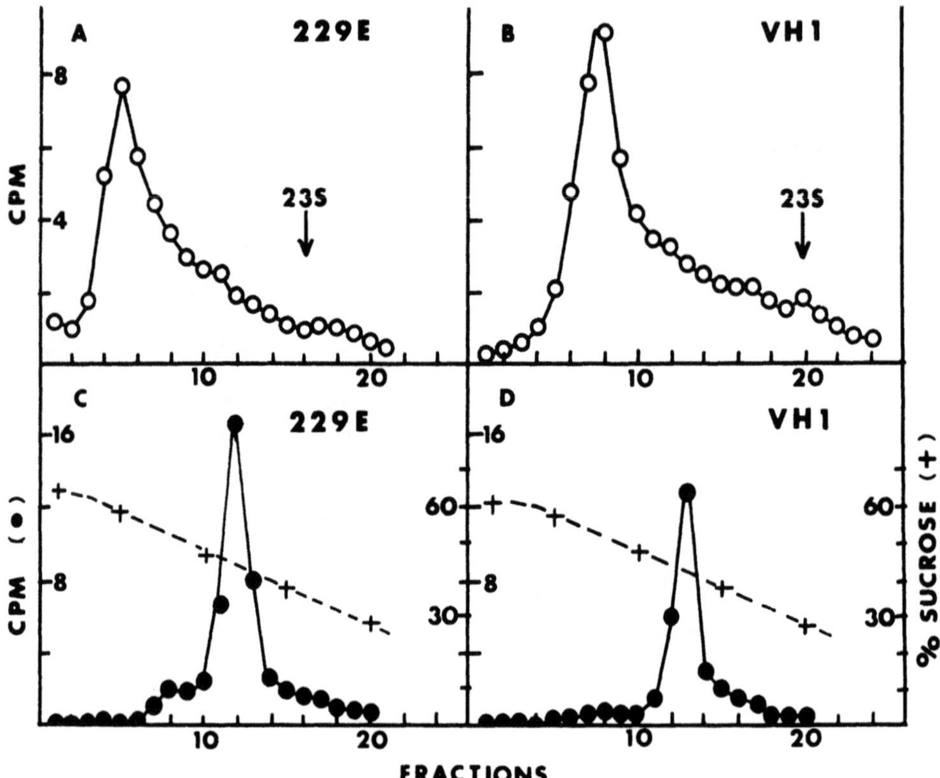

Fig. 3. Sucrose density gradient profiles of ^{3}H-uridine labelled virus and viral RNA. Isokinetic gradients of RNA extracted by proteinase K/SDS from 229E (A) and persistent VH virus (B) were spun at 43K g for 10 h through a 5-25% linear gradient containing SDS. Isopycnic gradients of purified 229E virus (C) and VH virus (D) were spun at 63K g for 18 h through a 25-65% linear gradient. Sedimentation in all cases was from right to left.

lated VH virus and the parental 229E replicate in L132 cells most efficiently at 33°C. And despite the lack of cytopathic effects of the VH viruses in the persistent cultures (at 37°C), they are apparently more cytocidal than the parent 229E virus in L132 cells at 33°C. In fact, from the earliest titrations of the VH viruses, there has been a consistent difference in plaque development and morphology: namely that, when isolated, the VH viruses produce clearer, slightly larger plaques which develop earlier (Figs. 4A and 4B). To date, this has been the only visible difference identified which could be regarded as a marker characteristic.

In further studies the increased cytocidal property was correlated to the earlier destruction of the L132 cell monolayer seen after infection with VH viruses. A comparison of the growth curves of the VH and

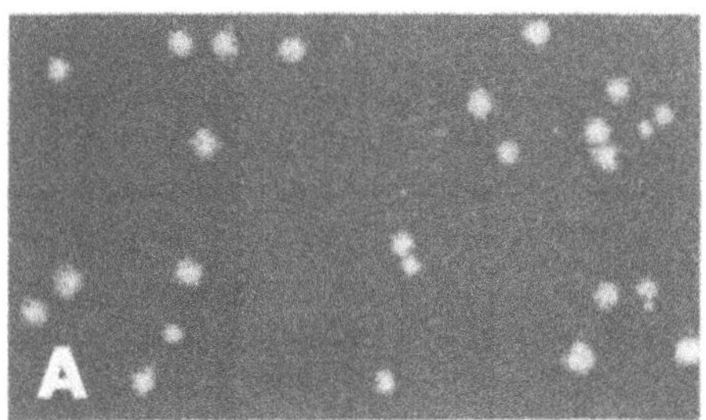

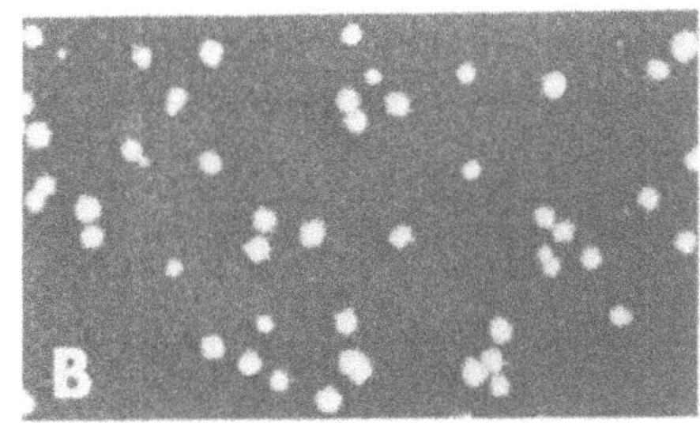

Fig. 4. Plaque morphology of 229E (A) and VH persistent (B) viruses. Dilutions of virus were inoculated onto L132 monolayers and plaques allowed to develop under agar for 6 days at 33°C. Plaques were visualized after fixation with formalin by staining with crystal violet. VH plaques developed earlier and were clearer than 229E virus plaques.

229E viruses revealed that the persistent VH virus did indeed replicate faster and to higher yields than did the stock virus (Fig.5).

The stability of this plaque morphology characteristic was evaluated by examining the yield of a number of serial infections of L132 cells with either stock 229E or the VH viruses at different multiplicities of infection. The results of these experiments are shown in Table 1. All infected cultures were incubated in parallel at 33°C following the initial 1 hour adsorption period at room temperature. Total virus yield was determined by plaque assay of frozen-thawed whole cultures[2]. The characteristics of the plaques produced by all the VH viruses regardless of the number of serial passages was indistinguishable from that originally described (Fig. 4A).

In the series A experiments, there was a 50% decrease in yield of 229E following three serial infections with the usual MOI used for 229E production. This is constrasted in series B by the gradual buildup in the yield of 229E during the six serial passages using at least tenfold lower multiplicities of infection. This result might be taken as an indication of the generation of defective interfering (DI) particles in series A by the stock 229E. However, in both series the VH1 isolate gave remarkably stable yields at both high and low MOI. In fact the yields were consistently one log higher throughout these experiments and appeared to correlate directly with the increase in MOI. The situation with VH4 was similar to VH1, especially at the higher MOI, but yields were somewhat lower in the B series. The reasons for this are unknown, however, in our experience growth characteristics of VH4 usually were found to lie somewhere between the VH1 and 229E results. It was concluded that, within the limits of these experiments, the plaque morphology of the VH viruses was a stable characteristic. Furthermore, the high yields of virus appeared to be stable.

Table 1. Yields of Serial Infection in L132 Cells

	Series A			Series B		
Virus	Pass.	MOI	Yield (pfu/mlx10^7)	Pass.	MOI	Yield (pfu/mlx10^7)
229E	1)	2.0	6.0	1)	0.2	1.29
	2)	2.0	4.0	2)	0.06	3.21
	3)	1.5	3.1	3)	0.16	2.73
				4)	0.13	3.96
				5)	0.2	4.05
				6)	0.2	5.07
VH1	1)	10	64.0	1)	0.2	5.9
	2)	20	68.0	2)	0.3	24.0
	3)	20	70.0	3)	1.2	24.0
				4)	1.2	24.0
				5)	1.2	21.0
				6)	1.0	24.0
VH4	1)	2	31.0	1)	0.2	0.06
	2)	10	30.0	2)	0.003	0.6
	3)	10	29.0	3)	0.03	3.0
				4)	0.15	4.02
				5)	0.2	3.96
				6)	0.2	8.76

We next examined the effect of temperature on the replication of the 229E and VH viruses. As stated earlier, though 37°C was optimal for cell growth and was required for the establishment of persistence both the isolated VH virus and 229E replicated most efficiently at 33°C. Virus replication at three temperatures, 33°C, 37°C and 39°C was evaluated on the basis of plaquing efficiency and virus yields at 40 hours post infection (h.p.i.). A preliminary, one-way temperature shift experiment was then performed to determine if the effect of temperature could be associated with an early event in replication. The results of these experiments are shown in Table 2. It is clear that virus replication is partially inhibited at 37°C and completely inhibited at 37°C and completely inhibited at 39°C for both 229E and the VH viruses.

The results of the temperature shift experiment demonstrate that residual virus inoculum is still detectable in relatively large quantities, a fact also noted in the growth curve experiment (Fig.5) where at 4 h.p.i., 10^3-10^4pfu/ml of residual infectious virus were detected.

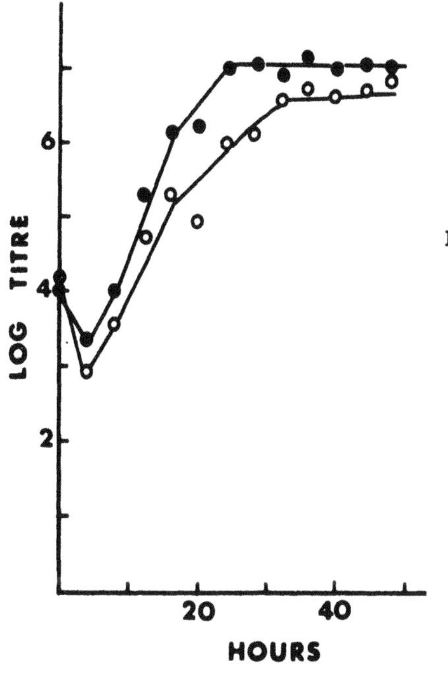

Fig. 5. Growth curves of 229E (o) and VH1 (•) viruses. Virus at 3-5 moi was adsorbed in replicate onto L132 cells for 1 h at rm temp. The inoculum was replaced with M199 and cultures incubated at 33°C. At 4 h intervals, sample cultures were removed, subjected to 3 freeze-thaw cycles and stored at -20°C. Samples were titrated in duplicate by plaque assay.
Titres are expressed as log pfu/ml.

After 24 hours incubation at 33°C, all three viruses showed two to three log increases in virus titres, the VH viruses having the greatest increase. Again, no virus was detectable after 24 hours incubation at 39°C which confirmed the observations of the previous experiments. When however, infected cells were shifted to 39°C after an initial 4 hour period of incubation at 33°C, there was a marked difference in the yields of the VH viruses compared to the standard 229E. In the latter case, no 229E was detected while in the former, small quantities of both VH viruses were found at concentrations about two logs lower than the residual virus inoculum found after the initial 4 hour, 33°C incubation.

Although these results do not show whether the VH viruses, when inside the cell were less susceptible to temperature inactivation or whether the VH viruses detected represented progeny virus synthesized at reduced rates, they do suggest once again, a temperature related difference between the standard and persistent viruses. Moreover, these results indicate the direction of further experiments necessary to the understanding of temperature involvement in this persistent system.

PROPERTIES OF THE PERSISTENTLY INFECTED CELLS

The establishment and maintenance of five parallel persistently infected cultures was achieved on the second attempt (Table 3). The cultures were numerically identified, two (HV1 and HV4) were chosen

Table 2. Effect of Temperature on Coronavirus Replication

Experiments	Virus	Incubation Temperature 33°	37°	39°
I Plaquing Efficiency	229E	$4.0x10^7$	$1.2x10^7$ (30%)	0
	VH1	$2.1x10^8$	$8.0x10^7$ (38%)	0
	VH4	$5.5x10^7$	$2.7x10^7$ (49%)	0
II Virus Yields 40 h.p.i.	229E	$3.9x10^7$	$3.7x10^6$ (9.3%)	0
	VH1	$2.1x10^8$	$2.1x10^7$ (10%)	0
	VH4	$1.2x10^8$	$1.2x10^7$ (10%)	0

III	Virus	33° 4 h	33° 24 h	39° 24 h	33°/4 h → 39°/20 h
Virus Yields Temperature Shift	229E	$1.6x10^5$	$1.9x10^7$	0	0
	VH1	$2.1x10^5$	$1.47x10^8$	0	$3.3x10^3$
	VH4	$7.8x10^4$	$7.5x10^7$	0	$3.0x10^2$

arbitrarily for further detailed study and the others were stored in liquid N_2. Since then, efforst have been made to repeat these experiments to help provide an understanding of the mechanisms involved in their establishment especially the temperature requirement. To date, five independent attempts have been made and the results are summarized in Table 3. In several trials, persistent VH virus was also used and it is of interest to note that with these, stable cultures were also successfully established but only on two occasions. On the basis of this experience, the only conclusions which we can draw are that while it was not difficult, we have not yet found a standard method by which one can predictably or readily establish a persistent infection of L132 cells with 229E except that a temperature of 37°C is a requirement.

Effect of Temperature on Virus Shed by Persistently Infected Cells

Further studies to explore the role of temperature in the persistent cell cultures were concerned with the effect of temperature on

Table 3. Attempts to Establish 229E Persistently Infected Cultures of L132 Cells

Trial	Number of Cultures	Virus	Duration	Result
1	5	229E	1 mo	Unstable
2	5	229E	24 mo	Stable
3	4	229E	2 mo	Unstable
4	2	VH1	1 wk	Acute
	2	VH4	1 wk	Acute
5	3	229E	1 mo	Unstable
	3	VH1	1 wk	Acute
	3	VH4	5 mo*	Stable
6	4	229E	1 mo	Unstable
7	3	229E	2 mo*	Stable
		VH1	2 mo*	Stable
		VH4	1 wk	Acute

* Stored in liquid N_2 for future study.

persistence. Routine maintenance of our two persistent culture (HV1 and HV4) consisted of a regular schedule of passaging at a split ratio of 1:3 every two days with incubation at 37°C. Virus shedding was monitored at intervals over the two day periods and the increase in titres of the persistent VH virus shed into the medium was found to correlate directly with the increase in number of cells in culture. However, when growth of the persistently infected cells was carried out at various temperatures different results were obtained. Stable cell growth and maximum virus shedding occurred at the optimal cell growth temperature of 37°C. But at 33°C cell growth deteriorated, virus shedding decreased and the cultures eventually died out even if returned to 37°C. At 39°C cell growth was aberrant (similar to uninfected cells) and splitting was continued only when the cells reached confluency (4-7 days). Virus shedding was erratic but both cell growth and virus shedding resumed at normal levels when the cultures were returned to 37°C incubation, even after periods as long as six weeks.

The results of these studies correlating the incubation temperature with the quantity of VH virus shed by the persistently infected cells are summarized diagrammatically in Fig.6. Since we have no firm evidence that replication of persistent VH virus occurs at 39°C, our tentative conclusion is that the virus must be protected in situ in the persistently infected cells. Further investigations of this phenomenon are necessary before final conclusions can be made.

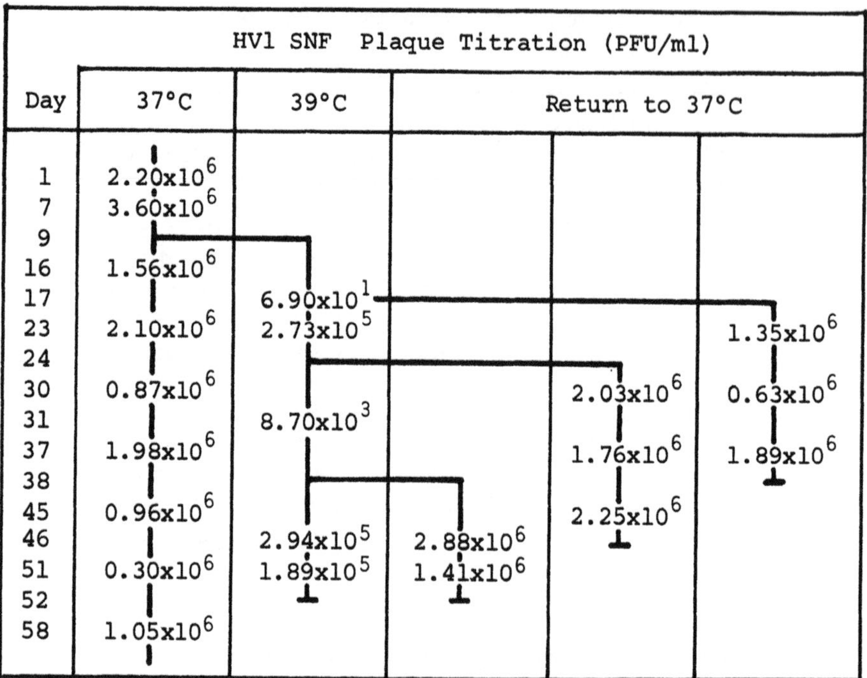

Day	HV1 SNF Plaque Titration (PFU/ml)				
	37°C	39°C	Return to 37°C		
1	2.20×10^6				
7	3.60×10^6				
9					
16	1.56×10^6				
17		6.90×10^1			
23	2.10×10^6	2.73×10^5			1.35×10^6
24					
30	0.87×10^6			2.03×10^6	0.63×10^6
31		8.70×10^3			
37	1.98×10^6			1.76×10^6	1.89×10^6
38					
45	0.96×10^6			2.25×10^6	
46		2.94×10^5	2.88×10^6		
51	0.30×10^6	1.89×10^5	1.41×10^6		
52					
58	1.05×10^6				

Fig. 6. Temperature effect on virus shed by persistently infected cells. Cells passaged regularly at 37°C were split on day 9 and some were incubated at 39°C. After passaging on days 17, 24, and 38, some of these 39°C cultures were returned to 37°C. At intervals samples of supernatant fluid were removed and titrated by plaque assay.

Comparison of Coronavirus Persistently Infected Cells with Uninfected L132 Cells

Comparative studies of the uninfected L132 cells and the persistent cell cultures have been performed to determine if detectable changes have occurred. Most of the characteristics, cell growth, full monolayer morphology and chromosome counts[3], were similar. The only consistent difference could be seen when the cells were growing at low density. This visual difference between the uninfected L132 and the persistently infected L132 cells was most apparent on the first day after passage when the pattern of spreading of the persistent cultures could be distinguished from the normal cell cultures. The process of spreading involved much less elongation of the persistent cells. At confluence, the monolayers were virtually identical.

Number of Virus-producing Cells in Persistently Infected Cultures

Infections centres assay was carried out to determine the number of virus-shedding cells in the cultures. Our results have shown that 50-100% of the cells were infected. Confirmation of this finding was sought by parallel studies involving cloning to determine whether all cells were infected and also whether other growth characteristics had been altered. Both persistently infected and uninfected L132 cells have been cloned and in all cases the cells showed essentially the same efficiency of cloning. Of interest however, was the finding that all the clones from the persistently infected cells initially did not shed virus but were resistant to superinfection by coronavirus 229E. After 25 passages of these cultures, virus shedding had resumed. (Data not shown). This indicated that the VH virus could be sequestered in the persistently infected cells.

Morphology of Persistently Infected Cells and of Normal Cells Acutely Infected with Persistent VH Virus

In addition to comparisons of the negatively stained virions in the electron microscope (Fig.1), thin sections of cell monolayers have been prepared for EM characterization. Monolayers of uninfected L132 cells, of persistently infected L132 cells and of L132 cells acutely infected with either 229E or VH viruses were fixed and Epon 812-embedded in situ (I.Dardick, personal communication). Thin sections were prepared, stained with lead citrate and uranyl acetate and examined in a Philips EM 300 electron microscope. In comparisons between the acute and persistently infected cells, though fewer virus particles were seen in the latter, in both cases virions were seen lined up along the surfaces of the cells and within cell vesicles (Figs.7A and 7B). The significance of the rather amorphous material regularly seen in association with the persistent VH virions is not known at this time.

When we compared the appearance of the L132 cells following acute infection with either 229E or VH viruses, no differences could be noted (Figs.7C and 7D). In both cases large numbers of virions were seen characteristically lined up along the cell surfaces and in the cell vesicles and intracellular spaces[4]. So far, in these preparations we have not seen the amorphous material referred to above in association with 229E or VH viruses either within vesicles or lined up along the cell surfaces.

We are presently engaged in further morphological studies using immune labelling techniques to locate and identify developing viral components within the cytoplasm and in association with the endoplasmic reticulum of the persistently infected cells. The results of these studies will be of value in further characterization of the persistent system but whether any relevant differences will be identified remains to be seen.

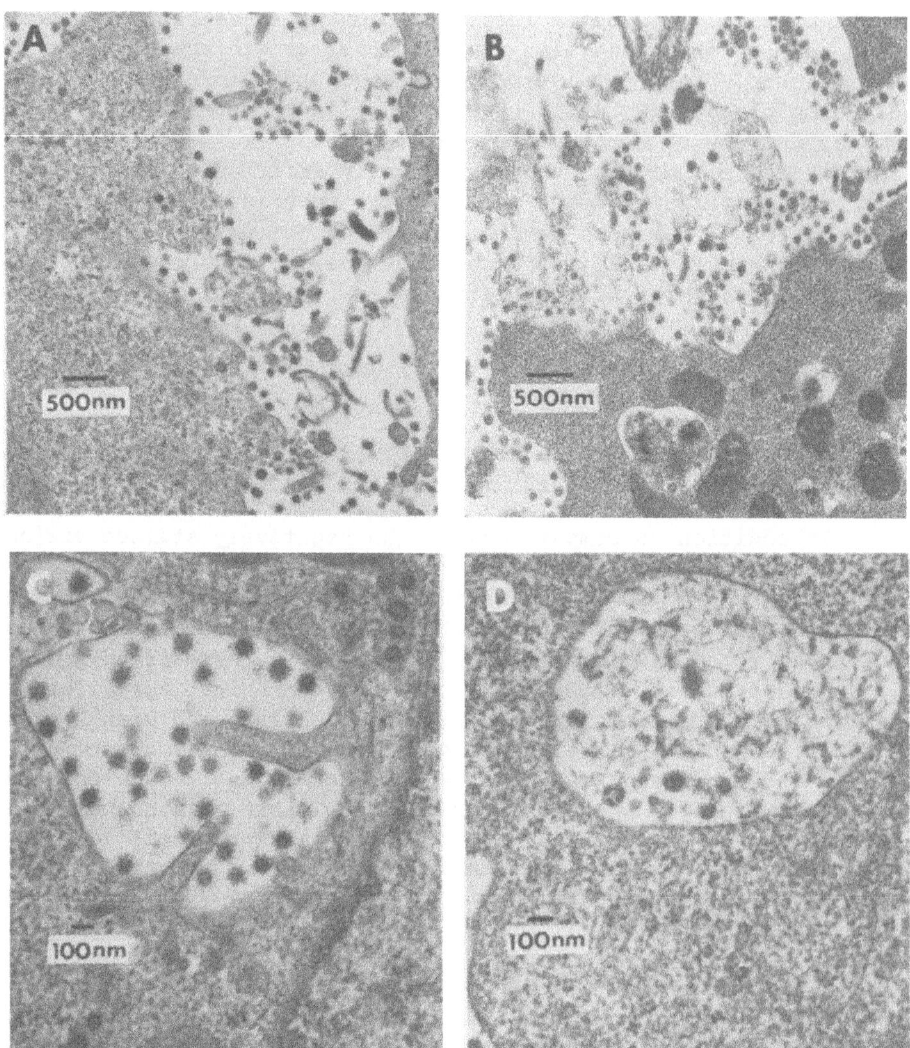

Fig. 7. Thin sections of cell monolayers embedded in situ showing coronavirus particles. Typical coronavirions are seen along the cell surfaces of L132 cells infected with 229E (A) or with VH persistent virus (B). Coronavirions are also seen in vesicles in the cytoplasm of 229E infected L132 cells (C) and HV1 persistently infected cultures (D).

CONCLUDING REMARKS

Our studies so far, have been aimed at the elucidation of the mechanisms involved in establishing and maintaining the coronavirus HCV/229E persistent infection of L132 cells. On the basis of the accumulated evidence, it seems clear that this human coronavirus: human cell persistent system belongs to the class of persistent noncytocidal infections transmitted through cell division[5]. This implies that all the cells contain copies of the viral genome and that expression of the genome requires host permissiveness.

To date our results have shown that the only difference between the acute and persistent infections of the same cell type with the same(?) virus were associated with temperature. Comparisons of the properties of standard 229E with the VH virus derived from the persistently infected L132 cultures have demonstrated no differences beyond an increased efficiency of replication of VH at the optimal temperature (33°C) with greater apparent cytopathic effect. Our experiments on the effect of temperature on virus shedding by persistently infected cultures have demonstrated that the expression of the viral genome along with normal cell replication was dependent on temperature (37°C). At higher temperatures (39°C) virus shedding diminished and the genome was not eliminated because virus shedding resumed normal levels once the cells were shifted back. However, when the persistently infected cells were incubated at the lower temperature (33°C) the cells were ultimately destroyed.

Our preliminary evidence seems to suggest that the effect of temperature is mediated through an alteration in host cell function implying the essential contribution of some host cell product to viral replication. The existence of such a host cell contribution was suggested by the effect of actinomycin D on 229E replication in L132 cells[6]. Further studies are aimed at an understanding of the role of temperature, including the effect of actinomycin D, and the identification of the essential component(s) contributed by the host cell.

REFERENCES

1. M.R. Macnaughton and M. H. Madge, The genome of human coronavirus strain 229E, J. gen. Virol. 39:497 (1978).
2. D. A. Kennedy and C. M. Johnson-Lussensburg, Isolation and morphology of the internal component of human coronavirus, strain 229E, Intervirol. 6:197 (1975/76).
3. R. G. Worton and C. Duff, Karyotyping, in "Methods in Enzymology vol LVIII", S. P. Colowick and N. O. Kaplan, eds., Academic Press, N. Y., (1979).
4. L. S. Oshiro, J. H. Schieble, and E. L. Lennette, Electron microscopic studies of coronavirus, J. gen. Virol. 12:161 (1971).

5. W. K. Joklik, Summary of mechanisms involved in persistent viral infections, in "Microbiology 1977", D. Schlessinger, ed. A. S. M. Washington, D. C. (1977).
6. D. A. Kennedy and C. M. Johnson-Lussenburg, Inhibition of coronavirus 229E replication by actinomycin D, J. Virol, 29:401 (1979).

(Supported by the Medical Research Council of Canada and the Multiple Sclerosis Society of Canada)

CORONAVIRUS ANTIBODIES IN PATIENTS WITH MULTIPLE SCLEROSIS

P.O. Leinikki, Kathryn V. Holmes, Isabel Shekarchi,
M. Iivanainen, D. Madden and J.L. Sever

Institute of Biomedical Sciences, University of Tampere, 33520 Tampere, Finland; Infections Diseases Branch, NINCDS, NIH, Bethesda, Md 20205 and Department of Pathology, Uniform Services University of the Health Sciences, 4301 Jones Bridge Road, Bethesda, Md 20014, USA

INTRODUCTION

Several strains of murine coronavirus are able to induce a demyelinative disease in laboratory animals. The disease is characterized by a chronic course with relapses after the initial phase of acute encephalitis (Herdon et al., 1975; Holmes et al., 1980). Recently a coronavirus has also been implicated in human demyelinative disease, multiple sclerosis (Burks et al., 1980). In order to determine whether a coronavirus etiology for MS could be demonstrated in analogy to the role of measles virus in SSPE, we have studied the occurrence of coronavirus antibodies in two collections of clinical material.

MATERIAL AND METHODS

The antibody levels for three different coronaviruses, OC43, 229E and A59 (a murine strain) were compared in 56 patients with multiple sclerosis (MS) in a clinically stable phase and their carefully matched controls (Madden et al., 1980). In the other collection we analyzed the levels of OC43 antibodies in a series of patients with acute clinical disease. Eighteen had MS, 8 had optic neuritis (ON), 27 had other neurological diseases (OND) and 88 were judged as controls without neurological disease by a careful clinical follow-up for more than a year after the samples were taken (Leinikki et al., 1980).

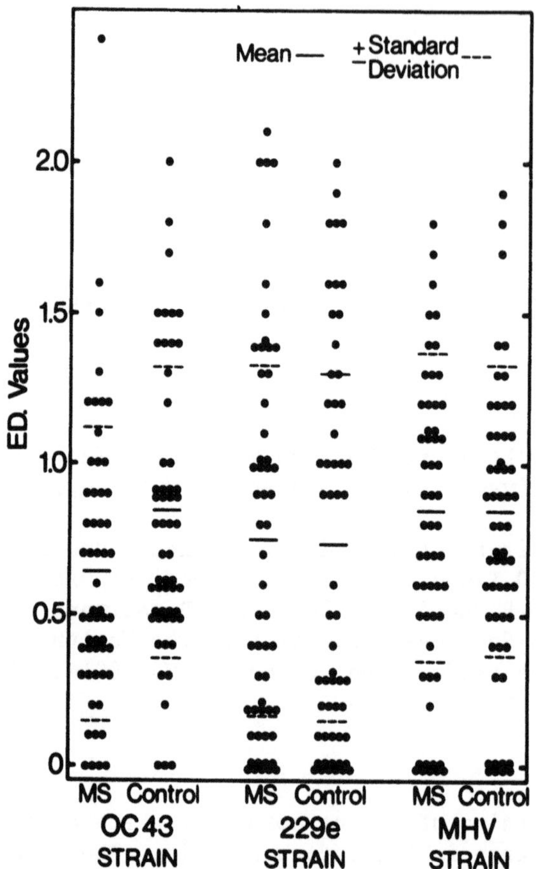

Figure. Occurrence of coronavirus OC_{43}, 229e and A59 antibody in 56 multiple sclerosis (MS) patients and matched controls.

The antibody assays were made by using ELISA as described (Leinikki and Pässilä, 1976). Tissue culture derived 229E and A59 viruses and mouse brain derived OC_{43} viruses were used for the sensitization of polystyrene cuvettes. Sera or cerebrospinal fluid (CSF) were incubated in the cuvettes and the amount of fixed IgG was determined by using alkaline-phosphatase conjugated anti-IgG. The results were calculated by comparing the optical density given by the sample with that of a standard curve and expressed as logarithmic ED-values (Leinikki and Pässilä, 1977).

RESULTS AND DISCUSSION

In the 56 MS patients with stable disease no difference was found in the distribution of antibody activities when compared to the controls with any of the three coronavirus antigens. (Figure). According to the ED-values, a very high number of patients and controls had various coronavirus antibodies. However, in a sensitive assay like ELISA the cut-off for seronegativity is often difficult to determine before a large clinical material has been analyzed. It is possible that part of the samples with low ED actually should be regarded as seronegatives. This however, does not alter the interpretation of the data from figure 1; the distribution of both high and low ED-values is quite similar for MS and controls. The high incidence of A59-antibodies both in MS and in controls suggest a strong cross reaction between murine and human coronavirus strains.

Table 1. Mean Values (ED±SD) of Serum Antibody Levels in different Patients Groups

	PATIENT GROUP			
VIRUS	MS	ON	OND	CONTR
CORONA	0.6±0.3	0.6±0.2	0.7±0.4	0.8±0.4
MEASLES	1.9±0.6	1.7±0.2	1.8±0.5	1.7±0.5
RUBELLA	1.6±0.4	1.6±0.5	1.9±0.6	1.7±0.5
VACCINIA	0.6±0.7	0.5±0.2	0.7±0.4	0.7±0.3
MUMPS	0.9±0.3	1.3±0.3	1.0±0.3	1.1±0.5

In the patients with acute disease the mean titres of serum antibodies were quite similar in the different study groups (Table 1). On the contrary, CSF antibody levels were significantly elevated in MS as judged from serum/CSF-antibody ratios (Table 2). However, a similar increase was found with several different viral antigens such as measles, rubella, vaccinia and mumps. Also the amount of increase of these unrelated viral antibodies was very similar in many individual patients. No correlation was found between the antibody levels and parameters for blood-brain-barrier condition such as serum and CSF albumin, IgG and total protein as measured by standard nephelometric techniques indicating that the antibodies are synthesized within the central nervous system.

The results indicate that seroepidemiologically no significant difference can be detected between MS and other patient groups or controls in their relationsip with coronaviruses. They also suggest that the elevation of coronavirus antibodies in CSF of MS patients

Table 2. Mean (±SD) of Serum/CSF Virus Antibody Ratios (ED serum - ED CSF) in Various Patient Groups

VIRUS	PATIENT GROUP MS	(N)[a]	ON	(N)	OND	(N)	CONTR	(N)
CORONA	1.5±0.1	(4)	-	(0)	2.1±0.2	(9)	2.3±0.2	(8)
MEASLES	1.6±0.2	(17)	2.0±0.3	(8)	2.2±0.3	(27)	2.5±0.2	(78)
RUBELLA	1.6±0.3	(18)	2.1±0.3	(6)	2.4±0.2	(26)	2.5±0.2	(74)
VACCINIA	1.3±0.7	(4)	1.5±0.2	(2)	2.2±0.3	(6)	2.3±0.2	(8)
MUMPS	1.8±0.1	(9)	2.1±0.2	(6)	2.3±0.1	(7)	2.5±0.3	(31)
ALL VIRUSES	1.6±0.3	(18)	2.1±0.2	(8)	2.3±0.3	(27)	2.5±0.2	(87)

[a]Number of patients with detectable CSF antibody levels.

in acute stage is caused by nonspecific stimulus which also increases the synthesis of several other viral antibodies within the central nervous system of these patients. These antibodies reflect an immunological disturbance rather than etiological relationship.

REFERENCES

Burks, J. S., DeVald, B. L., Jankovsky, L. D., and Gerdes, J. C., 1980, Two coronaviruses isolated from central nervous system tissue of two multiple sclerosis patients, Science, 209:933-934.

Herdon, R. M., Griffin, D. E., McCormick, U., Weiner, L. D., 1975, Mouse hepatitis virus-induced recurrent demyelination, Arch. Neurol., 32:32-35.

Holmes, K., Leinikki, P., Shekarchi, I., and Sever, J. L., 1980, A chronic neurological disease induced by murine coronavirus strain A 59. In preparation.

Leinikki, P., Shekarchi, I., Iivanainen, M., Taskinen, E., Holmes, K., Madden, D., and Sever, J., 1980, Virus antibodies in the cerebrospinal fluid in multiple sclerosis by using ELISA. Neurology, submitted.

Leinikki, P., Pässilä, S., 1976, Solid phase antibody assay by means of enzyme conjugated to anti-immunoglobulin, J. Clin. Pathol., 29:1116-1120.

Leinikki, P., and Pässilä, S., 1977, Quantitative, semiautomated entzyme linked immunosorbent assay for viral antibodies. J. Infect. Dis. 136:294-300, 1977.

Madden, D., Wallen, W., Houff, S., Shekarchi, I., Leinikki, P., Castellano, G., Holmes, K., and Sever, J., Humoral and cellular immune responses of multiple sclerosis patients.

JHM INFECTIONS IN RATS AS A MODEL FOR ACUTE AND SUBACUTE DEMYELINATING DISEASE

Helmut Wege, Makoto Koga, Hanna Wege and Volker ter Meulen
Institute for Virology and Immunobiology
University of Würzburg
D -8700 Würzburg,
Federal Republic of Germany

SUMMARY

An animal model with different central nervous system (CNS) disease processes associated with demyelination is described which provides a basis to analyse the pathogenetic mechanisms leading to these disorders. Intracerebral infection of rats with the murine coronavirus strain JHM can result in an acute encephalomyelitis with a short incubation period or in subacute to chronic encephalomyelitis occurring after prolonged incubation. The most prominent finding of the latter two diseases consists of typical demyelinated lesions distributed in selected areas of the CNS. The induction of high rates of animals with demyelination depends both on properties of the virus used for infection and host factors such as age and immune status. A high number of rats with demyelination was obtained by intracerebral inoculation of temperature sensitive mutants into suckling rats with maternal JHM antibodies.

INTRODUCTION

Subacute and chronic diseases of the central nervous system (CNS) in animal and man are often associated with a persistent virus infection (6). In such disorders a selective demyelination may occur which is a prominent neuropathological finding. The detection of virus particles in brain tissue has led to the assumption that the destruction of oligodendroglia cells by viruses may possibly be the underlying mechanism of demyelination.

However, available laboratory evidence suggest that the events leading to virus induced demyelination are probably of a more complex nature. Beside the genetic basis of the diseases as well as host reactions to the infections, the specific virus cell interactions which allow the agents to persist are of great interest in the studies to unreveal the pathogenesis of these diseases.

One model for virus induced demyelination is the infection of mice and rats with the neurotropic murine coronavirus strain JHM (1,2,3,4,5,13). In both animals an acute disseminated encephalomyelitis with areas of demyelination in brain and spinal cord can be induced. However, in contrast to mice, where it is difficult to obtain experimentally a subacute CNS disease, rats develop under defined conditions a high rate of marked demyelination without signs of an acute infection after prolonged incubation period (1,7,8,9).

The present communication describes the different CNS disease types observed in rats after JHM virus infection and the virological findings observed in these disorders.

TYPES OF CNS-DISEASES OBSERVED AFTER JHM VIRUS INFECTION

Acute Panencephalitis (APE). Intracerebral inoculation of suckling rats (outbred strain CHBB/Thom) leads after an incubation period of 2 - 8 days to an acute CNS disease which is neuropathologically characterized by widespread necrotic lesions and partly demyelination especially in the cerebral cortex, brainstem and spinal grey matter (7). Virus particles are easily detected in both neurons and glia cells. Inflammatory lesions are also found in the liver.

After intracerebral infection of weanling rats (age 20 -25 days) three different types of CNS-diseases can occur, which we designated as acute encephalomyelitis, subacute demyelinating encephalomyelitis and late demyelinating encephalomyelitis (8,9).

Acute Encephalomyelitis (AE). This disease develops after an incubation period of 7 - 12 days. The animals show incoordination, become motionless and die rapidly. Necrotic lesions are predominantly disseminated in the grey matter of the hippocampus, brainstem and spinal cord. Cell infiltrations are typical for acute inflammations consisting of granulocytes, lymphocytes and macrophages. By immunofluorescence, viral antigen can be found both in neurons and glia cells. Viral particles are detected only in degenerating oligodendroglia cells.

Subacute Demyelinating Encephalomyelitis (SDE). Diseased animals develop hind leg paralysis after an incubation period of 14 - 30 days (8). Similar observations were recently reported (11). The most prominent finding consists of demyelinating plaques distributed in the white matter of the optic nerve, midbrain, pons, cerebellum and spinal cord. As an example a section from the spinal cord of a rat which developed SDE 30 days p.i. is shown in Fig. 1. Within the demyelinated plaques axons and neurons are well preserved (Fig. 2). By immunofluorescence, no viral antigen can be detected in neurons. Cell infiltrations are consisting of lymphocytes, plasma cells and macrophages.

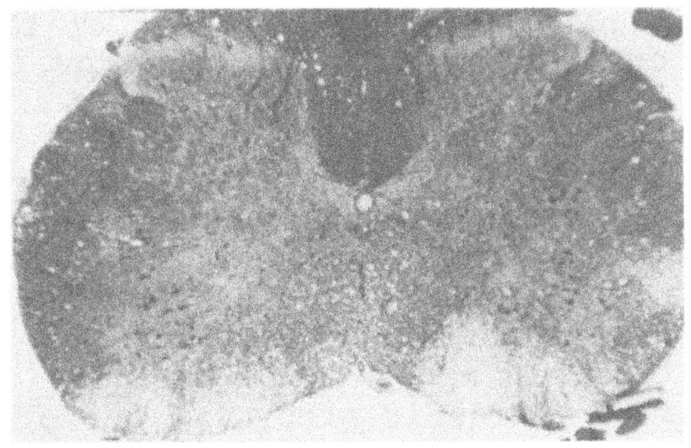

Fig.1: Demyelinated plaques in the spinal cord of a rat diseased with SDE 30 days p.i.

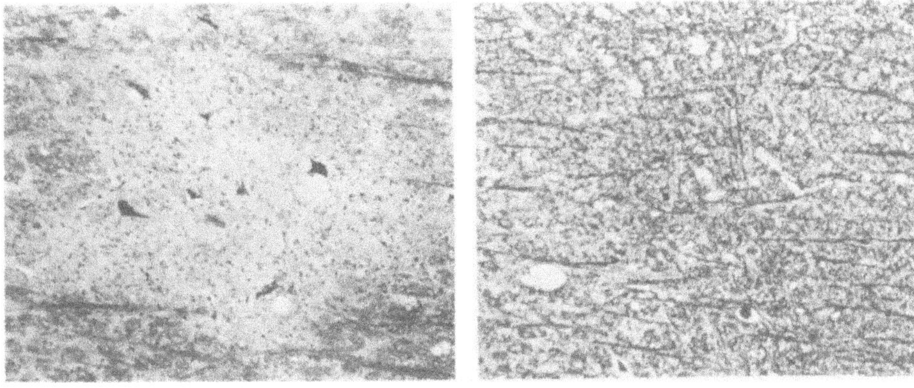

Fig.2: Preservation of neurons and axons within a demyelinated plaque (pons, 30 days, p.i.) a) stained with KB for myelin b) stained with GM for axons

Late Demyelinating Encephalomyelitis (LDE). After an incubation period of 2 - 8 months animals develop paralysis. The neuropathological lesions are typical plaques of primary demyelination as described for SDE. In addition, remyelination is detectable by electron microscopy (9). Infectious virus can be reisolated from diseased rats by conventional methods. Virus particles are detectable by electron microscopy in degenerating oligodendroglia cells.

VIROLOGICAL ASPECTS.

The above described disease types were only observed after intracerebral inoculation of JHM virus. Other murine coronaviruses are much less neurovirulent for weanling rats (12). Both weanling and suckling rats are relatively resistant against intraperitoneal infection. Furthermore, the type of clinical disease was not dependent on the amount of JHM virus injected but strongly influenced by the properties of the virus preparation inoculated as will be shown by the following experiments.

Comparison of uncloned and cloned JHM virus. Uncloned JHM-virus propagated in suckling mice induces in weanling rats the different types of disease as described above. From a virological point of view, the observation suggests that uncloned virus consists of a heterologous virus population. In order to investigate the course of AE and SDE, a time kinetic study was performed (Fig. 3). Beginning three days after infection with uncloned virus, groups of four clinically healthy rats were dissected for neuropathology, virus isolation and antibody determination at intervals of three days. Almost all clinically healthy animals revealed 6 - 14 days p.i. a latent AE. Infectious virus was easily recovered from brain and spinal cord during this acute stage. Later after infection, no infectious virus could be isolated, the latent AE disappeared, and in parallel to the raise of neutralizing antibodies clinically silent demyelinating lesions were found.

With the intention to obtain viruses with different neurovirulence, the JHM virus was cloned in tissueculture and tested for its capacity to induce demyelinating diseases. As shown in table 1, the cloned tissue

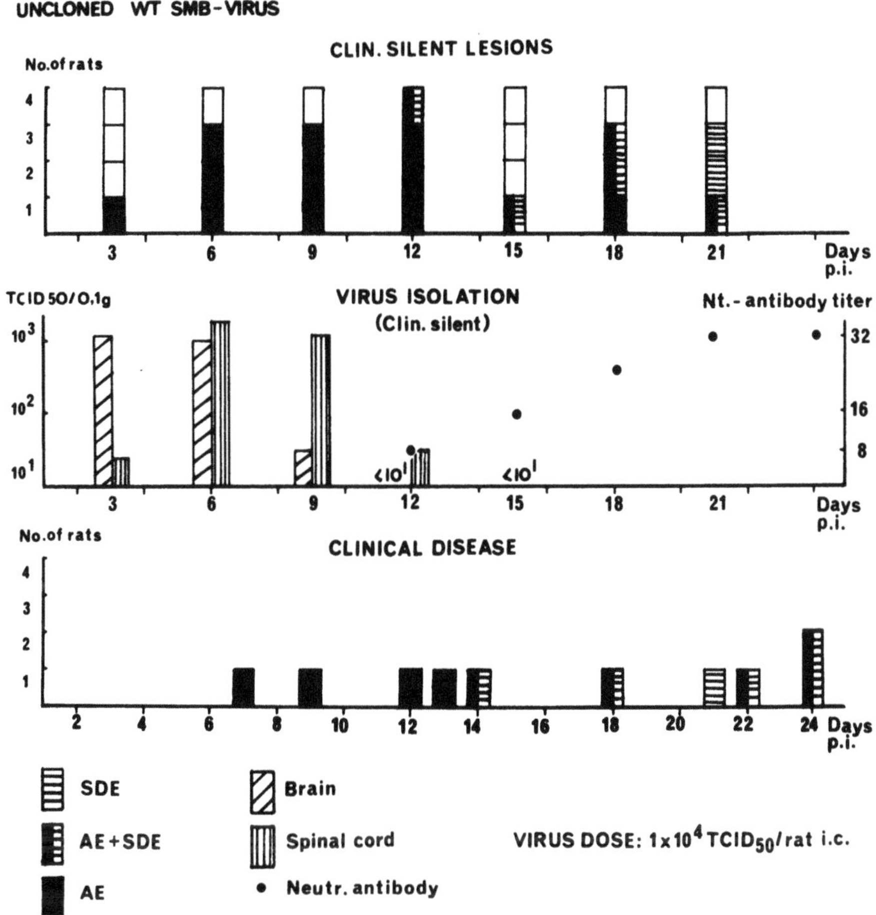

Fig.3: Time kinetics of clinically silent and overt encephalomyelitis, virus growth and development of neutralizing antibodies after infection of weanling rats with uncloned JHM virus.

culture adapted virus has lost its capacity to induce SDE or LDE in rats. Inoculation of uncloned virus resulted in about 15 % AE, 11 % of survivors developed SDE and 5 % of the remaining animals came down with LDE. Rats inoculated with the cloned, tissue culture adapted virus however, developed in 65 % AE. Survivors remained healthy without showing any clinical signs of a CNS disease.

Table 1. CNS-Diseases Induced by Uncloned and Clone Cloned JHM-Virus in Weanling Rats

VIRUS (I.C.) 4×10^3 $TCID_{50}$/RAT	CLINICAL DISEASE AE*	SDE**	LDE***
UNCLONED VIRUS (MOUSE BRAIN)	11/74	5/46	2/41
CLONED VIRUS (SAC(-)-CELLS)	29/45	0/16	0/16

* DISEASED / TOTAL

** DISEASED / UNDER FURTHER OBSERVATION

*** DISEASED / SURVIVORS OF SDE

As illustrated by Fig. 4, the survival rate of animals inoculated with cloned virus is dose dependent, whereas the type of clinical diseases is dose independent. All animals which died revealed neuropathologically a typical AE. Infectious virus could easily be isolated from diseased brain material with standard techniques or within two weeks p.i. from clinically healthy animals which revealed silent lesions.

Infection with temperature sensitive mutants. The failure to isolate from diseased animals a virus clone by tissue culture adaptation which induced SDE or LDE only, led to experiments in which the neurovirulence of cloned virus by selection of temperature sensitive mutants was changed. Mutants were induced by growth in presence of fluoruracil at 34,5 °C and selection of temperature sensitive mutants from the surviving fraction were carried out at 39,5 °C. A collection of mutants was obtained and biologically characterized by efficiency of plating, thermolability and leakiness.

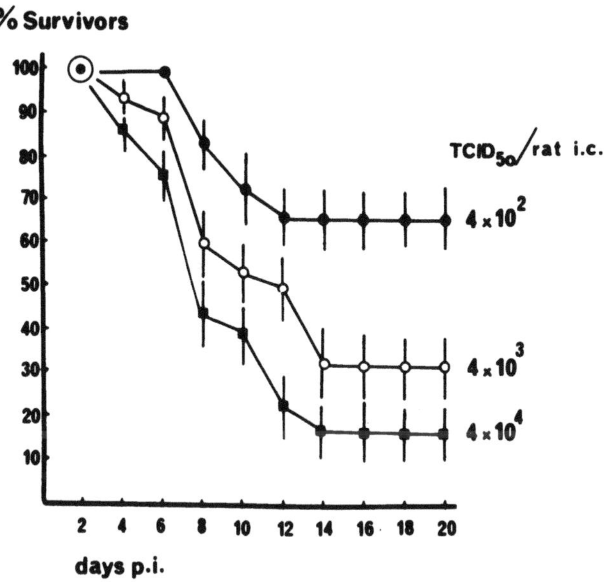

Fig.4: Dose dependent survival of weanling rats after i.c. injection of cloned JHM virus

Intracerebral inoculation of these mutants into weanling rats resulted either in no detectable disease at all or in SDE and LDE. A representative experiment with some of our mutants is summarized in table 2. The dose used for inoculation depended on the virus titre which was obtained in tissue culture. As can be seen in table 2 no AE was induced with this temperature sensitive mutants. Only different low rates of SDE and LDE developed. In addition, 10 - 30 % of clinical healthy animals revealed neuropathologically demyelinating lesions, an observation which demonstrates the property of these mutants to induce demyelination. However, inoculation of these mutants into suckling rats leads always to an acute encephalitis, suggesting that host factors such as the immune system in weanling rats contributes to the development of SDE.

Table 2. CNS-Diseases Induced by TS-Mutants Derived From Cloned JHM-Virus

	TCID50	CLINICAL DISEASE		
	DOSE/RAT	AE*	SDE**	LDE***
TS1	$1,4 \times 10^6$	0/37	0/28	1/28
TS6	$8,0 \times 10^3$	0/57	4/34	2/30
TS42	$1,0 \times 10^4$	0/31	0/26	2/26
TS43	$4,0 \times 10^4$	0/33	3/18	2/15

* DISEASED / TOTAL
** DISEASED / UNDER FURTHER OBSERVATION
*** DISEASED / SURVIVORS OF SDE

Infection of rats immunized by maternal antibodies. Adult, female rats were immunized by four intraperitoneal injections of cloned JHM-virus and thereafter mated. Litters of suckling rats born from these animals revealed neutralizing antibodies which were still present 30 days after birth. These litters were challenged by intracerebral injection of either cloned virus or temperature sensitive mutants at an age of 4 -6 days. The results obtained after intracerebral injection with ts mutants are shown in table 3 and summarized in table 4. Intracerebral infection of non immune suckling rats led to high rates of APE within 8 days p.i., whereas immune animals stayed healthy for 20 - 32 days after infection.Thereafter, these immune rats developed at a high rate paralysis and neuropathologically signs of SDE. In contrast, maternal JHM antibodies did not change the outcome of the disease in animals inoculated with cloned JHM virus.

Table 3. JHM Infection of Suckling Rats Possessing Maternal JHM Antibodies

CONTROL ANIMALS

DOSE	INCUBATION PERIOD (DAYS)				
PFU/RAT	8	16	24	32	40
2×10^4	10/11*	10/11	10/11	10/11	10/11
2×10^3	9/11	10/11	10/11	10/11	10/11
2×10^2	2/10	2/10	2/10	2/10	2/10

PREIMMUNIZED ANIMALS
(MATERNAL ANTIBODIES)

DOSE	INCUBATION PERIOD (DAYS)				
PFU/RAT	8	16	24	32	40
2×10^4	0/11*	0/11	3/11	5/11	•(CLIN.SIL.4/6)
2×10^3	0/12	0/12	5/12	5/12	5/12
2×10^2	0/9	0/9	2/9	2/9	2/9

NEUTRALIZING ANTIBODY TITRE 4 - 6 DAYS AFTER BIRTH: 1 : 32

PREIMMUNIZATION OF MOTHERS: CLONED VIRUS

CHALLENGE VIRUS (I.C.) : TS 6

*DISEASED ANIMALS/TOTAL

Table 4. JHM Infection of. Suckling Rats Possessing Maternal JHM (wt) Antibodies

CHALLENGE VIRUS	SUCKLING RATS (AGE 4 - 6 DAYS)	OCCURRENCE OF CLINICAL DISEASE	TYPE OF CLINICAL DISEASE
CLONED VIRUS	MINUS JHM MATERNAL ANTIBODIES	4 - 8 DAYS	APE
	PLUS JHM MATERNAL ANTIBODIES	4 - 8 DAYS	APE
TS 6	MINUS JHM MATERNAL ANTIBODIES	4 - 8 DAYS	APE
	PLUS JHM MATERNAL ANTIBODIES	23 - 40 DAYS	SDE WITH SCAR OF APE

DISCUSSION

The experiments carried out in this study reveal that after intracerebral inoculation of rats with JHM virus different CNS disorders of acute to chronic nature can be induced. Obviously, the development of these diseases depend on many parameters including biological properties of the virus preparation, age of the animals at the time of infection as well as the status of immunity of the host as summarized in table 5. In general, seronegative suckling rats always come down with an acute fatal CNS disease shortly after infection irrespective of the virus preparation used. Obviously, at this age virus spread cannot be limited either by the unmaturated immune system or by non-immune defence mechanisms.

However, already at the age of 20 days the disease type is determined by the virus preparation inoculated. Wild JHM virus induces acute, subacute or late diseases suggesting that different populations within this virus preparation are responsible for these diseases. In contrast, cloned JHM virus causes only an acute encephalomyelitis, whereas ts mutants predominantly lead to subacute or late disorders. In this case,

Table 5. Coronavirus JHM Infection in Rats

VIRUS	AGE OF ANIMALS UPON INFECTION	
	SUCKLING	WEANLING
UNCLONED WILDTYPE PASSAGED IN SUCKLING MICE (WT SMB)	• ACUTE PANENCEPHALITIS (4 - 8 DAYS) *	• ACUTE ENCEPHALOMYELITIS (7 - 12 DAYS) • SUBACUTE DEMYELINATING ENCEPHALOMYELITIS (14 - 30 DAYS) • LATE DEMYELINATING ENCEPHALOMYELITIS (2 - 8 MONTHS)
CLONED CELL ADAPTED (WT SAC CLONED)	• ACUTE PANENCEPHALITIS (4 - 8 DAYS)	• ACUTE ENCEPHALOMYELITIS (7 - 12 DAYS)
TS-MUTANTS	• ACUTE PANENCEPHALITIS (4 - 8 DAYS)	• SUBACUTE DEMYELINATING ENCEPHALOMYELITIS (14 - 30 DAYS) • LATE DEMYELINATING ENCEPHALOMYELITIS (2 - 8 MONTHS)
TS-MUTANTS (INOCULATED IN IMMUNIZED ANIMALS)	→ SUBACUTE DEMYELINATING ENCEPHALOMYELITIS (20 - 40 DAYS)	N.T.

* Incubation time p.i

the majority of animals do not develop clinical signs of illness, but reveal silent neuropathological lesions. It is of interest to note, that the neuropathological changes observed in animals with a subacute encephalomyelitis are proceeded by small clinically silent lesions of acute nature, consisting of focal necrosis and massive infiltration. Obviously in these instances virus spread is confined and an acute stage of the disease is prevented. However, the host fails to eliminate this infection which gradually proceeds developing into a subacute or late disorder with a prolonged incubation period of weeks or months.

The virus host relationship is certainly very complex in these diseases and at the present time poorly understood. Virological investigations have shown that after the initial infection in weanling rats infectious virus is easily isolatable from brain or spinal cord material even in those animals which look clinically healthy. However, after 12 - 14 days p. i., when JHM antibodies are present, no infectious virus can be recovered with standard techniques. Yet, in animals with clinical SDE or LDE infectious JHM virus is present. These findings indicate that a persistent JHM infection is established after inoculation which is probably activated at a later time before onset of clinical disease.

It is well established that humoral and cell-mediated immune reactions play a major role in a successful encounter with the virus infection. This defence system is still immature in newborn rats and it is therefore not surprising that in general these animals cannot overcome the JHM infection. However, maternal JHM antibodies influence the development of the disease processes. Whereas an acute fatal encephalomyelitis of unprotected control animals was observed in suckling rats, presence of JHM antibodies lead to a high rate of SDE after a prolonged incubation period when ts mutants of JHM virus were inoculated. Obviously, JHM antibody interferred with a spread of virus, prevented the acute disease and may have influenced replication of JHM virus as has been suggested for measles virus in the presence of antibodies (10). On the other hand, this protection was not sufficient in the case of infection with cloned JHM virus since these animals came down with an acute disease.

The described animal model of virus induced acute or subacute demyelinating encephalomyelitis reveals the complex virus host interaction underlying the different CNS diseases. Moreover, it offers the possibility to investigate the pathogenetic mechanisms of these diseases and provides the basis to understand the cell -virus interactions which lead to these disease processes. Especially the subacute and late demyelinating encephalomyelitis, caused by JHM virus in rats is of great interest in analogy to chronic CNS diseases of man associated with a virus infection.

ACKNOWLEDGEMENTS: We thank Mrs. Margarete Sturm for excellent technical assistance and Mrs. Helga Kriesinger for typing the manuscript. This work was supported by the Deutsche Forschungsgemeinschaft, Hertie Stiftung and Österreichische Gesellschaft zur Bekämpfung der Muskelerkrankungen.

REFERENCES

1. Bailey, O.T., Pappenheimer, A.M., Sargent Cheever, F. and Daniels, J.B. (1949). A murine virus (JHM) causing disseminated encephalomyelitis with extensive destruction of myelin: II. Pathology. Journal of Experimental Medicine 90, 195 - 212.

2. Cheever, F.S., Daniels, J.B., Pappenheimer, A.M. and Bailey, O.T. (1949). A murine virus (JHM) causing disseminated encephalomyelitis with extensive destruction of myelin: I. Isolation and biological properties of the virus. Journal of Experimental Medicine 90, 181 - 194.

3. Haspel, V.M., Lampert, P.W. and Oldstone, M.B.A. (1978). Temperature-sensitive mutants of mouse hepatitis virus produce a high incidence of demyelination. Proceedings of the national Academy of Science, USA, 75, 4033 - 4036.

4. Herndon, R.M., Griffin, D.E., McCormick, U. and Weiner, L.P. (1975). Mouse hepatitis virus induced recurrent demyelination. Archives of Neurology 32, 32 - 35.

5. Lampert, P.W., Sims, J.K. and Kniazeff, A.J. (1973). Mechanism of demyelination in JHM virus encephalomyelitis. Electron microscopic studies. Acta Neuropathologica 24, 76 - 85.

6. ter Meulen, V. and Hall, W.W. (1978). Slow virus infections of the nervous systems. Journal of General Virology 41, 1 -25.

7. Nagashima, K., Wege, H. and ter Meulen, V. (1978). Early and late CNS-effects of coronavirus infection in rats. Advances of experimental Medicine and Biology 100, 395 - 409.

8. Nagashima, K., Wege, H., Meyermann, R. and ter Meulen, V. (1978). Corona virus induced subacute demyelinating encephalomyelitis in rats. A morphological analysis. Acta Neuropathologica 44, 63 - 70.

9. Nagashima, K., Wege, H., Meyermann, R. and ter Meulen, V. (1979). Demyelinating encephalomyelitis induced by a long-term corona virus infection in rats. Acta Neuropathologica 45, 205 - 213

10. Fujinami, R.S. and Oldstone, M.B.A. (1979). Antiviral antibody acting on the plasma membrane allows measles virus expression inside the cell. Nature 279, 529 - 530.

11. Sorensen, O., Percy, D. and Dales, S. (1980). In vivo and in vitro models of demyelinating diseases. III. JHM virus infection of rats. Archives of Neurology 37, 478 -484.

12. Wege, H., Stephenson, J.R., Koga, M., Wege, Hanna and ter Meulen, V. (1981). Genetic variation of neurotropic and non neurotropic murine coronaviruses. Journal of General Virology, in press.

13. Weiner, L.P. (1973). Pathogenesis of demyelination included by a mouse hepatitis virus (JHM virus). Archives of Neurology 28, 293 - 303.

HOST AND VIRUS FACTORS ASSOCIATED WITH CNS CELLULAR TROPISM LEADING TO ENCEPHALOMYELITIS OR DEMYELINATION INDUCED BY THE JHM STRAIN OF MOUSE HEPATITIS VIRUS

Robert L. Knobler*†, Martin V. Haspel**, Monique Dubois-Dalcq***, Peter W. Lampert†, and Michael B.A. Oldstone*

*Department of Immunopathology, Scripps Clinic and Research Foundation, La Jolla, CA., **Laboratory of Oral Medicine, National Institute of Dental Research, Bethesda, MD., ***Infectious Disease Branch, NINCDS, Bethesda, MD., †Department of Pathology, UCSD College of Medicine, La Jolla, CA.

INTRODUCTION

Infection of mice with the neurotropic JHM strain (type 4) of mouse hepatitis virus (MHV), produces a spectrum of disease ranging from acute fatal encephalomyelitis (E+) to demyelination (D+) (Bailey et al., 1949; Haspel et al., 1978; Lampert et al., 1973; Weiner, 1973). The pattern of disease which prevails is affected by such factors as the age of the animal, the dose of virus administered, the route of infection (Weiner, 1973), the genetic strain of the mouse (Stohlman and Frelinger, 1978), and the nature of the virus (Haspel et al., 1978).

Intracerebral inoculation of two plaque forming units (PFU) of wild type (wt) MHV in susceptible four week old mice, produces a high frequency of fatal encephalomyelitis (E+), but infrequent demyelination (D-) due to virulence of the virus (Haspel et al., 1978). Intracerebral inoculation of 10^4 PFU of an attenuated mutant, designated ts8, rarely results in fatal encephalomyelitis (E-), but regularly produces demyelination (D+) (Haspel et al., 1978). We have developed a model system to dissect factors associated with the E+ and the D+ phenotypes.

GENETIC CONTROL OF SUSCEPTIBILITY TO MHV ENCEPHALOMYELITIS

To dissect factors associated with an E+ phenotype, we screened several inbred strains of mice for susceptibility to fatal disease:

A/J($H\text{-}2^{a/k}_{dd}$), A.SW($H\text{-}2^{ss}$), BALB/c($H\text{-}2^{dd}$), BALB/WEHI($H\text{-}2^{dd}$), B10.D2 OLD($H\text{-}2^{dd}$), B10.D2 NEW($H\text{-}2^{dd}$), C3H/ST($H\text{-}2^{kk}$), C57BL/6J($H\text{-}2^{bb}$), SJL/J($H\text{-}2^{ss}$) and SWR/J($H\text{-}2^{qq}$). The sex of the animal was found to have no influence on susceptibility to MHV (Haspel, unpublished data). The mice were obtained from Jackson Laboratories, Bar Harbor, ME, or from the breeding colony of the Research Institute of Scripps Clinic, and were screened for antibodies to MHV. The LD_{50} for each strain was calculated by the Reed-Muench method at the end of the 14 day assay period. Only SJL/J mice showed resistance to fatal encephalomyelitis.

To investigate the pattern of inheritance of susceptibility, BALB/c mice were selected as a susceptible strain and bred with resistant SJL/J mice to test the susceptibility of progeny to fatal encephalomyelitis in a 14 day assay. Hybrid F1 progeny of BALB/c x SJL/J, and SJL/J x BALB/c matings, F2 generation mice, and progeny of backcrosses of F1 mice to either BALB/c or SJL/J parental mice were studied at four weeks of age. In this experiment, the infecting dose of virus for intracerebral inoculation was 100 BALB/c LD_{50}. The results of these experiments support the conclusion that susceptibility is inherited as an autosomal dominant trait.

CELLULAR BASIS OF SUSCEPTIBILITY TO MHV REPLICATION

Although four week old SJL/J mice are resistant to fatal encephalitis compared to other strains, there is replication of MHV in brain tissue from SJL/J mice following intracerebral inoculation. Four week old SJL/J mice develop fatal encephalomyelitis only if very high infectious doses are used, but not under the conditions of these experiments. Table 1 contains virus titers expressed as PFU per gram of tissue from SJL/J and BALB/c mice at 1, 2 and 3 days after inoculation. Brain tissue from SJL/J mice, however, contains at least two logs less virus than brain tissue from similarly infected BALB/c mice. Deaths in BALB/c mice usually begin to occur on day 2 at this infectious dose. Since fatal encephalomyelitis is due primarily to neuronal involvement, it is important to determine whether the observed difference in mortalities and virus titers between SJL/J and the BALB/c mice reflects fewer infected neurons or less virus production per infected cell. In vitro systems were exploited to investigate this question.

Virus replication in thioglycollate stimulated macrophages or primary neuronal cultures from BALB/WEHI and SJL/J were compared, following infection with wt MHV at an MOI of 0.1. Table 2 contains the virus titers expressed as plaque forming units per ml from the supernatant culture fluids of the macrophages from each of the strains of mice. Macrophages derived from four week old BALB/WEHI mice produced 10^4 PFU/ml of MHV, while identical cell populations derived from four week old SJL/J mice had no detectable virus in the supernatant culture fluid. The phagocytic activity of macrophages from both strains was assessed with antibody coated sheep erythrocytes or zymogen granules, and found to be equivalent. It was possible to demonstrate MHV antigens by immunofluorescence in both SJL/J and BALB/WEHI derived macrophages. However, the labeling pattern of the SJL/J macrophages consisted of intracellular globules, while the BALB/WEHI macrophages were labeled diffusely, but homogeneously. Virus release from infected macrophages was also assessed by overlaying the SJL/J or BALB/WEHI macrophages with L-241 cells, which form multi-nucleated giant cells when infected with MHV. SJL/J macrophage cultures, so treated, had a contiguous sheet of L-241 cells (Figure 1), with only one giant cell per 10^6 plated L-241 cells demonstrated. In contrast, BALB/WEHI macrophage cultures contained numerous giant cells, and very few L-241 cells remaining intact. These findings indicate that macrophages from MHV resistant SJL/J mice, although infected, as indicated by positive immunofluorescence, do not readily release virus, and thus, may play a role in limiting the spread of MHV infection.

Table 1. The Replication of Wild Type MHV (JHM Strain) in Brain Tissue from BALB/c and SJL/J Mice Following Intracerebral Inoculation of 100 BALB/c LD_{50}*

Days Post-Infection	BALB/c	SJL/J
1	++++	++
2	+++++	+++
3	+++++	++++

*(+) signifies logs of PFU/gm

Primary neuronal cultures were established by the method of Peacock et al. (1973), from 11-12 day old embryonic spinal cords taken from A.SW($H-2^{ss}$), BALB/WEHI($H-2^{dd}$) and SJL/J($H-2^{ss}$) mice. Neuronal cells were identified by the binding of tetanus toxin (Mirsky et al., 1978), to their surfaces and subsequent demonstration by indirect immunofluorescence. Primary neuronal cultures derived from SJL/J mice had no detectable virus in the supernatant culture fluid (Table 3), although they did contain MHV antigens by immunofluorescence. In contrast, primary neuronal cultures derived from BALB/WEHI mice had 10^5 PFU/ml of MHV in supernatant culture fluid. The restriction of MHV replication in SJL/J derived neurons is not related to the $H-2^{ss}$ haplotype; primary neuronal cultures derived from A.SW mice, which are also of the $H-2^{ss}$ haplotype produced just under 10^5 PFU/ml of MHV in supernatant culture fluid. Restricted replication in neurons is the most probable cause for the resistance of SJL/J mice to fatal encephalomyelitis. Our data indicate that SJL/J neurons are capable of being infected with MHV, but that it is not a productive infection. Thus, the limited replication of MHV in the brains of SJL/J mice under the conditions of our experiments probably represents replication in non-neuronal cells.

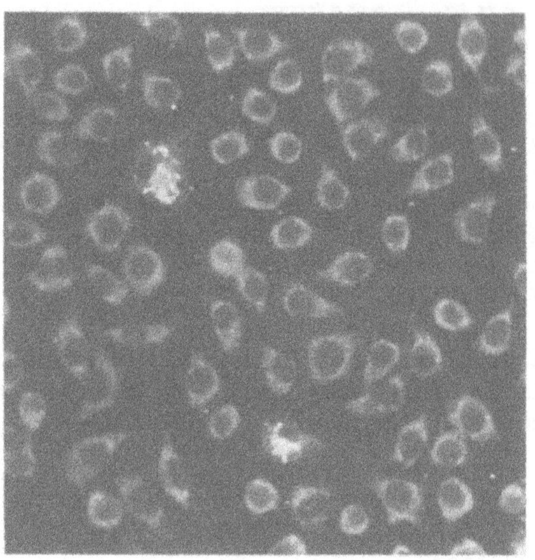

Fig. 1. There are two SJL/J macrophages with a globular pattern of MHV antigens demonstrated by immunofluorescence, surrounded by contiguous L-241 cells, which demonstrate autofluorescent granules. Light micrograph, 250x.

Table 2. The Replication of Wild Type MHV (JHM Strain) by Thioglycollate Stimulated Macrophages Derived from BALB/WEHI and SJL/J Mice, MOI = 0.1*

Days Post-Infection	BALB/WEHI	SJL/J
0	NIL	NIL
1	++++	NIL
2	++++	NIL
3	+++	NIL
4	+++	NIL

*(+) signifies logs of PFU/ml

Table 3. The Replication of Wild Type MHV (JHM Strain) by Primary Neuronal Cultures Derived from A.SW, BALB/WEHI and SJL/J Mice, Expressed as PFU/Ml of Supernatant Culture Fluid, MOI = 0.1*

Days Post-Infection	A.SW($H-2^{ss}$)	BALB/WEHI($H-2^{dd}$)	SJL/J($H-2^{ss}$)
1	++++	++++	NIL
2	+++++	+++++	NIL
3	+++++	+++++	NIL

*(+) signifies logs of PFU/ml

VIRUS TROPISM FOR DIFFERENT CNS CELLS CORRELATES WITH DISEASE PHENOTYPE

To dissect factors associated with a D+ (demyelinating) phenotype, we compared virus production and antigen localization following intracerebral inoculation of susceptible BALB/c mice with either wild type virus, which frequently produces fatal encephalomyelitis, or mutant ts8, which frequently produces demyelination. For this experiment, less than one PFU of wt virus (one half LD_{50}) was used, compared to 10^4 PFU of ts8. Animals were sacrificed at 2, 4, 7, 10 and 14 days after inoculation and tissues were taken for determination of virus titer or the animals were perfused for antigen localization studies. It should be noted that animals receiving wt virus did not survive past seven days after inoculation.

The infectious titers of virus produced in the brain or spinal cord following infection with either wt or mutant ts8 are equivalent (Table 4). Thus, the different pattern of disease with mutant ts8 is not due to a difference in the infectious titer produced in the tissues following infection. However, the localization of virus antigen by immunofluorescence in perfused (4% paraformaldehyde and 0.5% glutaraldehyde), vibratome sectioned spinal cords demonstrated an altered tropism for CNS cells of mutant ts8 compared to wt MHV, that closely correlated with the pattern of disease each produces. Animals inoculated with wild type MHV had MHV antigens localized principally in cells of the substantia gelatinosa and ventral horn neurons (Figure 2), as well as oligodendrocytes in the spinal cord. In marked contrast, animals inoculated with mutant ts8 had MHV antigens localized primarily in oligodendrocytes of the ventral median white matter of the spinal cord (Figure 3), while only rarely in neuronal cells. Thus, the high frequency of demyelination and infrequency of fatal encephalomyelitis observed with infection by mutant ts8 correlates with an altered cellular tropism within the CNS by ts8.

The demonstration of MHV antigens in oligodendrocytes processes extending to and surrounding intact myelin sheaths (Figure 3) is of further interest. The oligodendrocytes in MHV infection are hypertropic and have more notable connections to myelin sheaths than is usually observed (Powell and Lampert, 1975). Whether the MHV antigens are actually being incorporated into these myelin sheaths and the significance of this process for virus-induced demyelinating or immune-mediated demyelinating disease is under study.

SUMMARY AND CONCLUSIONS

1. Ten inbred strains of mice at four weeks of age were tested for susceptibility to fatal encephalomyelitis (E+) by intracerebral inoculation of ten-fold dilutions of wild type (JHM Strain) mouse hepatitis virus. Only SJL/J mice were resistant (E-) to fatal encephalomyelitis. This resistance is independent of the H-2^{ss} haplotype.

2. By testing appropriate crosses between BALB/c and SJL/J mice, susceptibility was determined to be an autosomal dominant trait.

3. Thioglycollate stimulated macrophages, and primary neuronal cultures from SJL/J mice did not produce infectious virus. In contrast, these cell populations derived from BALB/WEHI mice released 10^4-10^5 PFU of infectious virus/ml of supernatant culture fluid.

4. The labeling pattern of virus antigens by immunofluorescence was globular and moderately positive in SJL/J cells. The pattern in BALB/WEHI cells was diffuse and markedly positive.

Table 4. The Replication of Wild Type and Mutant ts8 MHV (JHM Strain) in Brain Tissue from BALB/ST Mice Following Intracerebral Inoculation*

Days Post-Infection	Wild Type	ts8
2	++++++	++++++
4	++++++	++++++
7	+++++	+++++
10		++++
14		+++

*(+) signifies logs of PFU/gm

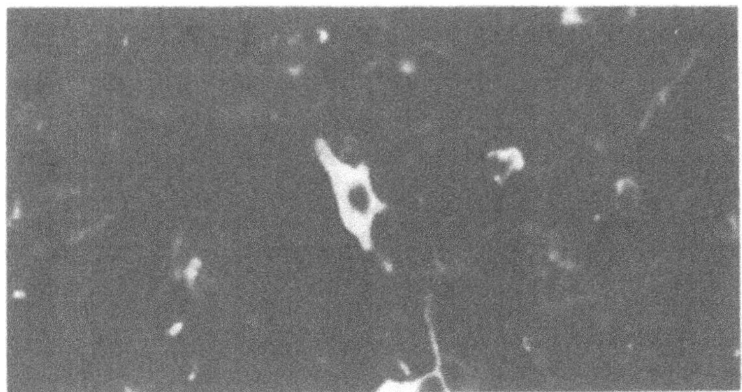

Fig. 2. Wild type mouse hepatitis virus antigens demonstrated in cervical spinal cord ventral horn neurons, two days after intracerebral inoculation by immunofluorescent staining of a vibratome section. Light micrograph, 400x.

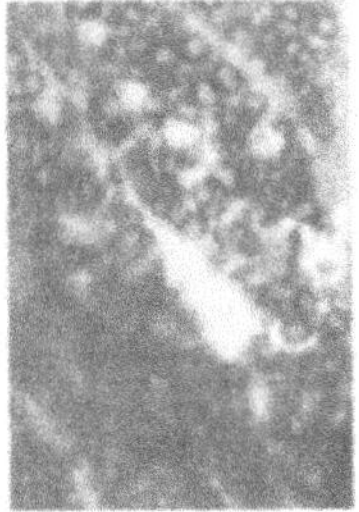

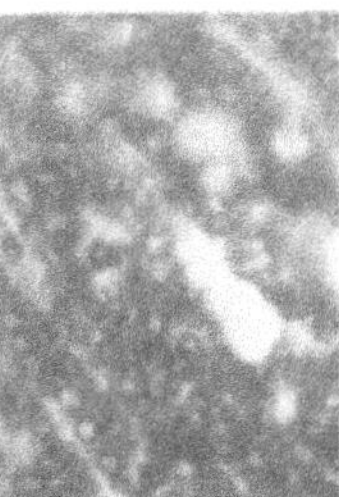

Fig 3. Mutant ts8 mouse hepatitis virus antigens demonstrated in cervical spinal cord ventral median white matter oligodendrocyte two days after intracerebral inoculation by immunofluorescent staining of a vibratome section. Two planes of focus on the same section are shown. Light micrograph, 400x.

5. Susceptibility to fatal disease from infection with wild type MHV (JHM Strain) correlates best with the ability of the virus to replicate in neuronal cells. Wild type viral antigens are localized in neuronal cells, as well as oligodendrocytes.

6. Mutant ts8 in contrast to wild type, produces a high frequency of demyelination without fatal encephalomyelitis. The viral antigens of ts8 are localized primarily in oligodendrocytes, and rarely in neuronal cells. This difference in CNS cell tropism correlates well with the different phenotype (D+,E-) produced by mutant ts8.

ACKNOWLEDGEMENTS

Dr. Knobler is a Postdoctoral Fellow of the National Multiple Sclerosis Society supported by fellowship FG 353 A1.

This is publication number 2278 from the Department of Immunopathology, Scripps Clinic and Research Foundation, La Jolla, California. This research was supported by NS 14068 and NS 12428, US Public Health grants. The authors thank Linda Tunison and Ruth Ott for technical assistance and Susan Edwards for preparation of the manuscript.

REFERENCES

Bailey, O.T., Pappenheimer, A.M., Cheever, F.S., and Daniels, J.B., 1949, A murine virus (JHM) causing disseminated encephalomyelitis with extensive destruction of myelin. II. Pathology, J. Exp. Med., 90:195.

Haspel, M.V., Lampert, P.W., and Oldstone, M.B.A., 1978, Temperature sensitive mutants of mouse hepatitis virus produce a high incidence of demyelination, Proc. Natl. Acad. Sci. (USA), 75: 4033.

Lampert, P.W., Sims, J.K., and Kniazeff, A.J., 1973, Mechanism of demyelination in JHM virus encephalomyelitis. Electron microscopic studies, Acta. Neuropathol., (Berl.), 24:76.

Mirsky, R., Wendon, L.M., Black, P., Stolkin, C., and Gray, D., 1978, Tetanus Toxin: A cell surface marker for neurons in culture, Brain Res., 148:251.

Peacock, J.H., Nelson, P.G., and Goldstone, M.W., 1973, Electrophysical study of cultured neurons dissociated from spinal cords and dorsal root ganglia of fetal mice, Devel. Biol., 30:137.

Powell, H.C., and Lampert, P.W., 1975, Oligodendrocytes and their myelin plasma membrane connections in JHM mouse hepatitis virus encephalomyelitis, Lab. Invest., 33:440.

Stohlman, S.A., and Frelinger, J.A., 1978, Resistance to fatal central nervous system disease by mouse hepatitis virus, strain JHM. I. Genetic analysis, Immunogenetics, 6:277.

Weiner, L.P., 1973, Pathogenesis of demyelination induced by a mouse hepatitis virus (JHM virus), Arch. Neurol., 28:298.

PATHOGENICITY AND PERSISTENCE OF MOUSE HEPATITIS VIRUS IN INBRED STRAINS OF MICE

Jean-Louis Virelizier

Groupe d'Immunologie et de Rhumatologie Pédiatriques
INSERM U 132, Hopital des Enfants Malades
75730 Paris Cedex 15

Typical virus infections are short in incubation, acute in course, and rapid in their progress to either death or recovery. Some viruses, however, are able to escape host defense mechanisms and persist for long periods of time, often indefinitely. The pathogenesis and mechanisms of virus persistency vary widely according to the type of model considered. With scrapie, mink encephalopathy, kuru and Creutzfeld-Jacob disease, the infection elicits no inflammatory response. Apparently, immunological factors neither control nor complicate the disease. In other models, the virus persists in the face of an active host immune response. Two situations may be distinguished : the virus may be actively replicated by host cells, and viremia persists until the death of the host. This is true, for example, of lactic dehydrogenase virus infection, Aleutian mink disease or equine infectious anemia. In these cases the virus circulates as infective immune complexes made of virus particles and specific antibody. Alternatively, like in herpes simplex and varicella-zoster infection, the virus remains latent and able to persist in cells of the nervous system. A permanent cell-mediated immune control is exerted on these infected cells, so that the virus is not actively replicated. Diminution of the effectiveness of T cell-mediated responses, for example during immunosuppressive therapy, allows reactivation of the infection.

An interesting aspect of mouse hepatitis virus type 3 (MHV-3) infection is that the severity and the type of infection produced depend entirely on the mouse strain experimentally used[1,2]. The susceptibility of animals to viruses is often genetically determined [3]. The early work of F.B. Bang and his colleagues[4,5] has shown that susceptibility to mouse hepatitis virus type 2 (MHV-2) is under genetic control at the cellular level. In the case of MHV-3, the natural resistance shows various degrees according to the mouse strain considered[6,7]. Most mouse strains show a full susceptibility leading to death within a few days. A unique strain, A/J, shows a full resistance with 100% survival of infected animals. In the course of an early study on the in vivo resistance to MHV-3, we found that old C3H/He mice resist the acute phase of the disease but develop a chronic illness with progressive neurological involvement[8]. Clearly, in this type of model, there are two variables : the virus and the host. The fate of the infection is not determined by the virus, which intrinsic virulence remains constant, but rather by host resistance factors which vary in efficiency in different mouse strains. The present communication intends to review the different pathogenetic aspects of MHV-3 infection and to discuss the possible mechanisms leading to virus persistence.

ACUTE MHV-3 INFECTION

MHV-3 is one of the most virulent strains of mouse hepatitis viruses. In the majority of mouse strains, including C57 BL/6 and 10, DBA/2, BALB/c and NZB, parenteral administration of as little as 10 LD 50 always leads to fulminant hepatitis and death. The first cycles of replication occur in macrophages, including Kuppfer cells of the liver. Infection is soon generalized and the virus can then be found in all organs tested, including blood, liver, spleen, lymph nodes, brain and kidney[9]. Giant cells actively replicating the virus are observed in the liver and lymphoid organs. Neighbouring cells, especially hepatocytes, are soon infected. Large, confluent areas of necrosis are seen in the liver. Lymphoid organs also show profound anatomical modifications, particularly in the thymus where the cortical, but not the medullary area is strikingly depleted of lymphocytes as early as 48 hours after intra-peritoneal virus inoculation[10]. Mice die in 5 to 10 days, the clinical picture suggesting acute hepatic failure.

In the A/J strain of mice, full resistance to MHV-3 is observed. Whatever the dose of virus used, all adult mice survive. The virus is cleared from liver, brain and serum within 7 days[6]. The virus titers found in all organs tested are less than 10^2 LD 50/0.1 ml, contrasting with titers of more than 10^4 found in susceptible animals at the time of death. Pathological sections show no tissue lesions. This full resistance of the A/J strain, however, is age-dependent. Up to 15 days of age, A/J animals regularly die even when injected with low doses of virus. Resistance develops suddenly during the third week of life[6]. Adult resistant mice always show, after recovery, a clear serum anti-MHV-3 antibody response.

PERSISTENT MHV-3 INFECTION

In contrast with the full susceptibility or the full resistance described above, mice of the C3H/He and the A2G strains show a genetically determined semi-resistance leading to virus persistence [11,12]. In these two strains, intraperitoneal administration is not followed by acute death, except in a minority of animals. The majority (75 to 95 %) of animals survive, but develop a chronic disease. Three to six weeks after infection, mice progressively begin to show loss of activity, failure to thrive, ruffled fur and neurological signs. Incoordination and paresis of one or more limbs, especially the hind limbs, are observed. When suspended by the tail, mice show circling movements. The date of appearance of paralysis and the intensity of the neurological disorder vary widely from one animal to another. The animals die between 1 and 12 months after infection. The semi-resistance of A2G mice appears to be less reproducible, however, since some batches show full susceptibility and early death in a majority of animals.

This chronic disease is associated with persistence of MHV-3 in its virulent, hepatotropic form. Indeed, most brain suspensions, and occasional liver, spleen and lymph node suspensions, induce a typical lethal hepatitis upon transfer into susceptible recipients. Thus parenteral inoculation of a non-neuro-adapted strain of MHV-3 leads to virus persistence and neurological signs. It should be noted that the virus titers are always very low (about 10^1 LD 50/g of tissue), and that the virus cannot be transferred from the blood.

An age-dependent resistance of a peculiar type is observed in C3H/He and in two other semi-resistant stains, CBA and AKR [12]. These animals are fully susceptible at 6 weeks of age, and it is only by the 12th week of age that animals escape the lethal hepatitis and develop the chronic neurological disease. Since host factors, rather than intrinsic MHV-3 virulence, are clearly involved in this age-dependent phenomenon, our observations indicate that the maturation of anti-MHV-3 effectors is slower and incomplete in semi-resistant strains, whereas it is early and complete in the resistant A/J strain.

PATHOLOGICAL EFFECTS OF PERSISTENT MHV-3 INFECTION

Persistence of MHV-3 is associated with severe lesions of the central nervous system and with systemic amyloid, as reported previously [11]. The neuropathological lesions are partially different in A2G and C3H mice, and will now be described successively. The neuropathological findings in persistently infected A2G mice are dominated by severe hydrocephalus and hydromyelia associated with chronic ependymitis and inflammatory cell cuffing of small blood vessels in the subependymal tissues and choroid plexus. C3H mice sacrified one to 8 months after infection had lesions both in the brain and the spinal cord. In the former, the lateral and third ventricles were moderately dilated. The predominant lesion was vasculitis, with polymorph infiltration, leukocytoclasis, and often fibrinoid necrosis. These vascular lesions were observed in both arteries and veins of large and small diameter. In most mice, nearby long ascending and descending tracts were damaged, both myelin and axis cylinders being destroyed by proliferative perivascular lesions. Such neural changes were seen more often around the root of the fifth cranial nerve, the choroid plexus in the third and fourth ventricles, and the basilar artery in the brain, widely throughout the leptomeninges of the cord and in many spinal nerve roots. It should be stressed that there was no extensive neuronal damage nor areas of selective demyelination other than the rims of spongy change around well-defined vascular lesions. This picture suggests that the neural damage was in fact the consequence of the vasculitis.

Amyloid was found in the kidneys, liver and spleen of C3H mice infected for more than 6 months. In the spleen, the amount of amyloid deposition was considerable, occupying up to 50 % of the organ. In the mouse, amyloidosis has been detected in survivors of acute reovirus type I and II infection, at a stage when infective virus is no longer recoverable [13]. In the MHV-3 model, it is likely that amyloidosis is the consequence of virus persistence in the face of an active immune response.

MECHANISMS OF NEUROLOGIC LESIONS

The mechanisms through which virus persistence leads to neurological lesions in the absence of direct cytopathic effects of the virus in neural cells has to be discussed. The severe hydrocephalus and hydromyelia observed in A2G are likely to be the consequence of the chronic inflammatory processes observed in ependyma and meninges. A role for chronic obstruction of the aqueduct by proliferating glial and ependymal cells, or disturbed cerebrospinal fluid absorption can be discussed, but has not been demonstrated. That acute viral ependymitis may be followed by hydrocephalus has also been demonstrated in the reovirus type I and the mumps model [14,15]. Lesions of the central nervous system in C3H mice appear to be secondary to the immunopathological, systemic vasculitis. Indeed, no evidence of primary demyelination was observed unlike what is seen with another coronavirus, JHM [16]. In chronically infected C3H mice, old fibrotic neurological lesions, or more recent destruction of neural structures, were almost always observed in close association with a perivascular infiltration of inflammatory cells, and these changes were predominant in the areas of the CNS with the richest vascularization.

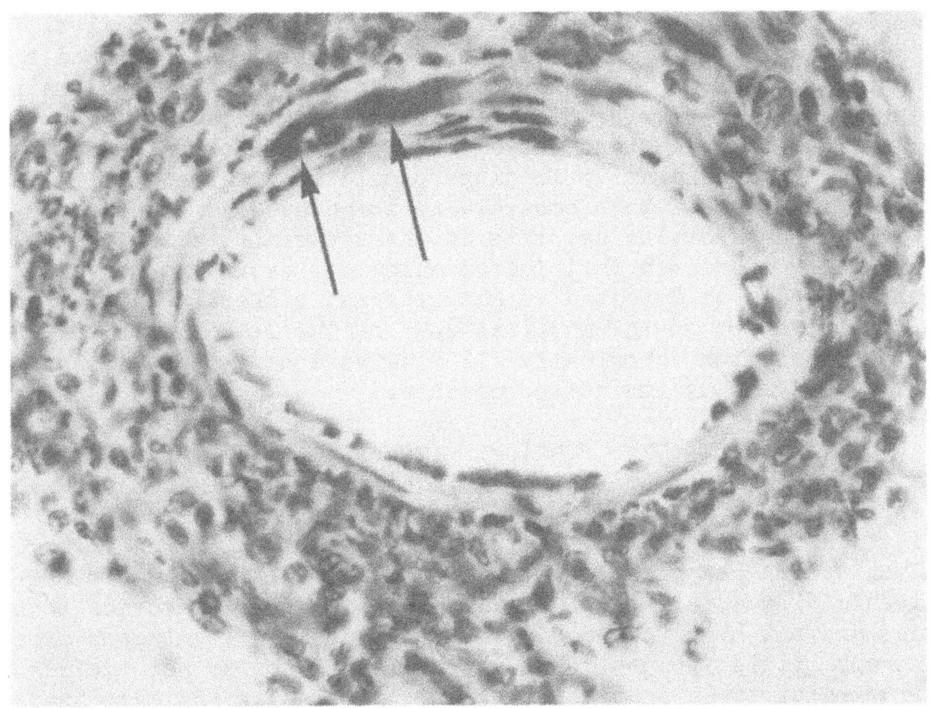

Fig. 1. Vasculitis observed in the basilar artery of a C3H/He mouse sacrified 150 days after intra-peritoneal injection of MHV-3. Note infiltration by polymorphs and areas of fibrinoid necrosis (arrows) in the wall of the vessel (Picro-Mallory staining, X 700)

SITES OF VIRUS PERSISTENCE

Direct and indirect immunofluorescence techniques have been used to detect MHV-3 antigens and immunoglobulin deposition in persistently infected animals [11]. In contrast to clinical and pathological evidence of neural damage, MHV-3 antigens could not be detected in any neural tissue. In A2G mice, a bright, patchy fluorescence of meningeal cells was found in large areas along the meninges. Many areas of the ependymal wall and choroid plexus contained groups of cells showing cytoplasmic fluorescence which indicated the presence of viral antigens. No fluorescence was seen in neurones. In C3H mice sacrificed 45 days to 8 months after infection, no viral antigens or immunoglobulin deposition could be found in neurones or meninges. However, in some parts of the ependyma and in all sections of the choroid plexus, bound immunoglobulins were detected, especially in choroid plexus vessels, suggesting the presence of immune complexes. In the same areas, direct staining with a fluorescein-conjugated anti-MHV-3 serum detected the presence of viral antigens. Spleen sections from the same animals showed appearances typical of immune vasculitis with detection of both viral antigens and bound immunoglobulins in the walls of most arteries, veins and small vessels. Virus-carrier mice persistently infected but without major neurological signs showed also some degree of immune vasculitis. Three negative findings should be stressed : firstly, kidney sections of both control and infected C3H mice showed slight immunoglobulin deposits in the glomeruli, which were not detectably increased in infected animals. Secondly, no viral antigen could be detected in macrophages, either in Kuppfer cells of the liver or in the marginal zone of the spleen. Thirdly, hepatocytes from chronically ill mice were never shown to contain viral antigens by immunofluorescence.

Altogether, these findings suggest that MHV-3 persists mainly, and may be exclusively, in ependymal and meningeal cells (especially in A2G mice), and in vessel wall structures of C3H mice. No evidence could be found of viral persistence in parenchymal cells (hepatocytes or neurones) or in tissue macrophages. It should be underlined, however, that immunofluorescence techniques are not highly sensitive and may miss viral antigens present in very little amounts. Our observations thus do not exclude virus persistence in other tissues, but clearly indicate that persistency takes place essentially in meninges and in vessel walls, probably in endothelial cells. This is consistent with the findings that infective virus can be transferred more easily from brain and lymphoid organs than from liver or kidneys, and that the titers of virus in all organs tested are always very low. Viruses which persist by replicating freely in many cell types, including macrophages, such as lymphochoriomeningitis or lactic dehydrogenase virus, are always recoverable in high titers. Chronic MHV-3 infection with chronic vasculitis resembles another type of experimental model, equine viral arteritis, in which the virus has been shown by electron microscopy to replicate in the endothelial cells of the damaged vessels [17]. Indeed, the contrast between the absence of glomerular damage and the existence of a widespread vasculitis further favors the hypothesis that vascular damage is not due to deposition of circulating immune complexes but rather to in situ formation of immune complexes within vessel walls where MHV-3 antigens persist.

POSSIBLE MECHANISMS OF VIRAL PERSISTENCE

Viral persistence implies that the virus is able to escape, at least partially but indefinitely, the immune surveillance of the host. MHV-3 does not loose its virulence in chronically infected mice, since its transfer into susceptible recipients always leads to acute, lethal hepatitis. Clearly, persistence depends on host factors, able to protect animals during the acute phase of the disease, but unable to clear completely the virus from the cells where it has found a refuge. Is this "semi-resistance" fundamentally different in its mechanisms from the full resistance observed in A/J mice ? The difference may only be a question of degree, since intermediate titers of virus are found in mice from semi-resistant strains during the first days of infection [12]. These titers are predictive, since virus titers in blood of C3H mice four days after infection show a clear correlation with the course of the disease. Most of the animals with high virus titers die of acute disease, whereas those that survive and subsequently develop a chronic disease show low virus titers. Thus early events appear to decide whether MHV-3 infection will be acute or chronic.

While antibody to MHV-3 seems to play very little role in resistance [6], two non specific early host factors appear to have a critical role in recovery : one is viral restriction in individual cells, including macrophages and hepatocytes. Indeed, macrophages are known to be the primary target cell of MHV-3 in vivo [9], and we have shown a precise correlation between in vivo resistance and a variable genetic ability of peritoneal macrophages to restrict virus growth, C3H macrophages being intermediate in this respect [7]. Moreover, primary monolayer cultures of hepatocytes isolated from adult, resistant A/J or partially resistant C3H/He mice exhibit resistance to MHV-3 as the respective macrophages do [18]. Thus, even if the virus were able to escape the macrophage blood-organ barrier, it would find resistance in individual hepatocytes. The second early host defense mechanism is interferon production, which neutralization in vivo with a potent anti-type I murine interferon serum potentiates strikingly MHV-3 infection in the C3H strain : all mice die of acute hepatitis [19]. Thus the fate of MHV-3 infection in C3H mice is decided at a stage (48 hours) when the specific immune response is unlikely to be operative. Classical (type I) interferon and macrophages are likely to collaborate in host defense against MHV-3, since macrophages are susceptible to the antiviral effect of interferon and also are able to produce interferon themselves. Furthermore, it is possible that lymphocytes and macrophages cooperate through immune (type II) interferon. Indeed, we have shown that the latter type of interferon, a product of activated leucocytes, can protect cultures of mouse peritoneal macrophages against MHV-3 [20]. In C3H mice, however, interferon production is not fully effective, since the virus persists in the face of permanent (although low) titers of circulating interferon [10]. As discussed previously [2], it should be envisaged that sensitivity to interferon action, rather than interferon production, is genetically deficient in C3H mice. According to this hypothesis, some body cells in this strain (especially meningeal and endothelial cells) would not be fully sensitive to the antiviral effects of interferon and would serve as permanent refuge for the virus.

T lymphocytes also are likely to participate in host defense against MHV-3 infection, since it has been reported that the protective capacity of spleen cells transferred from adult, resistant to neonatal, susceptible A/J mice is abolished after treatment with anti-θ serum [21]. Finally, it should be remembered that persistent MHV-3 infection is associated with a profound, permanent state of immunodepression [10]. This may further diminish the ability of the host to eradicate the infection. Clearly, no single mechanism is likely to underlie the complex host-virus relationship leading to MHV-3 persistence.

REFERENCES

1. J. L. Virelizier, Pathogenesis of mouse hepatitis virus (MHV-3) infection in various inbred strains of mice, in: "Mechanisms of viral pathogenesis and virulence", P. B. Bachmann, ed., WHO Collaborating Centre for Collection and Evaluation of Data on Comparative Virology, Munich (1979).
2. J. L. Virelizier, Role of macrophages and interferon in natural resistance to mouse hepatitis virus infection, in: "Natural resistance to viruses and tumors", Current Topics in Microbiology and Immunology, Springer Verlag, Berlin, Heidelberg, in press (1980).
3. A. C. Allison, Genetic factors in resistance against virus infection, Arch. Ges. Virusforsch., 2:280 (1965).
4. F. B. Bang and A. Warwick, Mouse macrophages as host cells for the mouse hepatitis virus and the genetic basis of their susceptibility, Proc. Nat. Acad. Sci. (Wash.), 46:1065 (1960).
5. I. Shif and F. B. Bang, In vitro interaction of mouse hepatitis virus and macrophages from genetically resistant mice. I. Adsorption of virus and growth curve, J. Exp. Med., 131:843 (1970).
6. C. Le Prevost, E. Levy-Leblond, J. L. Virelizier, and J. M. Dupuy, Immunopathology of mouse hepatitis virus type 3 infection. I. Role of humoral and cell-mediated immunity in resistance mechanisms, J. Immunol., 114:221 (1975).
7. J. L. Virelizier and A. C. Allison, Correlation of persistent mouse hepatitis virus (MHV-3) infection with its effect on mouse macrophage cultures, Arch. Virol., 50:279 (1976).
8. J. L. Virelizier, Etude virologique et immunologique d'une virose persistante chez la souris infectée par le virus de l'hépatite murine (MHV-3), Thèse de

Doctorat en Médecine. Faculté de Médecine Paris-Sud, Paris (1972).
9. M. Piazza, G. Pane, and F. De Ritis, The fate of MHV-3 after intravenous injection into susceptible mice, Arch. Ges. Virusforsch., 22:472 (1967).
10. J. L. Virelizier, A. M. Virelizier, and A. C. Allison, The role of circulating interferon in the modification of immune responsiveness by mouse hepatitis virus (MHV-3), J. Immunol., 117:748 (1976).
11. J. L. Virelizier, A. D. Dayan, and A. C. Allison, Neuropathological effects of persistent infection of mice by mouse hepatitis virus, Infect. Immun., 12:1127 (1975).
12. C. Le Prevost, J. L. Virelizier, and J. M. Dupuy, Immunopathology of mouse hepatitis virus type 3 infection III. Clinical and virologic observation of a persistent viral infection, J. Immunol., 115:640 (1975).
13. P. A. Phillips, M. N. I. Walters, N. F. Stanley, and D. Keast, Amyloidosis, immunocompetence and the chronic murine diseases induced by reovirus type I and II, Pathology, 3:267 (1971).
14. L. Kilham and G. Margolis, Hydrocephalus in hamsters, ferrets, rats and mice following inoculation with reovirus type I, Lab. Invest., 21:183 (1969).
15. R. T. Johnson and K. D. Johnson, Hydrocephalus following viral infection : the pathology of aqueductal stenosis developing after experimental mumps virus infection, J. Neuropathol. Exp. Neurol., 27:591 (1968).
16. P. W. Lampert, J. K. Sims, and A. J. Kniazeff, Mechanism of demyelination in JHM virus encephalitis. Electron microscopic studies, Acta Neuropathol., 24:76 (1973).
17. P. C. Estes and N. F. Cheville, The ultrastructure of vascular lesions in equine viral arteritis, Am. J. Pathol., 58:235 (1970).
18. H. Arnheiter and O. Haller, Inborn resistance of mice to mouse hepatitis virus type 3 (MHV-3) : Liver parenchymal cells express phenotype in culture, (1980), see the proceedings of this symposium on the biochemistry and biology of coronaviruses.
19. J. L. Virelizier and I. Gresser, Role of interferon in the pathogenesis of viral diseases of mice as demonstrated by the use of anti-interferon serum.V. Protective role in mouse hepatitis virus type 3 infection of susceptible and resistant strains of mice, J. Immunol., 120:1616 (1978).
20. J. L. Virelizier, A. C. Allison, and E. De Maeyer, Production by mixed lymphocyte cultures of a type II interferon able to protect macrophages against virus

infections, Infect. Immun., 17:282 (1977).
21. E. Levy-Leblond and J. M. Dupuy, Neonatal susceptibility to MHV-3 infection in mice. I. Transfer of resistance, J. Immunol., 116:1219 (1977).

THE USE OF A GENETICALLY INCOMPATIBLE COMBINATION OF HOST AND VIRUS (MHV) FOR THE STUDY OF MECHANISMS OF HOST RESISTANCE

Frederik B. Bang

Department of Pathobiology
The Johns Hopkins University
School of Hygiene and Public Health
Baltimore, M.D. 21205

In 1960 when we found that mouse hepatitis virus (MHV) could grow in, and would destroy, macrophages in tissue culture, and that macrophage behavior in vitro reflected the single gene for susceptibility in the mouse,[1,2] we constructed a simple model of how genetic resistance and susceptibility to this virus functioned. Today, the basic experimental findings remain unchanged, but new findings have compelled a very different interpretation of the same data. We believe that this re-interpretation applies to many host-virus genetic systems. It may be useful to first follow each item that has been re-interpreted, and then illustrate how the more complex model can clarify one way in which the environment affects host-parasite interrelations. We believe that the effects of environmental pollutants could be tested in this system. The original view of the system and the change in viewpoint between 1960 and 1980 are shown in Table 1.

We will present below the data which have caused each change in interpretation. It is of primary importance to recognize that from the start we have used an unusual medium developed originally by Y. Chang to study the growth of rat leprosy bacilli in mouse macrophages[3]: 90% horse serum with 5% beef embryo extract. The macrophages do well in this medium, but to the uninitiated the cells do not look as beautiful because they are spread out on the glass as well as when grown in fetal calf serum or in other diluted sera. However, we continue to use it as a standard because cells grown in it show the maximum difference in genetic susceptibility and resistance without altering the absolute susceptibility of the susceptible cells. This medium has several disadvantages. We have not found commercial lots useful, so we bleed individual horses, and strictly

Table 1. Changing Concepts on Mouse Hepatitis: 1960→1980

1. Genetic resistance and susceptibility due to one single character

   GENETICALLY COMPATIBLE AND INCOMPATIBLE FOUR-FOLD PAIR OF HOST AND VIRUS; OTHER GENETIC EFFECTS

2. Mouse and macrophages resistant to MHV in general

   MOUSE AND MACROPHAGES RESISTANT TO SPECIFIC STRAIN OF MHV

3. Virus is absorbed into and dies in resistant cells

   INITIAL GROWTH OF VIRUS (ONE-STEP) EQUAL IN RESISTANT AND SUSCEPTIBLE CELLS

4. Resistance of macrophages absolute: 10^7 log

   RESISTANCE OF MACROPHAGES RELATIVE: 2×10^1 TO 10^7

5. Macrophage acting alone

   MACROPHAGE/LYMPHOCYTE IMMUNE INTERACTION

6. No evidence of interferon in resistant cells

   PROBABLE INTERFERON-LIKE MECHANISM

ensure that antibodies to MHV are not present in the sera.

An important caveat is that the 'purity' of the virus must be constantly checked. The agent which is adapted to the susceptible mouse may have varying proportions of a mutant which is highly virulent for the genetically resistant strain of mice.[4] Thus a basic requirement for the studies is to keep the proportion of this mutant virus below $1:10^6$ of the standard agent. This means that the stock virus destroys genetically resistant cells at no greater a dilution than 10^{-2}, whereas the same virus titers to more than 10^{-8} in genetically susceptible cells. Finally, despite the extensive knowledge of the metabolism of macrophages in culture, there are no data available on the biochemical changes of macrophages maintained under these conditions so important to our studies.

We will now discuss each of the points in Table 1 and will try to demonstrate the reason for the re-interpretation.

The original idea was that the standard virus obtained from PRI mice simply did not grow in the resistant C_3H cells, and for some time I dismissed the fact that low dilutions of stock virus did kill resistant cells, attributing it to a toxic effect. However, when Shif was working in my laboratory, he showed that the supernatant taken from the cells that are destroyed by 10^7 or 10^8 infectious doses of virus contains a new virus which is able to destroy C_3H macrophages and kill C_3H mice even at low dilutions.[4] This adaption to a new host forces us to recognize, as did the students of bacteriophage a long time ago,[5] that host resistance and virus virulence can be described only in terms of specific pairs. Plant geneticists had also recognized this in the case of fungal infections. Flor[6] combined genetic analysis of the virulence of a rust fungus with a similar analysis of the genetics of resistance of the flax plant, and established that there is a one to one relationship of genes of host and parasites which regulates the resultant disease.[6] If the genes of host and parasite are matched, or compatible, then severe disease results, whereas if they are incompatible, then very mild disease results. Flor constructed the diagram presented in Fig. 1, which he called a quadratic check.[6] For us, the quadratic check has become an essential instrument for the study of factors which influence the adjustment between host and virus. We will concentrate particularly on the incompatible system in dealing with the effects of malnutrition and cortisone, and it is this system which in vitro is susceptible to the effect of agar and agarose,[7] while the compatible system serves as an excellent control showing that the basic health of the cells has not been altered.

In order for the genetic comparison between resistant and susceptible strains of mice eventually to have a specific biochemical

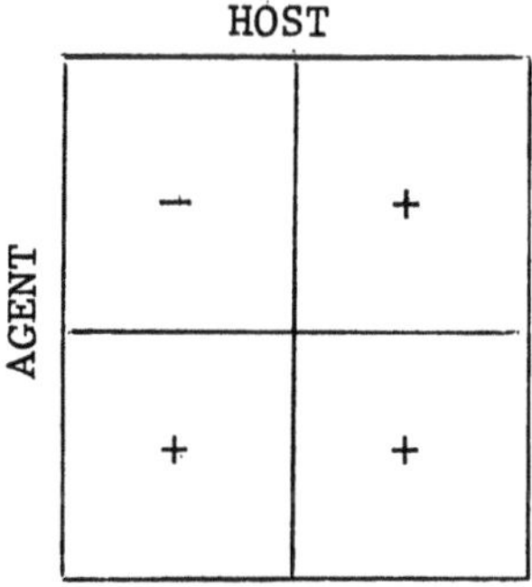

Fig. 1. Quadratic check.

meaning, we have introduced the gene for susceptibility into the inbred C_3H resistant mice, and now deal with two host strains: the original C_3H and a C_3H_{SS},[8] which are kept in isolation and from which we draw our animals as they are used. Using this system, and using a further cloned virus, Cody[7] analyzed the mechanism of the virus change and found, by fluctuation analysis, that the new virus arises from the stock by mutation at a rate of $3\text{-}5\times10^{-7}$. Thus we must constantly ensure that the agent we use is overwhelmingly of one type, and to maintain the standard cloning and dilution passes. To summarize the first two points: Although genetic resistance and susceptibility to MHV do follow typical mendelian patterns of inheritance, this is true only for the specific strain of MHV with which we started our work, and this virus can easily be changed, not only in its capacity to grow in so-called resistant mice and macrophages but also, as Cody again has shown,[7] in different types of tissue. Thus the necessity of the quadratic check.

In Shif's original work,[4] only PRI and C_3H mice were available, and the virus had not been selected for adaptation to macrophages.

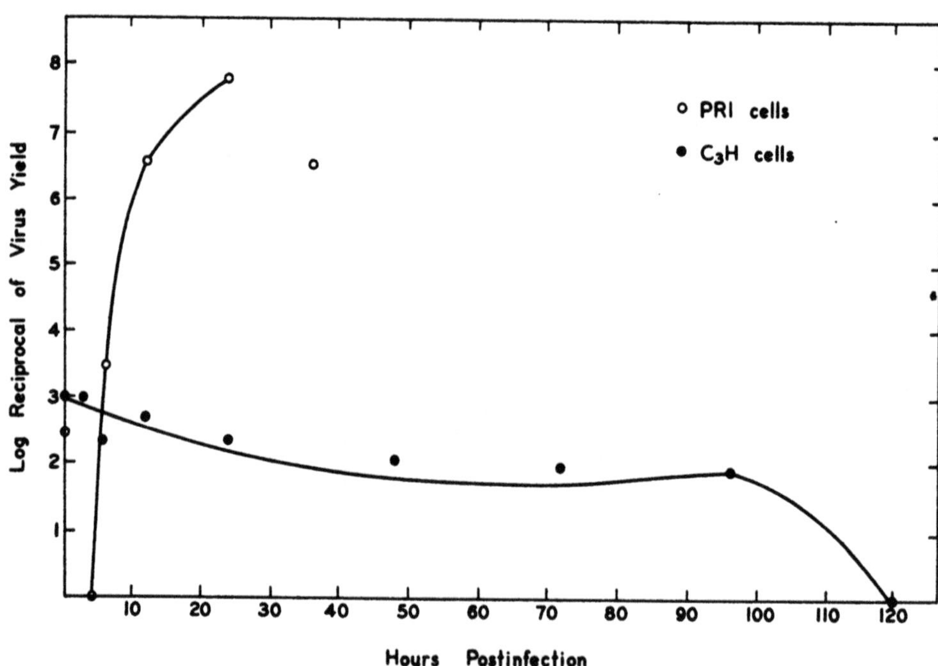

Fig. 2. Disappearance of infectious virus from C_3H resistant cells in macrophage cultures as compared to growth in PRI susceptible cells (Shif).

He found that following exposure of resistant macrophages to MHV(PRI), there was no apparent difference in the rate of absorption of the virus between the incompatible and the compatible pair, but that adsorption onto the resistant cells was followed by a loss of infectious virus titer (Fig. 2). The idea that the incompatible virus is absorbed into, and gradually dies within, the resistant cell had to be re-interpreted when Cody showed that the virus grows equally well in the resistant and susceptible cell, but is infective at about 1/20 the rate in resistant cells (Fig. 3).[7] This further demonstrates the value of the quadratic check and the selection of mutants that are specifically adapted to macrophages. Between the original findings[4] and the present ones[7,9] lie: (i) the development of congenic strains of mice so that the genetically resistant and susceptible differ by only one gene; (ii) the selection of a virus strain specifically adapted to growth in macrophages of the C_3H_{SS} mouse; and (iii) the development of one-step growth curve techniques in macrophage cultures. The considerable difference between the original findings and present data suggests that virus adaption occurs through a continuous series of steps, that virus stocks may well be somewhat polymorphic, and that tissue adaption (liver _vs._ macrophages) may be included in these steps. Recent electron-

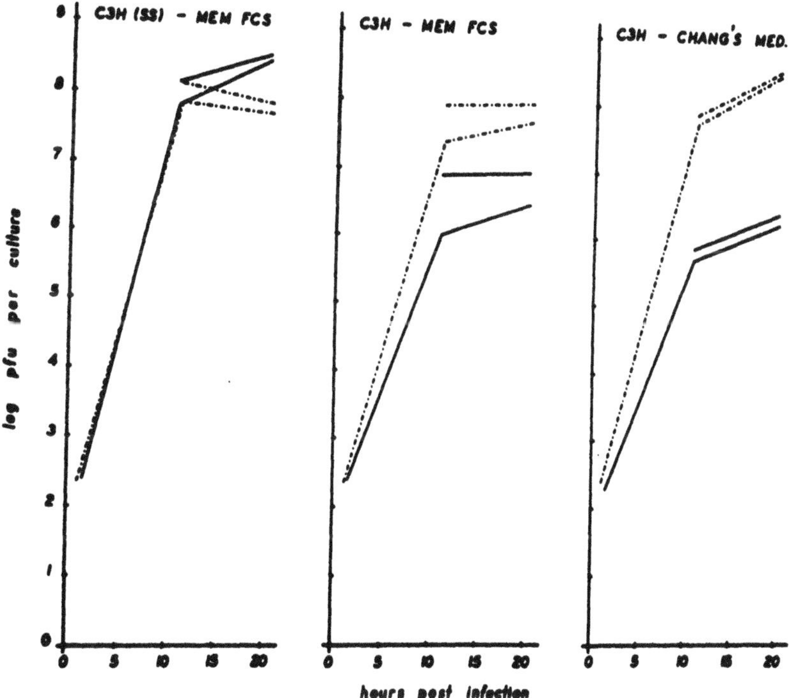

Fig. 3. One-step growth curves of macrophage adapted virus in C_3H and C_3H_{SS} cells (Cody).

microscopic studies by Dr. Reissig in our department support the evidence of initial growth during the first 24 hours, but with only 1/10 as many cells infected.[10] We will return to possible mechanisms of resistance later.

We have dealt sofar with the quadratic check system as if it were uninfluenced by the environment, that is, by physiological changes within the mouse, or by changes in tissue culture media or metabolism. But we have known from the beginning that this is not so because virus titer differed in macrophages which grew in small numbers from liver explants on glass, and when different numbers of liver explants were inoculated in collagen slants. In addition, whenever 20% fetal calf serum, which produces much more attractive spreads of macrophages, was substituted for 90% horse serum, there was a decrease in the difference between resistant and susceptible cells (Table 2).[11] This difference, which is usually 10^6 or a million-fold, is reduced to $10^{2.5}$ in fetal calf serum to or about 300-fold, and in subsequent studies has been shown not to be due to a change in the virus, but to a greater permissiveness of the cells. In turn, the permissiveness is greatly inhibited by the addition of mouse serum.

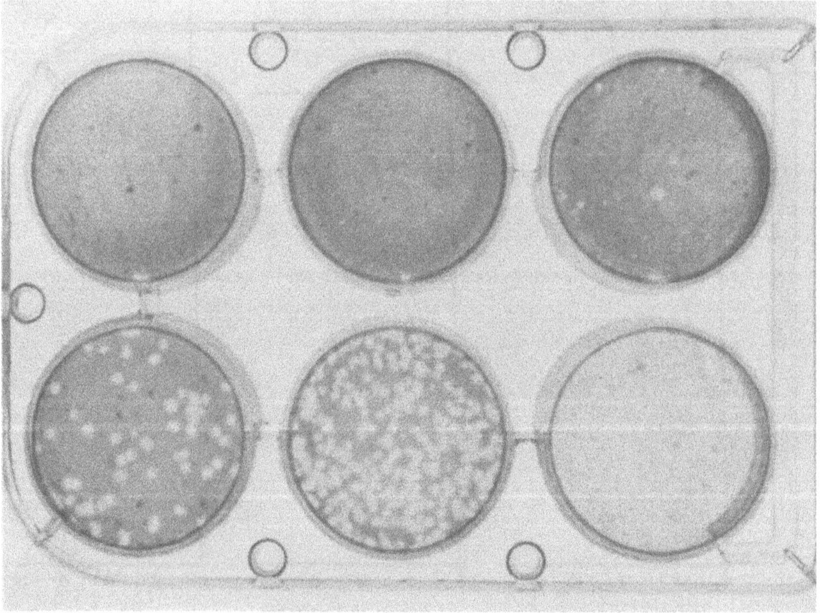

Fig. 4. Plaques of incompatible virus-cell system under agar and agarose (Cody). Top row: agar; bottom row: agarose.

Table 2. Influence of Type and Concentration of Serum on Titration of MHV(PRI) Virus in Cultures of C_3H and PRI Macrophages

% and type of sera in medium	Infectivity of virus (log TCD_{50}/0.05 ml)*	
	on C_3H cells	on PRI cells
90, horse	1.3, 2.5, < 1.0	7.3, 7.6
20, horse	3.8, 4.8, 4.5	8.3, 7.8
10, C_3H mouse	< 1.0, < 1.0	7.8, 8.0
20, horse+C_3H mouse	< 1.0, < 1.0	not done
10, PRI mouse	< 1.0	6.9
10, fetal calf	5.0	not done
10, rat	3.3	not done

*results of 3 different experiments

Obviously, variation in susceptibility of macrophages in culture may be of great significance if our theory that the macrophage regulates the susceptibility of the host is correct. Cody[7] studied susceptibility of macrophages of the C_3H and C_3H_{SS} mice by determining the numbers of plaques that develop under agar and agarose. The results are of great practical and theoretical importance. As seen in Fig. 4, cells from the resistant (C_3H) strains of mice show a striking difference in susceptibility if they are kept under agar or agarose with fetal calf serum. However, if the C_3H_{SS} susceptible cells are placed under agarose and fetal calf serum, they are equally susceptible. The C_3H resistant cells then differ from the genetically susceptible cells by only 10-fold when under agarose. Thus the genetically resistant cell is only potentially resistant and manifests this resistance only under the appropriate conditions. We were extremely fortunate in choosing the unusual medium, 90% horse serum and 5% beef embryo extract, for under these conditions the genetically resistant cells function at their maximum level of resistance.

To bring point 5 of Table 1 up to date, we must re-examine our quadratic check, and recognize that it is incomplete. When phenotypic changes are introduced, the model becomes a cube, for the role that lymphocytes and the immune response may play in genetic resistance must be incorporated (Fig. 5). Two other early findings were involved in this change of concept. One was Kantoch's finding that when resistant macrophages were treated with a crude extract of susceptible peritoneal exudate cells, they were "converted" to become

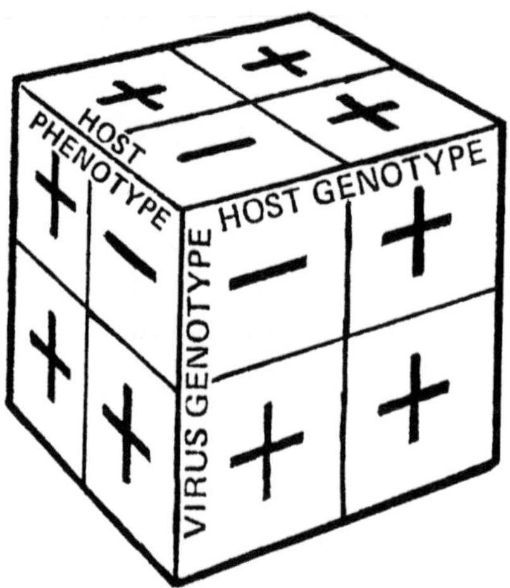

Fig. 5. Three-dimensional representation of interaction of genotypes of host and virus with environmental factors.

more susceptible.[12] The other was that a variety of environmental factors, such as cortisone,[13] cytoxan,[14] and concomitant Epierythrozoon infection[15] make the resistant mice susceptible. Kantoch's "conversion" of resistant macrophages to susceptible ones[12] utilized PRI and C_3H mouse strains which are of course allogeneically different. It turned out that the "conversion" was due to the allogeneic stimulus imposed on the C_3H peritoneal exudate cells, which comprised both macrophages and lymphocytes. Treatment with exudate cells, including lymphocytes from the congenic susceptible mice resulted in no such stimulus.[16] This induced us to examine the way in which susceptibility of both macrophages and mice might be altered by putative lymphokines.

From the start, the question of an interferon effect has been raised. I first learned about mouse hepatitis from Gledhill, when working at the National Institute for Medical Research, Mill Hill, England. In a laboratory across the corridor, Isaacs and Lindenmann had just discovered interferon. A year or so later when we found that mouse macrophages were susceptible to the virus of mouse hepatitis, it was impossible to ignore interferon and interference. But several sets of experiments made us postpone careful study of this group of substances. First, when explants of resistant and susceptible livers were placed together on the same collagen substrate, only about half of the migrating macrophages (presumably those from the susceptible strain of mice) were destroyed (Figs. 6 and 7).[17] Next, when a mixed culture of resistant and susceptible peritoneal macrophages is set up, the virus apparently kills the susceptible and spares the resistant.[18,19] Finally, this held true even when the two congenic strains of mice were used, and the clarity of the plaque depends upon the proportion of susceptible and resistant cells (Figs. 6 and 7). Thus in no case did the resistant cells protect the susceptible cells.

Nonetheless, there are at least three reasons _not_ to accept this apparent negative evidence. The first is the indirect evidence of Virelizier et al.[20] that interferon plays a role in response to mouse hepatitis virus type 3 (MHV-3); the second is the striking experiments of Virelizier and Gresser,[21] which show that antibodies to interferon convert a mild infection with MHV-3 to a virulent one; and thirdly, our own results with Concanavalin A (ConA), which is a well known stimulus to interferon production. Genetically susceptible mice (and their macrophages), in our hands, can be protected by the administration of ConA to the mice.[22] Finally (see later), the effect of cortisone on macrophage susceptibility is neutralized by supernatants from ConA-treated cells. Thus we tend more and more

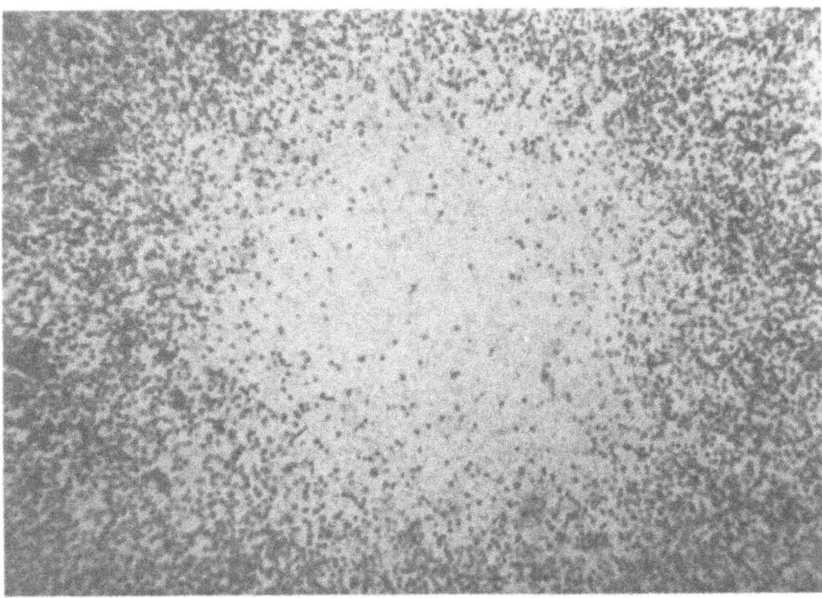

Fig. 6. Complete plaque of MHV on susceptible cells (Cody).

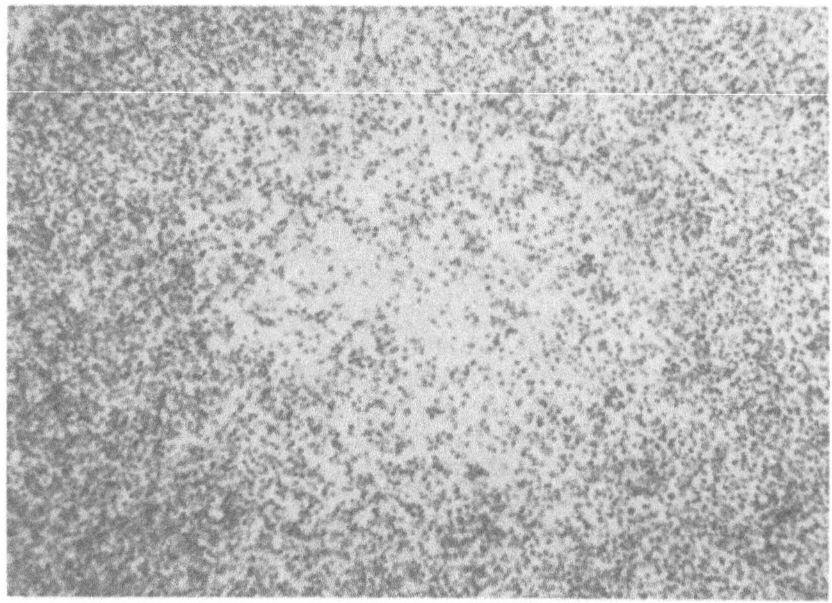

Fig. 7. Incomplete plaque of MHV on mixture of susceptible and resistant cells (Cody).

to think of some mechanism involving an interferon (Table 3) which is evoked in, and bound to, the resistant cell but cannot get to the susceptible cell.

Table 3. Reversal of Cortisone Effect by Supernatant of ConA-Treated Spleen Cells (Taylor)

	LD_{50}
C_3H alone	2.3
$HC\text{-}R_x$	5.7
$HC\text{-}R_x$ + ConA supernatant	1.5
$HC\text{-}R_x$ + normal supernatant	3.5

The major thrust of this presentation is the proposal that a genetically defined incompatible system of host and parasite which allows for the development of a mild infection is an ideal system on which to study the mechanisms of host resistance and is a system which may be of value in testing the effects of various environmental factors on susceptibility to infection. An understanding of how the system seems to work is a necessary prelude to discussion of two examples which are currently under study in our laboratory. Our incompatible (mild) system of mouse hepatitis, like so many other experimental infections, can be made into a fatal infection by administration of cortisone.[13] Over the years, we have used cortisone to produce either minor or zero effects on susceptibility of resistant macrophages.[13,23] But when it was recognized that lymphokines are probably involved in changing the susceptibility of macrophages in vitro, Weiser[24] was able to show that spleen cells from cortisone-treated mice caused the resistant cells to become susceptible. Following up on this, Taylor[25] has now shown that macrophages taken from mice that receive three doses of cortisone over a 3-day period yield macrophages that are 1000-fold more sensitive to the virus (Table 4). This increased sensitivity lasts only a few days in tissue culture; it is produced by dexamethazone and prednisalone, as well as cortisone, but not by testosterone or progesterone. Increased susceptibility, judged by the destructive effect of the virus, is accompanied by greater growth of the virus. Finally, this increased susceptibility is counteracted by supernatant obtained from ConA-treated spleen cell cultures (Table 3). Thus the in vivo effect of cortisone on susceptibility of the mouse may be mimicked

Table 4. Susceptibility of C_3H Macrophages to MHV(PRI) after In Vivo Administration of Hydrocortisone (HC) (Taylor)

	LD_{50}
C_3H control	2.4
3 doses of:	
1.0 mg HC	4.6
2.5 mg HC	5.4
5.0 mg HC	4.8
10.0 mg HC	3.5
1 dose of:	
2.5 mg HC	2.6
C_3H_{SS} control	7.7

by in vitro results.

Nutrition. There is a tremendous literature on the effect of nutritionally inadequate diets on susceptibility to infection.[26,27] We can be fairly sure that the multiplicity of types of infection results in a spectrum of effects of different dietary components. One way to define the role of dietary factors is to selectively deprive the host of a nutrient which allows the immune system to react immediately to prevent a lethal outcome to a potentially serious infection. Dr. Shams Zaman came to our laboratory from Bangladesh, where the interactions of undernutrition and infectious disease take a heavy toll in infants after weaning. She studied the effect of a low protein diet on susceptibility of mice to MHV.[28] Her work and our continued studies are summarized in Table 5. Pathological studies suggest that the early destruction of liver cells and the later lesions in the thymus and the spleen involve the same cell types, and that the low protein diet is destructive of the macrophage-lymphocyte system. We have not as yet been able to obtain consistent in vitro results, so the mechanism of changed susceptibility can only be inferred.

SUMMARY

A unigenic and major difference in susceptibility of two strains of inbred mice (PRI and C_3H) to mouse hepatitis virus seemed initially to be simple and uncomplicated. In vitro macrophage susceptibility matched in all details the genetic and ontogenic constitution of the mice. Subsequently, combined use of a quadratic check system and in vitro analysis of macrophage susceptibility has produced a sophisticated system for testing the mechanisms of genetic

Table 5. Effect of Diet on Mortality of Incompatible Pair of Host and Virus

Diet	# of expts.	Total # of mice	# of deaths	%
Purina chow	9	54	1	2
Low (8%) protein	6	47	47	100
High (27%) protein	8	49	20	41

resistance to this one coronavirus.

The large (10^6) in vitro difference in susceptibility of resistant and susceptible macrophages to the original virus depends upon maintaining these cells in 90% horse serum, or in lower concentrations of sera to which mouse serum has been added.

The quadratic check system designates those pairs of host and virus in which infection is not full-blown as genetically incompatible and those in which a successful lethal infection is established as genetically compatible. Since genetic resistance of the host may be experimentally modified both in vitro and in vivo, it is necessary to diagram the host-virus system in a three-dimensional quadratic check, or a cube.

The original finding that virus is absorbed into and dies in resistant cells was based on a comparison of cells from PRI and C_3H mice. With further adaption of the virus to macrophage cultures of the congenic susceptible C_3H_{SS} mice, and the comparison of one-step growth in congenic C_3H and C_3H_{SS} macrophages, it is shown that the genetically resistant cells are 1/20 as susceptible as the susceptible, and that infection in both is initially the same.

Macrophage resistance is dependent upon associated lymphocyte action. Despite the absence of direct evidence that interferon is operating in protecting the genetically resistant cell, increasing evidence supports the idea that cell-bound interferon protects the genetically resistant cell.

The genetically incompatible system of host and virus seems ideal for both the study of the mechanism by which resistance is altered and as a test system on which to survey the effects of environmental factors on susceptibility to infection.

REFERENCES

1. F. B. Bang and A. Warwick, Macrophages and mouse hepatitis, Virology 9:715 (1974).
2. F. B. Bang and A. Warwick, Mouse macrophages as host cells for the mouse hepatitis virus and the genetic base of their susceptibility, Proc. Natl. Acad. Sci. 46:1065 (1960).
3. Y. T. Chang, Transactions of the Symposium on Research on Leprosy 1961, Sponsored by the Leonard Wood Memorial (American Leprosy Foundation) and the Johns Hopkins University School of Hygiene and Public Health, Baltimore, Maryland (1961).
4. I. Shif and F. B. Bang, In vitro interaction of mouse hepatitis virus and macrophages from genetically resistant mice. I. Adsorption of virus and growth curves. II. Biological

characterization of a variant virus MHV(C_3H) isolated from stocks of MHV(PRI), J. Exp. Med. 131:843 (1970).
5. W. Hayes, "The Genetics of Bacteria and Their Viruses. Studies in Basic Genetics and Molecular Biology," 2nd edition, Blackwell Scientific Publications, Oxford (1968).
6. H. H. Flor, The complementary genic systems in flax and flax rust, Adv. Gen. 8:29 (1956).
7. T. S. Cody, "Factors Governing the Response of Macrophages to MHV In Vitro," Doctor of Science thesis, The Johns Hopkins University School of Hygiene and Public Health, Baltimore, Maryland (1980).
8. W. Weiser, I. Vellisto and F. B. Bang, Congenic strains of mice susceptible and resistant to mouse hepatitis virus, Proc. Soc. Exp. Biol. Med. 152:499 (1976).
9. F. B. Bang and T. S. Cody, Is genetic resistance to mouse hepatitis based on immunological reactions? in: "Proceedings of the International Symposium on Genetic Control of Natural Resistance to Infection and Malignancy, Montréal, March 18-20, 1980," Academic Press, Inc., New York (in press).
10. M. Reissig, Unpublished.
11. G. C. Lavelle and F. B. Bang, Influence of type and concentration of sera in vitro on susceptibility of genetically resistant cells to mouse hepatitis virus, J. Gen. Virol. 12: 1 (1971).
12. M. Kantoch and F. B. Bang, Conversion of genetic resistance of mammalian cells to susceptibility to a virus infection, Proc. Natl. Acad. Sci. 48:1553 (1962).
13. R. Gallily, A. Warwick and F. B. Bang, Effect of cortisone on genetic resistance to mouse hepatitis virus in vivo and in vitro, Proc. Natl. Acad. Sci. 51:1158 (1964).
14. D. O. Willenborg, K. V. Shah and F. B. Bang, Effect of cyclophosphamide on the genetic resistance of C_3H mice to mouse hepatitis virus, Proc. Soc. Exp. Biol. Med. 141:762 (1973).
15. G. C. Lavelle and F. B. Bang, Differential growth of MHV(PRI) and MHV(C_3H) in genetically resistant C_3H mice rendered susceptible by eperythrozoon infection, Arch. ges. Virusforsch. 7:918 (1973).
16. W. Weiser and F. B. Bang, Macrophages genetically resistant to mouse hepatitis virus converted in vitro to susceptible macrophages, J. Exp. Med. 143:690 (1976).
17. F. B. Bang and A. Warwick, Unpublished.
18. I. Shif and F. B. Bang, Plaque assay for mouse hepatitis virus (MHV-2) on primary macrophage cell cultures, Proc. Soc. Exp. Biol. Med. 121:829 (1966).
19. I. Shif, "In Vitro Interaction between Mouse Hepatitis Virus and Macrophages from Genetically Resistant Mice," Doctor of Science thesis, The Johns Hopkins University School of Hygiene and Public Health, Baltimore, Maryland (1968).
20. J.-L. Virelizier, A.-M. Virelizier and A. C. Allison, The role of circulating interferon in the modifications of immune

responsiveness by mouse hepatitis virus (MHV-3), J. Immunol. 117:748 (1976).

21. J.-L. Virelizier and I. Gresser, Role of interferon in the pathogenesis of viral diseases of mice as demonstrated by the use of anti-interferon serum. V. Protective role in mouse hepatitis virus type 3 infection of susceptible and resistant strains of mice, J. Immunol. 120:1616 (1978).
22. W. Y. Weiser and F. B. Bang, Blocking of in vitro and in vivo susceptibility to mouse hepatitis virus, J. Exp. Med. 146: 1467 (1977).
23. D. O. Willenborg, "The Effect of Chemical and Physical Agents on the Genetic Resistance of Mice to Mouse Hepatitis Virus (MHV-PRI)," Doctor of Science thesis, The Johns Hopkins University School of Hygiene and Public Health, Baltimore, Maryland (1970).
24. W. Y. Weiser, "Macrophage-Lymphocyte Interaction in Mouse Hepatitis Virus Infection," Doctor of Philosophy dissertation, The Johns Hopkins University, Baltimore, Maryland (1978).
25. C. E. Taylor, Unpublished.
26. N. S. Scrimshaw, C. E. Taylor and J. E. Gordon, "Interactions of Nutrition and Infection. WHO Monograph Series No. 57," World Health Organization, Geneva (1968).
27. I. Gontzea, "Nutrition and Anti-Infectious Defence," S. Karger, Basel (1974).
28. S. N. Zaman, "Protein Deficiency and Susceptibility to Mouse Hepatitis Virus Infection," Master of Science thesis, The Johns Hopkins University School of Hygiene and Public Health, Baltimore, Maryland (1979).

INFLUENCE OF THE IMMUNE SYSTEM ON THE COURSE OF INFECTION WITH MURINE CORONAVIRUS JHM IN SUCKLING MICE

Karin Pickel, Maria Anna Müller and
Volker ter Meulen

Institute for Virology and Immunobiology
University of Würzburg
D-8700 Würzburg
Federal Republic of Germany

INTRODUCTION

JHM-virus, a neurotropic strain of murine corona virus, has been shown to induce various diseases of the central nervous system in rats which are influenced by the age of the animals at the time of infection (1-3). Infection early in life always results in acute disease while subacute or chronic diseases develop when adult animals are infected. In this connection it appears to be of importance to analyze the factors determining the different reactions of young and adult animals to infection with JHM virus. It has been shown for various viruses, that resistance to infection can occur, based either on the genetics or on the age of the animal (4-11). In this study experiments were carried out to investigate age dependent resistance by analyzing the influence of components of a competent immune system on the course of JHM virus infection in suckling mice.

MATERIALS AND METHODS

VIRUS: JHM-virus, originally derived from suckling mouse brain (1) was propagated in the C3H mouse fibroblast cell line L 929 to titres of 1 -5 x 10^5 plaque forming units (PFU)/ml. The titre was evaluated by plaque assay on L 929 cells. Inactivation of JHM-virus was obtained by UV-irradiation of 2×10^5 PFU/ml with 30.000 erg/mm^2.

MICE: C3H mice were purchased from Bomholtgart (Ry, Denmark). The expression "baby mice" was used for mice younger than 25 days, "adult mice" for mice older than 2 months.

CELLS: Spleen and thymus cell suspensions were prepared in MEM containing 5 % FCS, and injected intraperitoneally if not quoted otherwise.
Normal spleen cells (NSC) were derived from non-immune adult C3H mice, immune spleen cells (ISC) from adult C3H mice, which were immunized i.p. once with 10^5 PFU of JHM virus. Immune spleen cells were obtained 4 days, 14 -30 days, or 50 - 100 days after immunization. All ISC populations were tested for the presence of infectious virus *in vitro* by plaque assay, and *in vivo* by injecting the cells into susceptible baby mice. Both assays always worked comparably: injection of cell samples which turned out to be positive in the plaque assay killed suckling mice.

DESIGN OF EXPERIMENTS: To circumvent maturation differences between different litters, experiments were set up in the following way: When differently treated groups were compared in an experiment, in which more than one litter was used, the animals of the different litters were dispensed in such a way that each experimental group was represented in each litter. The virus was injected intraperitoneally throughout the experiments.

RESULTS

Age Dependence of the Outcome of JHM-Virus Infection in C3H mice

The outcome of an infection with respect to the age of the animals was followed up by injecting virus into suckling mice at different intervals after birth. As shown in Table 1A it was found that intraperitoneal infection with 20 PFU per mouse was always lethal for mice up to the age of 20 days. The rate of mortality was reduced when mice were 21 or 22 days old. Older animals were resistant to infection. There was hardly any time shift when higher virus doses were given (Table 1B). Table 1A and 1B show the results of distinct representative sets of experiments. Comparing different sets, the occurrence of resistance was shifted by maximally 2 days

days, probably reflecting the variation in the maturation of different litters. These findings demonstrate that natural resistance to JHM infection is an all or none effect. It does neither develop gradually over a longer period of time nor by showing clinical symptoms of changing severity. Paralysed hind legs and impaired balance could only be detected 8 - 4 hours before the animals died.

Table 1. Outcome of JHM Infection in C_3H Mice

A) AGE DEPENDENCE

TIME OF INFECTION (20 PFU[1)]/MOUSE) DAYS P.P.[2)]	SURVIVORS OF INFECTION / TOTAL GROUP	OCCURRENCE OF DEATH DAYS P.I.[3)]
14	0/1	4 - 8
16	0/6	5 - 6
18	0/5	6 - 8
20	0/5	5 - 7
21	3/5	8 - 11
22	7/9	9
23	7/7	-
24	8/8	-

1) PFU plaque forming units
2) P.P. postpartum
3) P.I. post infection

Table 1. Outcome of JHM Infection in C_3H Mice

B) DOSE DEPENDENCE

TIME OF INFECTION DAYS P.P.	PFU/ MOUSE	SURVIVORS OF INFECTION / TOTAL GROUP	OCCURRENCE OF DEATH DAYS P.I.
14	2×10^1	0/10	4 - 8
	2×10^2	0/10	4 - 6
	2×10^3	0/5	4 - 5
22	2×10^2	3/4	7
	2×10^3	2/3	7
	2×10^4	1/3	7
24	2×10^2	3/3	-
	2×10^3	1/2	7
	2×10^4	4/7	7 - 11
25	2×10^5	49/50	18

This development of natural resistance to intraperitoneal JHM virus infection parallels in time the development of competence of the immune system in mice (12). We therefore investigated whether or not immunological factors can influence the course of JHM virus infection in suckling mice.

Influence of Spleen Cells from Adult Mice on the Course of JHM Infection in Suckling Mice

Normal spleen cells from adult mice as a source of mature lymphocytes were injected intraperitoneally into baby mice together with or before application of virus (Table 2). Although up to 6 x 10^7 cells were transferred protection was found only in a few cases.

Table 2. Effect of Normal Spleen Cells on JHM Virus Infection in Baby Mice

TIME OF INFECTION (20 PFU/MOUSE) DAYS P.P.	CELL TRANSFER: DAYS BEFORE INFECTION	NUMBER OF NSC[1)] TRANSFERRED	SURVIVORS / TOTAL GROUP	OCCURRENCE OF DEATH DAYS P.I.
14 - 16	0	6 x 10^7	1/6	5 - 8
		3 x 10^7	3/8	5 - 10
	2	6 x 10^7	1/8	5 - 11
		3 x 10^7	1/10	5 - 8
	4	6 x 10^7	0/9	6 - 12
		3 x 10^7	0/5	5 - 7
14 - 16	-	-	0/20	4 - 12

1) NSC Normal Spleen Cells

To see if any immune protection at all could occur in suckling mice immune spleen cells from adult mice, which had been immunized with JHM virus for various periods were injected into baby mice on the day of infection (Table 3). By this transfer - in contrast to the transfer of non-immune spleen cells- the majority of baby mice could be protected from death of infection, when at least 10^7 spleen cells were applicated. Protection by these cells did not depend on the priming period of the immune mice. These results show that immunological events can play a protective role , however, priming of the transplanted lymphocytes was a prerequisite for protection.

Table 3. Effect of Immune Spleen Cells on JHM Virus Infection in Baby Mice

TIME OF INFECTION (20 PFU/MOUSE) DAYS P.P.	PRIMING PERIOD IN DAYS	NUMBER OF ISC[1)] TRANSFERRED	SURVIVORS / TOTAL GROUP	OCCURRENCE OF DEATH DAYS P.I.
14	50	3×10^7	2/3	7
		1×10^7	6/8	7
14	14 - 30	3×10^7	5/6	11
		1×10^7	2/3	8
		3×10^6	0/2	5 - 6
14	4	3×10^7	8/8	-
14	-	-	0/15	4 - 8

1) ISC IMMUNE SPLEEN CELLS

Influence of Baby Lymphocytes on the Course of Infection in Adult Mice

As primed lymphocytes were not inhibited to exert their function in suckling mice the question was asked whether the lack of protection by normal spleen cells was due to suppression of their priming by the baby host. Immune suppression by lymphocytes from suckling mice has been shown in several other systems (13-15). As a first approach we tested this possibility by injecting thymocytes or spleen cells of 14 days old mice intraperito neally or intravenously into adult mice one day before infection with 10^5 PFU per mouse (Table 4). None of the injected animals showed any clinical symptoms. Thus the resistance of adult mice to JHM virus infection could not be abolished by lymphocytes from suckling mice. These findings could suggest that baby lymphocytes did not interfere with the anti-JHM immune response of adult mice. On the other hand it could well be possible that the immune response was affected but the effect was masked because defense mechanisms other than the immune system, or a lack of appropriate target cells prevented the conversion from resistant to susceptible mice.

It further cannot be excluded that lymphocytes from suckling mice were only able to suppress adult spleen cells when they were allowed to operate in their own surrounding, namely the baby's body.

Table 4. Effect of Baby Lymphocytes on the Infection in Adult Mice

CELL TYPE TRANSFERRED	MODE OF CELL TRANSFER	NUMBER OF CELLS TRANSFERRED	PFU PER MOUSE	SURVIVORS / TOTAL GROUP
THYMOCYTES	I.V.[1]	4×10^8	1×10^5	2/2
"	"	2×10^8	"	3/3
"	"	1×10^8	"	2/2
"	I.P.[2]	2×10^8	"	3/3
"	"	1×10^8	"	2/2
SPLEEN CELLS	I.V.	1×10^8	"	3/3
"	I.P.	1×10^8	"	3/3

1) I.V. INTRAVENOUSLY

2) I.P. INTRAPERITONEALLY

Priming of Non-Immune Adult Spleen Cells in Baby Mice

The lack of protection of baby mice by unprimed spleen cells from adult mice as a consequence of suppression by the host was investigated in the following way: normal spleen cells from adult mice were injected into baby mice together with UV-inactivated JHM virus at different times before challenge with live virus. If the antigen-dependent differentiation -induced by the inactivated virus -were suppressed a priming of the injected lymphocytes would not occur. Consequently the rate of survivors should not extend the rate of survivors of those groups which were supplemented with NSC or UV-inactivated virus alone. Table 5 shows that application of UV-inactivated virus did not change the fate of 14 days old baby mice after infection, but that it slightly enhanced the rate of survivors when the animals were infected at the age of 19 - 21 days. Thus priming of the babies' own

Table 5. Effect of UV-Inactivated JHM-Virus on JHM-Virus Infection in Baby Mice

TIME OF INFECTION (20 PFU/MOUSE) DAYS P.P.	APPLICATION OF UV-JHM DAYS BEFORE INFECTION	SURVIVORS / TOTAL GROUP		OCCURRENCE OF DEATH DAYS P.I.
14 - 16	0	0/10		5 - 10
	2	1/8		4 - 8
	4	0/6		4 - 9
19 - 21	0	3/4		11
	1 - 2	6/10	16/31	6 - 13
	3 - 4	5/17		4 - 12
	5 - 6	6/8		5 - 13
14 - 16	-	0/15		5 - 8
19 - 21	-	6/18		5 - 12
NO INFECTION	14 - 16 DAYS P.P.	7/7		

lymphocytes did not occur in 2 weeks old animals, but seemed to become possible in 3 weeks old mice. On the other hand, when UV-inactivated JHM-virus was injected into 14 - 16 days old mice together with spleen cells from adult mice (Table 6) more than 50 % of the baby mice were protected against death of a subsequent infection. It made no difference whether the mice were challenged with live virus 2 or 4 days after cell transfer.

CONCLUSION

The experiments suggest that the lack of protection by normal spleen cells alone is not due to suppression by the host, because normal spleen cells can be primed in suckling mice. Thus the discrepancy is still unexplained that the presence of normal spleen cells in adult mice

Table 6. Priming of Normal Spleen Cells from Adult Mice in Baby Mice

TIME OF INFECTION (20 PFU/MOUSE) DAYS P.P.	CELL TRANSFER AND APPLICATION OF UV-JHM (DAYS BEFORE INFECTION)	NUMBER OF CELLS TRANSFERRED	SURVIVORS / TOTAL GROUP	OCCURRENCE OF DEATH DAYS P.I.
14 - 16	2	6×10^7	4/7	5 - 8
	2	3×10^7	4/8	4
	2	1×10^7	2/5	7 - 9
	3	6×10^7	2/3	7
	3	3×10^7	8/12	4 - 10
	4	6×10^7	6/7	5
	4	3×10^7	9/14	7 - 8
	4	1×10^7	5/10	4 - 6
	4	3×10^6	0/5	5 - 6
14 - 16	-	-	0/20	4 - 9
NO INFECTION	14 - 16 DAYS P.P.	6×10^7	5/5	-

is sufficient to cope with a JHM virus infection, while suckling mice, when supplemented with normal spleen cells from adult mice, are not able to control an infection successfully. It is therefore suggestive that the different course of infection with JHM virus in suckling mice and in adult mice is not only due to the different stages of immune competence, but that additional factors must play a role.

It is well known that dissemination of virus in the adult animal can also be prevented by non-immunological defence mechanisms. These might not yet be fully developed in a baby mouse. Findings reported by Taguchi et al. (16) for the interferon system would be in line with these interpretations. Comparing suckling and weanling mice these authors showed that, after infection, the production of interferon was delayed in suckling mice. In addition, target cells for JHM-virus might change during development. Baby mice might have relatively more target cells for JHM-virus than adult mice, and the change during maturation might reflect a reduction of target cells by loss of virus receptors, or by alteration of the cellular competence for virus replication. An age-related conversion from susceptibility to resistance has been shown for infection of mouse fibroblasts with Sindbis virus (10), and for infection of mouse macrophages with MHV 2 (17). In addition, the relevant cells, namely the potential target cells, might change with respect to their importance for the organism.

SUMMARY

The course of infection with murine corona virus JHM in C3H mice depends on the age of the animals. Mice up to 20 days of age are fully susceptible while mice older than 23 days resist the infection. Protection of suckling mice from death of infection can be provided by intraperitoneal administration of immune spleen cells but not by non-immune spleen cells from adult mice. The immune spleen cells can be generated by priming adult mice, or by priming non-immune spleen cells from adult mice in baby mice with inactivated JHM virus. Thus the immune system might well be involved in the different outcome of infection with JHM-virus in suckling and adult mice, but it does not seem to be the exclusive factor responsible for the achievement of natural resistance.

ACKNOWLEDGEMENTS

We thank Mrs. Helga Kriesinger for typing the manuscript. This work was supported by the Deutsche Forschungsgemeinschaft.

REFERENCES

1) Nagashima, K., H. Wege, R. Meyermann, V. ter Meulen. 1978.
Corona Virus Induced Subacute Demyelinating Encephalomyelitis in Rats: A Morphological Analysis.
Acta Neuropathol. (Berl.) 44, 63 - 70.

2) Nagashima, K., H. Wege, R. Meyermann and V. ter Meulen 1979,
Demyelinating Encephalomyelitis Induced by a Long-term Corona Virus Infection in Rats. Acta Neuropathol. (Berl.) 45, 205-213.

3) Wege, H., M. Koga, Hanna Wege and V. ter Meulen JHM Infections in Rats As A Model for Acute and Subacute Demyelinating Disease, Plenum Press, in press

4) Bang, F.B., Warwick, A. (1960). Mouse Macrophages as Host Cells for the Mouse Hepatitis Virus and the Genetic Basis of their Susceptibility. Proc. Natl. Acad. Sci. USA 46, 1065 -1075.

5) Goodman, T., Koprowski, H. (1962). Study of the Mechanism of Innate Resistance to Virus Infection. J. Cell. Comp. Physiol. 59, 333 -373.

6) Chalmer, J.E., Mackenzie, J.S., Stanley, N.F. (1977). Resistance to Murine Cytomegalovirus linked to the Major Histokompatibility Complex of the Mouse. J. Gen Virol. 37, 107 - 114.

7) Lopez, C. (1975). Genetics of Natural Resistance to Herpes Virus Infecitons in Mice. Nature 258, 152 -153.

8) Lennette, E.H., H. Koprowski (1944). Influence of Age on the Susceptibility of Mice to Infection with Certain Neurotropic Viruses. J. Immunol. 49, 175 -191.

9) Johnson, R.T. (1964). The Pathogenesis of Herpes Virus Encephalitis. II. A Cellular Basis for the Development of Resistance with Age. J. exp. Med. 120, 359-373.

10) Johnson, R.T., H.F. McFarland, S.E. Levy (1972). Age Dependent Resistance to Viral Encephalitis: Studies of Infections due to Sindbis Virus in Mice. J. Infect. Dis. 125, 257 - 261.

11) Hirano, N., S. Takenaka, K. Fujiwara (1975). Pathogenicity of Mouse Hepatitis Virus for Mice Depending upon Host Age and Route of Infection. Japan. J. Exp. Med. 45, 285 - 292.

12) Spear, P.G., G.M., Edelman (1974).
Maturation of the Humoral Immune Response in Mice.
J. exp. Med. 139, 249 - 263.

13) Mosier, D.E., B.M., Johnson (1975).
Ontogeny of Mouse Lymphocyte Function. II. Development of the Ability to Produce Antibodies is Modulated by T-Lymphocytes.
J. exp. Med. 141, 216 - 226.

14) Rodriguez, G. G. Andersson, H. Wigzell, A.B. Peck, 1979.
Non-T Cell Nature of the Naturally Occurring, Spleen-Associated Suppressor Cells Present in the Newborn Mouse.
Eur. J. Immunol. 9, 737-746.

15) Durandy, A., A. Fischer, C. Griscelli (1979).
Active Suppression of B Lymphocyte Maturation by two Different Newborn T Lymphocyte Subsets.
J. Immunol. 123, 2644-2650.

16) Taguchi, F., A. Yamada, K. Fujiwara (1979).
Factors Involved in the Age-Dependent Resistance of Mice Infected with Low-Virulence Mouse Hepatitis Virus.
Arch. Virol. 62, 333-340.

17) Gallily, R., A. Warwick, F.B. Bang (1967).
Ontogeny of Macrophage Resistance to Mouse Hepatitis Virus in vivo and in vitro.
J. exp. Med. 125, 537-548.

Macrophages and Resistance to JHM Virus CNS Infection

Stephen A. Stohlman and Jeffrey A. Frelinger

University of Southern California School of Medicine

2025 Zonal Avenue, Los Angeles, CA 90033

INTRODUCTION

The macrophage is an important cell in determining the outcome of viral infections, especially those due to herpes and mouse hepatitis viruses (Morgensen, 1979). Mouse hepatitis virus (MHV), is a member of the coronavirus group which are positive stranded RNA viruses (Lai and Stohlman, 1978) and produce a wide spectrum of diseases in their natural hosts (McIntosch, 1973). The principle organs attacked by MHV during infection are the liver and the central nervous system (CNS). Bang and co-workers have demonstrated a genetic basis for the resistance of mice to fatal hepatitis caused by MHV and that *in vitro* macrophages from resistant animals exhibit resistance parallel to that determined *in vivo* (Bang, 1978). They have shown that MHV can only replicate *in vitro* in macrophages from susceptible animals. This type of resistance appears to be analogous to the intrinsic resistance described for herpes viruses (Johnson, 1964). Intrinsic resistance to viral replication limits virus dissemination thereby affording protection to the target organ and the host. Recently, we have demonstrated the ability of passively transferred macrophages to confer resistance to the JHM strain of MHV (MHV-JHM) induced acute CNS disease (Stohlman et al, 1980). However, macrophages from both susceptible and resistant animals exhibited intrinsic resistance to MHV-JHM replication.

We have examined the ability of macrophages to exhibit extrinsic anti-viral activity, the ability of macrophages to suppress MHV replication in another cell, correlated this with intrinsic anti-viral activity, and examined the macrophages from resistant and susceptible mice for a number of macrophage markers.

ABSTRACT

Thioglycollate elicited peritoneal exudate cells from resistant SJL mice, younger susceptible SJL mice, and susceptible ASW, BALB/c, and C57/BL6 mice all exhibit extrinsic antiviral activity. The active cell was characterized as a Thy 1.2 negative, Ia negative, radiation resistant adherent cell. The antiviral activity was not due to nonspecific cellular cytotoxicity directed against the susceptible cell nor interferon. Adherent PE cells from resistant and susceptible SJL mice were similar with respect to the number of phagocytes, nonspecific esterase containing, Fc, and C_3b receptor bearing cells. Finally, extrinsic antiviral activity was not dependent upon intrinsic antiviral activity.

MATERIALS AND METHODS

Mice: SJL, $C_{57}BL/6$, and BALB/c were all purchased from Jackson Laboratories, Barr Harbor, Maine. ASW mice were obtained from the Immunogenetics Mouse Colony, USC.

Effector Cell Preparation: Peritoneal exudate (PE) cells were elicited by the intraperitoneal injection of thioglycollate broth 3 days prior to peritoneal lavage with Hanks balanced salt solution containing 10 IU of heparin/ml. The PE cells were removed, washed and the viability determined as previously described (Stohlman et al, 1980). In some experiments, PE cells were subjected to 2000 R with a 60_{Co} source emitting at 1000 R/min. Nonadherent cells were prepared as previously described (Stohlman et al, 1980).

Assay for Extrinsic Anti-Viral Activity: To test for extrinsic anti-viral activity, DBT cells, a continuous mouse astrocyte cell line (Stohlman and Weiner, 1978) were grown in 24 well (16 mm) plates using Dulbecco's modified MEM containing 5% Newborn calf serum (Biocell, Carson, California). Monolayers contained approximately 5×10^5 cells. All wells were infected with 10-15 pfu of the DL plaque size variant of MHV-JHM for 1 hr at 37°C.

Following removal of the inoculum, 0.5 ml of RPMI-1640 containing 2% NBC serum and 10 mM Hepes was added to each well. At 2-4 hr after inoculation, the effector PE cells at final concentration of from 10^4 to 5×10^6 cells per well were added in quadruplicate in a 0.5 ml volume. Control wells received medium only. Cultures were incubated for 18 hr and the supernatants from the 4 wells were pooled before the samples were frozen at -70°C. Released progeny virus was determined by plaque assay on monolayers of DBT cells as previously described (Stohlman and Weiner, 1978). The average virus yield in the 4 wells was determined in either triplicate or quadruplicate assays.

Antisera Depletion: T cells were depleted by treating 2 x 10^7 cells/ml with congenic anti-Thy 1.2 serum PL/J x B6-Thy1^a) F_1 anti-B6 and rabbit complement (C). Ia bearing cells were removed as described by treatment with A.TL anti A.TH serum and C (Niederhuber, et al, 1975). Cells were reconstituted to 10^7 viable cells/ml.

Nonspecific Cytotoxicity: Nonspecific cytotoxicity was determined by adding 5.0 uCi of ^{3}H-thymidine (ICN Pharmaceuticals) to 1 x 10^6 L929 or DBT in 75 cm^2 flasks. After 24 hr at 37°C the targets were trypsinized, washed, and counted. Target cells were added to 24 well plates at 4 x 10^4 cells per well in 0.5 ml. Dilutions of the test PE cells at the quantities used in the extrinsic anti-viral assay in 0.5 ml were also added in quadruplicate. Total release was determined by adding 0.5 ml of 1.0% SDS in place of PE cells. After 48 hrs, 0.2 ml of the supernatant was removed and counted as previously described (Stohlman and Lai, 1979).

ADCC and ADP: Antibody dependent cellular cytolysis (ADCC) and antibody dependent phagocytosis (ADP) were determined simultaneously using the method of Walker (1977). TNP-coated SRBC were labeled with ^{51}Cr (NEN) and incubated with PE cells at an effector to target ratio of 5:1 for 2 hrs at 37°C with constant rocking.

Intrinsic Antiviral Activity: PE cells were placed in 35 mm plates at 4 x 10^6 viable cells/plate. After 2-3 hrs the cultures were washed vigorously 3x with serum free DMEM. The remaining adherent cells were infected with 0.2 ml of MHV-JHM for 1 hr at 37°C. At various times post infection the cells were scraped into DMEM 2% fetal calf serum and then disrupted by two cycles of freezing and thawing. The virus content was determined by plaque assay on DBT cells (Stohlman and Weiner, 1978).

RESULTS

Extrinsic anti-viral activity: SJL mice exhibit an age-dependent resistance to intracranial (i.c.) challenge with MHV-JHM. We have previously shown that PE cells from non-immune SJL donors confer resistance to syngenic susceptible animals (Stohlman et al, 1980). To determine if extrinsic macrophage-mediated anti-viral activity was a protective mechanism operating under these circumstances, an assay for extrinsic antiviral activity was established similar to those developed for herpes virus (Morahan et al, 1980). Table 1 shows that the addition of thioglycollate elicited PE cells from 12 week old SJL mice to cultures of infected cells effectively suppresses virus replication at effector to target ratios in excess of 1:1.

TABLE 1

Extrinsic anti-viral activity of PE cells,
PE cells depleted of Ia bearing cells, and heat killed PE cells

TREATMENT	EFFECTOR TO TARGET RATIO	PERCENT RELEASED VIRUS
None		
	10:1	0
	5:1	0
	1:1	26
	None	100
Anti-Theta + C[2]	10:1	0
	5:1	0
	1:1	28
Anti-Ia + C[2]	10:1	0
	5:1	2
	1:1	33
NMS[1] + C[2]	10:1	0
	5:1	2
	1:1	31
Irradiation (1000 R)	10:1	0
	5:1	0
	1:1	30
Heat Killed	10:1	94
	5:1	100
	1:1	98

[1] NMS = normal mouse serum

[2] C = complement

Suppression of the release of virus into the supernatant was not dependent upon T cells since treatment of the PE cell population with congenic anti-Thy 1.2 serum had no effect. Protection from lethal i.c. challenge is mediated by a PE cell population lacking Ia antigen (Stohlman et al, 1980). Therefore, PE cells depleted of Ia bearing cells were tested for anti-viral activity. Table 1 also shows that removal of the Ia bearing cells did not significantly reduce the anti-viral activity of the remaining cell population. Furthermore, the activity was also not decreased by irradiation of the effector PE cell population. Heating at 56°C for 30 min. completely abolished protection. In addition, the nonadherent PE cell population exhibited markedly reduced protection. Partial protection in the nonadherent population is probably due to contamination with a cell population that is able to adhere in an additional two hr inoculation (approximately 10%). This residual population contains nonspecific esterase, Fc and C_3b receptor positive cells (data not shown). Experiments were run in parallel comparing thioglycollate elicited and resident peritoneal cells to determine if thioglycollate treatment enhanced the protective capacity. Table 2 shows that resident cells were as effective in suppressing virus replication as thioglycollate elicited PE cells, which is in agreement with our previous finding that splenic macrophages are also effective in confirming protection (Stohlman et al, 1980).

TABLE 2

Comparison of extrinsic anti-viral activity of Resident and Thioglycollate elicited PE cells

	EFFECTOR TO TARGET RATIO	PERCENT RELEASED VIRUS
Elicited PE cells		
	10:1	0
	5:1	4
	2:1	32
	1:1	26
Resident PE cells		
	10:1	0
	5:1	9
	2:1	41
	1:1	28

To insure that the apparent anti-viral activity was not due to nonspecific cytotoxic activity resulting in the destruction of the host cells, DBT and L929 cells were tested as targets. SJL PE cells exhibited nonspecific cytotoxicity against L929 cells. No killing of DBT cells was detectable at any effector to target ratio (data not shown).

Age-Dependent Activity: PE cells from 4, 6, and 12 week old SJL were tested for extrinsic anti-viral activity to determine if the basis of the age-related change in resistance to MHV-JHM could be correlated with an inability of PE cells from mice younger than 12 weeks of age to suppress viral growth. Table 3 shows that there was essentially no difference in anti-viral activity between the three age groups tested. To insure that the cells responsible for the anti-viral activity of the PE cells from 4 and 6 week old animals was similar to that described above, these PE cells were also tested following irradiation. In addition,

PE cells from 6 week old animals were tested following Ia and Th 1.2 depletion. No loss of anti-viral activity was found following these treatments (data not shown). PE cells from 6 week old SJL were also tested for nonspecific cyotoxicity against DBT and L929 cells. Similar to the results with PE cells from 12 week old SJL, there was no nonspecific cytotoxic activity against the DBT cells. The level of activity against L929 cells was comparable to that found for PE cells from 12 week old SJL, a maximum of approximately 30% of the total counts released.

TABLE 3

Comparison of the anti-viral activity of PE cells from 4, 6 and 12 week old SJL mice

AGE	EFFECTOR TO TARGET RATIO	PERCENT RELEASED VIRUS
12 weeks	10:1	0
	5:1	0
	2:1	2
	1:1	31
	0.5:1	64
6 weeks	10:1	0
	5:1	0
	2:1	0
	1:1	28
	0.5:1	70
4 weeks	10:1	0
	5:1	0
	2:1	3
	1:1	27

Histochemical Analysis: Adherent PE cell populations from 6 and 12 week old SJL were examined for the number of nonspecific esterase positive, phagocytic, Fc and C_3b receptor bearing cells. The number of adherent cells in any particular PE cell preparation varied from 50-80%, however, in any given experiment the number of adherent cells from 6 and 12 week old cells varied no more than ± 5%, and the variation was not consistent with age.

Table 4 shows that the adherent PE cells from 6 week old and 12 week old mice are slightly different with respect to the number of cells able to phagocytize 1.0 u latex beads, and in the number of cells with C_3b receptors. The difference is probably not large enough to be correlated with the dramatic change in the ability of these cell populations to prevent acute CNS disease. The two populations were similar with respect to the number of cells positive for nonspecific esterase and Fc receptor.

TABLE 4

Macrophage marker associated with the adherent PE cell population from 6 and 12 week old SJL mice

MARKER	PERCENTAGE ADHERENT CELLS POSITIVE	
	6 week	12 week
Phagocytosis[1]	91.9 ± 0.1	87.4 ± 0.6
Nonspecific Esterase	88.3 ± 3.1	91.6 ± 1.7
Fc Receptor	91.6 ± 1.06	92.5 ± 0.1
C_3b Receptor	68.4 ± 0.9	72.1 ± 1.40

[1] Determined by uptake of latex beads

ADCC and ADP: Antibody dependent cellular cytolysis (ADCC) and antibody dependent phagocytosis (ADP) of TNP-modified sheep red blood cells were examined using 6 and 12 week old SJL PE cells as effectors. Table 6 shows three of these experiments. There is no difference in the ability of the PE cells from the 6 or 12 week old SJL to lyse TNP-coated SRBC or to phagocytize antibody coated SRBC. Increased ADCC activity with increased dilution of antibody is a regular finding in ADCC systems (Lovchik and Hong, 1977).

Intrinsic Viral Resistance: MHV stains replicate in PE cells obtained from susceptible animals (Bang, 1980; Virelizier and Allison, 1976). However, MHV-JHM would not replicate in adherent PE cells from either resistant 12 week old SJL, susceptible 6 week old SJL or from susceptible B10.S mice (Stohlman et al, 1980). Adherent PE cells from 6 week old SJL and BALB/c were tested for their ability to support MHV-JHM replication. Table 6 shows that the adherent PE cells from BALB/c mice would support MHV-JHM while those from SJL mice would not support virus replication.

Extrinsic Activity in Susceptible Strains: Thioglycollate elicited PE cells from ASW, BALB/c, and $C_{57}BL/6$ mice were examined for extrinsic antiviral activity in parallel experiments with PE cells from SJL. Table 7 shows that PE cells from these three strains of mice which are all susceptible to i.c. challenge with MHV-JHM (Stohlman and Frelinger, 1978) are as efficient as PE cells from SJL mice in suppressing viral growth in DBT cells.

TABLE 5

Antibody dependent cellular cytolysis and phagocytosis of PE cells from 6 week old and 12 week old SJL mice

EXPERIMENT NUMBER	AGE WEEKS	ANTIBODY DILUTION (RECIPROCAL)	PERCENT OF TOTAL ADCC	ADP
1	6	100	6.0	30.0
		1000	6.7	35.4
	12	100	5.3	41.6
		1000	6.3	36.0
2	6	100	7.7	36.0
		1000	10.7	24.2
	12	100	7.7	32.4
		1000	11.4	24.0
3	6	100	17.0	29.2
		1000	24.7	16.9
	12	100	18.6	27.1
		1000	22.6	17.1

TABLE 6

Replication of MHV-JHM in adherent PE cells from SJL and BALB/c mice

MOUSE STRAIN	HOURS POST INFECTION	TITER
BALB/c	6	0[1]
	12	3×10^2
	24	1.1×10^3
	48	2.9×10^4
	72	3.9×10^3
SJL	6	0[1]
	12	0[1]
	24	0[1]
	48	0[1]
	72	0[1]

[1]) No virus deleted

TABLE 7

Extrinsic anti-viral activity of thioglycollate elicited PE cells from different strains of mice.

MOUSE STRAIN	EFFECTOR TO TARGET RATIO	PERCENT RELEASED VIRUS
SJL	10:1	0
	5:1	0
	2:1	9
	1:1	40
ASW	10:1	0
	5:1	0
	2:1	6
	1:1	42
C_{57}BL/6	10:1	0
	5:1	2
	2:1	2
	1:1	19
BALB/c	10:1	0
	5:1	0
	2:1	11
	1:1	40

DISCUSSION

Cells of the macrophage series play a major role in the hosts ability to defend against viral infection. Macrophages exhibit both "intrinsic" and "extrinsic" anti-viral effects as part of the hosts immune defense. Intrinsic resistance is the inability to support virus replication (Morahan and Morse, 1979). It is related to the ability either to phagocytize viruses, thereby rendering them noninfectious, or to adsorb virus at the cell surface and restrict a complete replication cycle within the milieu of the cellular cytoplasm. Extrinsic antiviral activity, on the other hand, is the ability to suppress virus replication in another cell susceptible. The mechanism of this suppression, which can be demonstrated with in vitro systems in the absence of other cells of the immune system, is not clear (Morahan et al, 1980). It is expressed by both circulating monocytes and PE cells that have properties attributable to macrophages (Morahan and Morse, 1979).

Intrinsic antiviral activity of macrophages has been implicated in resistance to both herpes virus and MHV infections (Morahan and Morse, 1979; Bang, 1978; Virelizier and Allison, 1976). In the case of herpes simplex virus, the intrinsic resistance is correlated with an age-dependent acquisition of host resistance (Johnson, 1964; Stevens and Cook, 1971). Intrinsic resistance to MHV has been related to the genetic basis of resistance to acute viral hepatitis (Bang, 1978). JHM, the neurotropic strain of MHV, causes an acute encephalomyelitis with both acute and chronic demyelination in mice (Weiner, 1973; Herndon et al, 1975). CNS disease in SJL mice can be prevented by the passive transfer of PE cells (Stohlman et al, 1980). However, *in vitro*, macrophages from mice that are both susceptible and resistant to i.c. challenge with MHV-JHM exhibit extrinsic anti-viral activity which clearly sets these results apart from the results reported for both HSV and other strains of MHV.

In this communication we report the first evidence of extrinsic anti-viral activity for a virus other than a member of the herpes virus group. PE cells from SJL mice resistant to i.c. challenge with MHV-JHM exhibit extrinsic anti-viral activity. The cell responsible was characterized as a macrophage based on refractiveness to irradiation, negative selection for adherence, and the absence of Thy 1.2 antigen. In addition to these properties, all in common with the cell type capable of confirming resistance to susceptible young SJL (Stohlman et al, 1980), the active cell type lacked suface Ia antigens similar to the cells active in the *in vivo* model. The anti-viral activity was dependent on the effector to target ratio and was not related to either interferon or the lysis of the infected cells by nonspecific cytotoxicity.

We examined the extrinsic anti-viral activity of PE cells from 12 week old SJL mice to help understand its possible role in macrophage mediated age-dependent resistance to i.c. challenge. Intrinsic anti-viral activity had previously been ruled out since macrophages from both susceptible and resistant SJL mice were refractory to infection with MHV-JHM (Stohlman et al, 1980). Evidence presented indicates that PE cells from 4, 6 and 12 week old SJL all have equal ability to suppress viral growth in a second cell type.

In addition to trying to correlate extrinsic antiviral activity with the age-dependent change in resistant of SJL mice we have also examined the PE cell populations from these two age groups for other markers associated with macrophages. No differences significantly large to account for the dramatic change in resistance were noted in the percent adherent cells, the number of adherent cells that were phagocytic, contained nonspecific esterase, Fc or C_3b receptor, or in the ADCC or ADP activity of PE cells from these two age groups.

Since we have previously shown that SJL is the only strain of mice capable of surviving a lethal i.c. challenge with MHV-

JHM (Stohlman and Frelinger, 1978), we examined other strains of susceptible mice for their ability to express macrophage mediated extrinsic anti-viral activity against MHV-JHM. We found that PE cells from BALB/c, ASW, and C_{57}BL/6 mice, which are susceptible to MHV-JHM, suppressed virus replication to the same extent as PE cells from the resistant SJL strain. This observation is in contrast to the apparent differential expression of intrinsic anti-viral activity. SJL adherent cells show complete intrinsic anti-viral activity, while the adherent cells from BALB/c are permissive. This indicates that macrophages can exhibit extrinsic anti-viral activity quite apart from intrinsic anti-viral activity and that these two functions may not be directly correlated with the ability to survive an acute CNS viral infection or an *in vivo* model of protection based on the passive transfer of macrophages.

ACKNOWLEDGEMENTS

This work was supported by grants RG 1233-A-1 from The National Multiple Sclerosis Society, NS 12967, NS 15079, and CA 22662 from the National Institutes of Health. J.A.F. is recipient of American Cancer Society Faculty Research Award FRA-179.

REFERENCES

Bang, F.B. 1978. Genetics of resistance of animals to viruses: 1. Introduction and studies in mice. Adv. Virus Res. 23:270-349.

Herndon, R.M., Griffin, D.E., McCormick, U., and L.P. Weiner. 1975. Mouse hepatitis virus-induced recurrent demyelination. Arch. Neurol. 32:32-35.

Johnson, R.T. 1964. The pathogenesis of herpes virus encephalitis. II. A cellular basis for the development of resistance with age. J. Exp. Med. 120:359-374.

Lai, M.M.C., and Stohlman, S.A. 1978. The RNA of mouse hepatitis virus. J. Virol. 26:236-242.

Lovchik, J.C., and R. Hong. 1977. Antibody-dependent cell-mediated cytolysis (ADCC): Analysis and projections. Prog. Allergy 22:1-44.

McIntosh, K. 1973. Coronaviruses: A comprehensive review. Curr. Top. Microbiol. Immunol. 68:85-129.

Morahan, P.S., and S.S. Morse. 1979. Macrophage-virus interactions. In Proffitt ed. "Virus-lymphocyte Interactions Implications for Disease". Elsevier, North Holland, Inc.

Morgensen, S.C. 1979. Role of macrophage in natural resistance to virus infections. Microbiol. Rev. 43:1-26.

Stevens, J.G. and M.L. Cook. 1971. Restriction of herpes simplex virus by macrophages. An analysis of the cell-virus interaction. J. Exp. Med. 133:19-38.

Stohlman, S.A., and L.P. Weiner. 1978. Stability of neurotropic mouse hepatitis virus (JHM strain) during chronic infection of neuroblastoma cells. Arch. Virol. 57:53-61.
Stohlman, S.A., and J.A. Frelinger. 1978. Resistance to fatal central nervous system disease by mouse hepatitis virus, strain JHM. I. Genetic analysis. Immunogenetics 6:277-281.
Stohlman, S.A., and M.M.C. Lai. 1979. Phosphoproteins of murine coronaviruses. J. Virol. 32:672-675.
Stohlman, S.A., Frelinger, J.A., and L.P. Weiner. 1980. Resis tance to fatal central nervous system disease by mouse hepatitis virus, strain JHM. II. Adherent cell-mediated protection. J. Immunol. 124:1733-1739.
Virelizier, J.R., and A.C. Allison. 1976. Correlation of persis tent mouse hepatitis virus (MHV-3) infection with its effect on mouse macrophage cultures. Arch. Virol. 50:279.
Walker, W.S. 1975. Antibody-dependent cytolysis of chicken erythrocytes by an in vitro established line of mouse peri- toneal macrophages. J. Immunol. 114:765-769-.
Weiner, L.P. 1973. Pathogenesis of demyelination induced by a mouse hepatitis virus (JHM virus). Arch. Neurol. 28:298- 303.

VOMITING AND WASTING DISEASE,

A CORONAVIRUS INFECTION OF PIGS

K. Andries and M. Pensaert

Laboratory of Virology, Faculty of Veterinary Medicine
State University of Gent, Casinoplein 24
B-9000 Gent, Belgium

I. THE DISEASE

In 1957, an epizootic disease of nursing pigs characterized by high morbidity, vomiting, anorexia, constipation and severe progressive emaciation was observed in Canadian swine herds.[1] In acute cases, vomiting and severe depression were the only symptoms noted before death. More frequently the disease tended to become chronic. The affected suckling pigs became emaciated and usually died of starvation after a few weeks. Pigs that survived were permanently stunted. The condition was called "vomiting and wasting disease" because of its salient characteristics.

A second condition, called viral encephalomyelitis, appeared almost concurrently and caused some confusion as to whether one or two disease entities existed.[2] The initial clinical signs also consisted of anorexia, vomiting and constipation, but in this second condition, they progressed after one to three days to an acute encephalomyelitis. At that time hyperesthesia, muscle tremor, ataxia, blindness and paddling of the legs could be observed. The mortality rate was low in older litters (over 3 weeks of age) but it often approached 100 % in very young litters. The Canadian workers Greig et al.[3] isolated in 1961 a virus from the brains of such pigs with encephalomyelitis. It was called hemagglutinating encephalomyelitis virus (HEV) because of its hemagglutinating properties.

In 1969, Cartwright et al.[4] isolated a virus from pigs in England with vomiting and wasting disease. This isolate was later classified as a coronavirus[5] which turned out to be antigenically similar if not identical with HEV.[4] In repeated trials, Mengeling and Cutlip could reproduce the vomiting and wasting syndrome as well as the motoric disorders, using American field isolates.[6] It was, therefore, concluded that the two diseases are different manifestations of the same virus.

Meanwhile, outbreaks of vomiting and wasting disease (VWD) were reported in many European countries.[7-11] However, the epizootic character of the disease seems now to have disappeared. Clinical outbreaks on larger breeding farms are rare and usually occur only in a few litters from gilts. Only on very small breeding farms, outbreaks are still observed in pigs from sows of all ages.[12]

II. EPIZOOTIOLOGY

The spread of VWD virus in the pig population has been studied in several countries by means of serological surveys. In fattening swine, 31 per cent of the sera were positive in Canada,[13] 49 per cent in England,[14] 46 per cent in N.-Ireland,[15] 52 per cent in Japan,[16] 0 to 89 per cent in the United States[17] and 75 per cent in W. Germany.[18] The percentage of sows with antibodies at slaughter varied from 43 per cent in N.-Ireland[15] to 98 per cent in the United States.[17]

From these data, it can be concluded that VWD virus is widely spread among the swine population in different countries. To determine the incidence of infection in Belgium, 140 sow sera were collected in slaughterhouses in 1974 and again in 1979.[12] Seroneutralising antibodies were present in about 93 per cent of these sera. This indicates that most Belgian breeding farms either become regularly infected or harbour the virus persistently. To obtain a better understanding of the normal pattern of infection by the VWD virus, the seroepizootiologic study was extented to younger animals, kept under various circumstances.

The rate of decline of maternal antibodies, was examined in three litters consisting of 29 pigs which were suckling their immune mothers, while kept in isolation. During 4 months, 464 sera were collected at various time intervals after birth. The geometric mean seroneutralisation titer was 192 during their first week of life. At the age of 8 weeks, 4 out of 27 pigs had become negative and at the age of 14 weeks all the pigs were seronegative.

The decline of maternal immunity was also studied in twenty-one weaned pigs, housed in a small stable at the age of 7 weeks. They represented the only pigs on the farm. The geometric mean titer declined until the age of 15 weeks. Four weeks later, the geometric mean titer had risen to 64. The infection which apparently had taken place, passed without clinical signs. The source of infection remained unknown.

On two breeding farms with animals of different ages and a high turnover of pigs, the course of development of seroneutralising antibodies was different from that in the former group of animals. The titers first declined until the age of ten to twelve weeks, but the animals did not become seronegative. A gradual increase in average titer indicated that the passive immunity subsequently was converted into active immunity. On one of these farms, the VWD virus was isolated from nasal discharge of healthy pigs at the age of 2 to 5 weeks. These observations confirmed that the VWD virus was continuously present on these farms and that the pigs became subclinically infected in the presence of maternal antibodies.

Field outbreaks of VWD in piglets seldom occur on conventional breeding farms. This observation can be explained by the fact that most sows have seroneutralising antibodies and that their litters obtain a colostral immunity which protects them against clinical signs during the susceptible period. Suckling pigs will only become sick if they are born from seronegative mothers. On large breeding farms, clinical outbreaks are usually limited to a few litters from gilts. These gilts have probably, through circumstances, insufficient active immunity at the time of parturition. On very small breeding farms, outbreaks are observed in pigs from sows of all ages. These sows can be seronegative, because viral persistence is not likely to occur in such a small animal populations.

III. THE SPREAD OF VWD VIRUS IN PIGS

Preliminary studies on the pathogenicity of VWD virus using different routes of inoculation provided evidence that viral spread occurs along nerve pathways.[9] Typical disease was obtained in pigs after the virus was inoculated into oral and nasal cavities or into the infraorbital nerve but not after intravenous inoculation. In oronasally inoculated pigs killed during the incubation period, the virus could be isolated regularly from the tonsils and the respiratory tract, irregularly from the digestive tract, rarely from the blood and never from lymph nodes, spleen and kidney. In pigs which were killed when ill, the brainstem practically always contained virus while other parts of the brain and the vagal nerve were inconsistently positive.[20]

In a recent experiment, the route of viral spread and the exact sites of viral replication in oronasally infected pigs were examined in detail.[21] Fourteen colostrum deprived pigs were inoculated oronasally within 6 hours after birth with a Belgian VWD virus isolate earlier described.[22] They were killed between post inoculation day (PID) 1 and 7 and frozen sections of different tissues were examined using the direct fluorescent antibody technique.

The incubation period lasted four days in all the pigs which were not yet killed at that time. Illness was characterised by inappetence and listlessness, accompanied or quickly followed by vomition.

In the respiratory tract and tonsils, fluorescent antigens were detected in epithelial cells of the nasal mucosa, tonsillary crypts and greater bronchi of a pig killed on PID 1. The epithelium of terminal and respiratory bronchioli and the pneumocytes of the alveoli became positive starting at PID 2.

In the gastrointestinal tract viral antigens could be detected in the small intestine starting at PID 2. They were located in the cytoplasm of a few cells in the epithelial layer on the villi and in neurons of the submucosal plexus. Neurons of the myenteric plexus became infected at PID 4. Fluorescence was not present in the submucosal and myenteric plexuses of colon and rectum of pigs killed during the incubation period but was found in a pig killed at PID 7. The stomach remained also negative during the incubation period but was positive in 6 of the 7 pigs which were killed when ill. The fluorescence in the stomach was always restricted to the perikaryon of neurons.

In the peripheral nervous system, the trigeminal ganglion became infected at PID 2. The inferior vagal ganglion, the superior cervical ganglion and the solar ganglion (fig. 1) contained viral antigens starting at PID 3. The fluorescence in these ganglia was always restricted to the perikaryon of neurons.

In the lower thoracic region (Th 12-16), a few dorsal root ganglion cells exhibited cytoplasmic fluorescence starting at PID 3. Ganglia at higher and lower levels of the spinal cord were negative in a pig killed at PID 4 but had become positive in a pig killed at PID 7, together with a few neurons of the cervical cord and the thoracic spinal cord.

In the brain, the viral infection started in the sensory nuclei of the trigeminal and the vagal nerve, located in the medulla oblongata. In pigs killed at PID 3 and PID 4, viral antigens were mainly found in neurons of the nucleus spinalis nervi trigemini. In pigs killed after the appearance of the clinical signs, the sensory nucleus of the vagal nerve, the nucleus solitarius, also contained several infected neurons. In pigs killed 2 to 3 days later, the virus had spread into other parts of the brainstem, and sometimes also into the cerebrum and the cerebellum. The medulla oblongata remained, however, the most heavily infected part of the brain. Fluorescence in the brain always remained restricted to the neurons.

Based on the results of the studies presently reported, the following concepts on the spread of VWD virus in pigs can be put forward. After the oronasal inoculation of the virus, the nasal

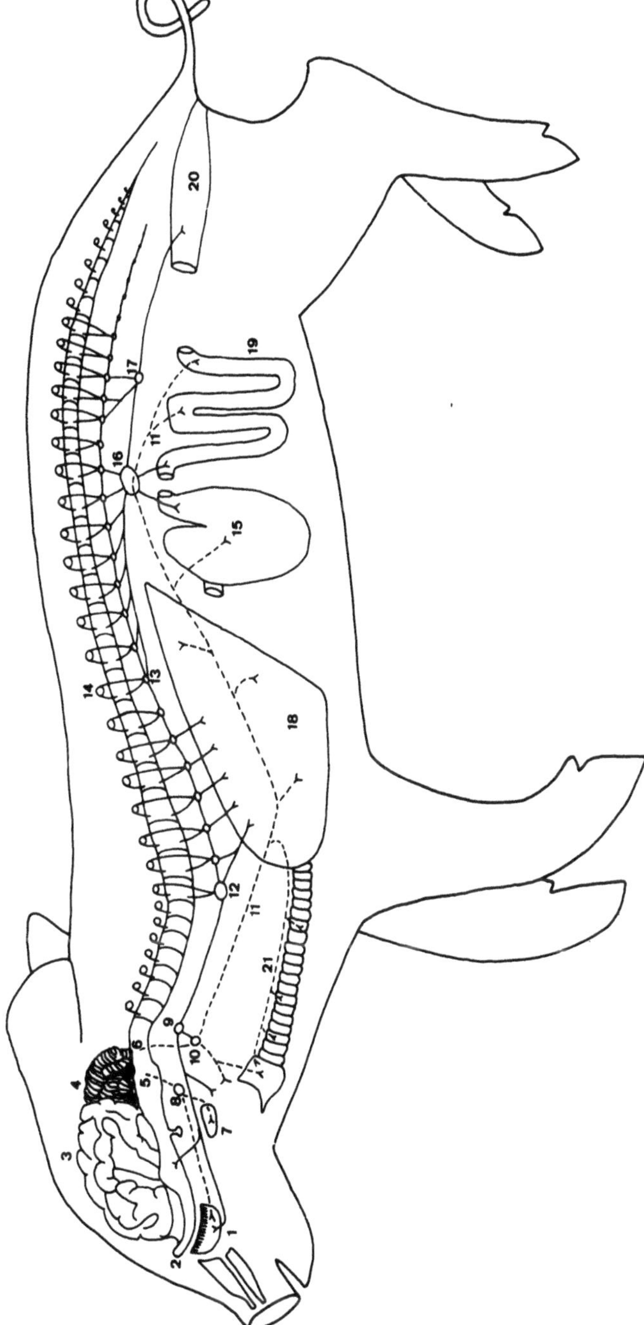

Fig. 1. Scheme of the tissues, nerve paths and ganglia involved in the pathogenesis of Vomiting and Wasting disease
1. nasal mucosa, 2. olfactory bulb, 3. cerebrum, 4. cerebellum, 5. pons varoli, 6. medulla oblongata, 7. tonsils, 8. trigeminal ganglion, 9. cranial cervical ganglion, 10. inferior vagal ganglion, 11. vagal nerve, 12. stellate ganglion, 13. sympathic trunc, 14. dorsal root ganglia, 15. stomach, 16. solar ganglion, 17. caudal mesenteric ganglion, 18. lungs, 19. small intestine, 20. rectum, 21. recurrent vagal nerve.

mucosa, the tonsils, the lungs and the small intestine served as primary sites of replication. The VWD virus then progressed via nerves corresponding to these areas towards the associated peripheral ganglia and further to the central nervous system. At least three pathways appeared to be involved (fig. 1). A first pathway to the central nervous system led from nasal mucosa and tonsils to the trigeminal ganglion and to the nucleus spinalis nervi trigemini in the medulla oblongata. A second pathway occurred along the vagal nerves via the inferior vagal ganglion, towards the nucleus solitarius in the medulla oblongata. A third pathway led from the intestinal plexuses to the spinal cord, either by way of sensory fibers which have their cell bodies in the dorsal root ganglion or after viral replication in the solar ganglion. In the central nervous system, the infection started in well defined nuclei of the medulla oblongata but progressed later into the entire brainstem, the spinal cord and sometimes also into the cerebrum and the cerebellum.

The question whether the vomition is induced centrally by viral replication in the brainstem or is due to viral replication in the peripheral nervous tissue (gastric or intestinal plexuses, solar ganglion, dorsal root ganglia, distal vagal ganglion) remains unanswered after these experiments. In fact, the invasion of the neurons in these tissues almost coincided with the start of the clinical signs.

IV. THE PATHOGENESIS OF THE VOMITING

From the results of the oronasally inoculated pigs, it was concluded that there are six possible target-tissues : the brainstem, the stomach plexuses, the intestinal plexuses, the dorsal root ganglia in the lower thoracic region, the solar ganglion and the distal vagal ganglion. The vomiting is induced by viral replication in one or more of these target-tissues. Further experiments were performed to study the relation between viral replication in these tissues and the appearance of clinical signs. Eleven colostrum deprived piglets were inoculated at one of the following sites : intragastrally (wall) or intraintestinally (wall + lumen) or intramuscularly (neck) or into the cerebrospinal fluid. They were always killed within 12 hours after the appearance of the clinical signs. Viral replication in the candidate target-tissues was examined by immunofluorescent tracing. The results are presented in table 1. All the inoculated piglets developed typical clinical signs after an incubation period of 3 to 5 days. Several candidate target-tissues were consistently negative by immunofluorescence after inoculation at a particular site. In the brainstem,fluorescing neurons were never found after the intraintestinal inoculation. In the stomach plexuses, no fluorescence was seen after the inoculations

Table 1 - Fluorescence in candidate target tissues of pigs sick upon inoculation of vomiting and wasting disease virus at different sites

Inoculation sites	Candidate Target Tissues					
	Brainstem	Stomach Plexuses	Intestinal Plexuses	Dorsal Root Ganglia	Solar Ganglion	Distal Vagal Ganglion
Intraintestinal	0/3	1/3	3/3	2/3	3/3	3/3
Intramuscular	2/2	0/3	2/3	1/3	2/3	2/3
Cerebrospinal fluid	1/1	0/2	1/2	2/2	1/2	2/2
Intragastral (wall)	3/3	3/3	0/3	1/3	2/3	3/3

Data are expressed as No. pigs positive / No. tested

in the cerebrospinal fluid or in the neck muscles. Finally, the intestinal plexuses contained no viral antigens after inoculation into the gastric wall. However, also the three remaining candidates were sometimes negative. Fluorescence was not found in the dorsal root ganglia of five piglets, in the solar ganglion of three piglets and in the vagal ganglion of one piglet.

The present results do not allow a definite conclusion concerning the target-tissue for the vomiting. Nevertheless, they demonstrate that at least five of the six candidates were regularly negative for viral antigens at the time the pigs were sick. Two explanations are still possible. First, the distal vagal ganglion, which was only once negative in the eleven pigs, can still turn out to be the "one and only" target-tissue. However, it is also possible that the vomiting is not induced by viral replication in one target-tissue only. Infected neurons at different sites could give impulses to the vomiting center. The phenomena of emesis could be induced at the moment that sufficient afferent stimuli reach this center. In this hypothesis, it is not necessary that the same target-tissue is infected in each vomiting pig. Vomiting might be induced when a sufficient number of infected neurons are present in one or more target-tissues. Further studies on this question are in progress.

V. THE PATHOGENESIS OF THE WASTING

Chronically affected pigs have lost their appetite and rapidly become emaciated. They suffer from a paralytic ileus and often present a large distended abdomen.[23] This unthrifty state may persist for several weeks until they die of starvation or secondary disease.[1] The stomach of such pigs is dilated and contains much gas, together with a yellow-green fluid.[23]

Recent experiments showed that the wasting syndrome can be experimentally reproduced by inoculating colostrum deprived pigs around the fifth day of age. Radiologic studies were performed to follow the passage of food through the alimentary tract of two chronically infected pigs and one control animal. Thirty-five to fifty ml of micropaque were brought into the stomach lumen via a gastric tube. In the control pig the stomach was empty after 13 to 17 hours whereas the barium was retained in the stomach lumen for 5 to 7 days in the two diseased pigs. Although only a few animals were tested until now, the difference can be considered as remarkable.

Based on the present knowledge, the following concepts on the pathogenesis of the wasting can be put forward. After infection of certain neurons in the brainstem, the stomach itself and/or the associated ganglia, the gastric emptying mechanism is greatly disturbed. The food stagnation in the stomach reduces the appetite and can cause gastric dilation. Furthermore, the few swallows of milk which are taken up are retained in the stomach for several days and its nutritive value may have become very low when entering the intestine. The pigs have to use their own body protein and glycogen to stay alive, but die of emaciation after a few weeks.

REFERENCES

1. C.K. Roe and T.J.L. Alexander, A disease of nursing pigs previously reported in Ontario, Can.J.Comp.Med.22 : 205 (1958).
2. T.J.L. Alexander, W.P.C. Richards and C.K. Roe, An encephalomyelitis of suckling pigs in Ontario, Can.J.Comp.Med. 23 : 316 (1959).
3. A.S. Greig, D. Mitchell, A.H. Corner, G.L. Bannister, E.B. Meads and R.J. Julian, Can.J.Comp.Med. 26 : 49 (1962).
4. S.F. Cartwright, M. Lucas, J.P. Cavill, A.F. Gush, and T.B. Blandford, Vomiting and wasting disease of piglets, Vet.Rec. 84 : 175 (1969).
5. J.I.H. Phillip, S.F. Cartwright, and A.C. Scott, The size and morphology of TGE and vomiting and wasting disease of pigs, Vet.Rec. 88 : 311 (1971).
6. W.L. Mengeling, and R.C. Cutlip, Pathogenicity of field isolants of hemagglutinating encephalomyelitis virus for neonatal pigs, J.Am.Vet.Med.Assoc. 128 : 236 (1976).
7. D. Schlenstedt, H. Barnikol, and H. Plonait, Erbrechen und Kümmern bei Saugferkeln, Dtsch.Tierärztl.Wschr. 76 : 781 (1969).
8. W.M. Gotink, G.M. Lambers, H. van Soest, and F.W. van Ulsen, Vomiting and Wasting disease in piglets, Vet.Rec. 84 : 445 (1969).
9. M. Pensaert, J. Derijcke, P. Callebaut, H. Thoonen, and J. Hoorens, Virologisch en pathologisch onderzoek van biggen met braakziekte, Tijdschr.Diergeneesk. 99 : 557 (1974).
10. G. Chappuis, J. Tektoff, and Y. le Turdu, Isolement en France et identification du virus de la maladie du vomissement et du dépérissement des porcelets (corona-like virus), Rec.Méd. Vét. 151 : 557 (1975).
11. F. Steck, B. Scharen, R. Fatzer, M. Vandevelde, E. Scholl, and H. Häni, "Vomiting and wasting disease" bei Ferkeln in der Schweiz, Schweiz.Arch.Tierheilk. 117 : 617 (1975).
12. M. Pensaert, and K. Andries, A seroepizootiologic study of vomiting and wasting disease virus in pigs, Vet.Quat. 2 : 142 (1980).
13. A. Girard, A.S. Greig, and D. Mitchell, Encephalomyelitis of swine caused by a hemagglutinating virus. III. Serological studies, Res.Vet.Sci. 5 : 294 (1964).

14. S.F. Cartwright, and M. Lucas, Vomiting and wasting disease in piglets, Vet.Rec. 86 : 278 (1970).
15. J.B. McFerran, J.K. Clarke, T.J. Connor, and E.R. Knox, Serological evidence of the presence of hemagglutinating encephalitis virus in Northern Ireland, Vet.Rec. 88 : 339 (1971).
16. K. Hirai, C. Chang, and S. Shimakura, A serologic survey on hemagglutinating encephalomyelitis virus infection in pigs in Japan, Jap.J.Vet.Sci. 36 : 375 (1974).
17. W.L. Mengeling, Incidence of antibody for hemagglutinating encephalomyelitis virus in serums from swine in the United States, Am.J.Vet.Res. 36 : 821 (1975).
18. R.H. Hess, and P.A. Bachmann, Erbrechen und Kümmern der ferkel. Vorkommen und verbreitung in suddeutschland, Tierärztl. Umschau 33 : 571 (1978).
19. K. Andries, M. Pensaert, and P. Callebaut, Pathogenicity of hemagglutinating encephalomyelitis (vomiting and wasting disease) virus of pigs, using different routes of inoculation, Zentralbl.Veterinärmed. (B) 25 : 461 (1978).
20. K. Andries, and M. Pensaert, Virus isolation and immunofluorescence in different organs of pigs infected with hemagglutinating encephalomyelitis virus, Am.J.Vet.Res. 41 : 215 (1980).
21. K. Andries, and M.B. Pensaert, Immunofluorescence studies on the pathogenesis of hemagglutinating encephalomyelitis virus in pigs after oronasal inoculation, Am.J.Vet.Res. 41 : 1372 (1980).
22. M.B. Pensaert, and P.E. Callebaut, Characteristics of a coronavirus causing vomiting and wasting in pigs, Arch.gesamte Virusforsch.44 : 35 (1974).
23. K. Tuch, Pathologisch-anatomische befunde bei einer der "Vomiting and wasting disease" (Erbrechen und Kümmern) vergleichbaren erkrankung der saugferkel, Dtsch.Tierärztl. Wschr. 78 : 496 (1971).

INBORN RESISTANCE OF MICE TO MOUSE HEPATITIS VIRUS TYPE 3 (MHV_3): LIVER PARENCHYMAL CELLS EXPRESS PHENOTYPE IN CULTURE

Heinz Arnheiter and Otto Haller

Institute for Immunology and Virology
University of Zürich, POB,
8028 Zürich, Switzerland

SUMMARY

Primary monolayer cultures of hepatocytes isolated from adult resistant A/J or partially resistant A/Sn or C3H/HeJ mice exhibited resistance to MHV_3 as the respective macrophages do: Compared to susceptible C57BL/6 hepatocyte cultures, cytopathic effect occurred later and was restricted to small foci, coinciding with areas specifically labelled by immunofluorescence. Production of infectious particles was delayed, titers being 100 to 1000 fold lower at the moment of maximal yields in susceptible cultures. Pretreatment with interferon could reduce the titers in susceptible cultures to a level as seen in resistant cultures not treated with interferon. Nevertheless, interferon was not responsible for the genetic resistance of hepatocytes: it reduced virus titers in susceptible and resistant cultures to the same extent and the addition of specific antibodies to interferon after infection did not augment susceptibility of resistant cultures. We assume that intrinsic resistance of liver parenchymal cells is an important facet of inborn resistance of mice in vivo.

INTRODUCTION

Inbred strains of mice can be ranked for their degree of innate resistance to MHV_3: A/J mice survive infection even with high virus doses. C57BL/6 mice, on the other hand, die with severe hepatitis soon after infection and are representative for several highly susceptible strains (1). Other strains, such as C3H/HeJ or A/Sn, show intermediate susceptibility: a certain percentage of animals survives infection, but survivors may become chronic virus carriers and show signs of a progressive neurologic disease (1,2,3). The fate of the adult mouse during the early phase of infection seems to be determined by 2 non H-2 linked genes (3); a coherent picture of how these genes may operate has not yet emerged.

Mononuclear phagocytes decisively determine pathogenicity of viruses for the liver: viruses undergoing productive replication in macrophages may cause viral hepatitis, whereas those incapable of growing in these cells in general do not express hepatotropism (4). Isolated macrophages of resistant animals show a certain degree of resistance to MHV_3 infection in vitro (5). They are considered to play an important role in mediating resistance in vivo.

Resistance at the cellular level may be restricted to cells of the mononuclear phagocyte system. Alternatively, macrophages could represent but one exemplary cell type displaying resistance by mechanisms common to all potential target cells. Our findings support the latter view. Hepatocytes, the main parenchymal target cells within the liver, isolated from resistant adult animals and kept in chemically defined media, exhibited resistance in vitro, whereas those from susceptible animals were fully permissive for MHV_3. This resistance was virus specific and appeared to be independent of the action of interferon.

MATERIALS AND METHODS

The method of isolating hepatocytes from adult mice by in situ collagenase perfusion of the liver and the procedures to establish primary hepatocyte monolayer cultures have been described in detail (6,7). Mice were purchased from the Jackson Laboratory, Bar Harbor, Maine, and were kept under conventional conditions.

Stock MHV_3 virus, originally obtained from Jean-Louis Virelizier, Hôpital Necker-Enfants-Malades, Paris, France, was prepared in C57BL/6 peritoneal macrophages. Virus was plaque purified and assayed in mouse DBT cells (kindly provided by A. Kirn, Groupe de Recherches sur la Pathogénie des Infections Virales, Strasbourg, France) exactly as described (8). Stock virus preparations and assays of the avian influenza A virus M-TUR (A/TUR/Engl/63, Hav1Nav3) adapted to grow in mouse liver cells, vesicular stomatitis virus (VSV) and herpes simplex virus type 1 (HSV-1) were as previously described (7).

For immunofluorescence, an antiserum obtained from A/Sn mice after infection with MHV_3 or a rabbit antiserum prepared against purified JHM virus (kindly supplied by Kathrin Holmes, Department of Pathology, USUHS, Bethesda, Md) were used. Indirect immunofluorescent labelling was done by treating with antiserum, washing and adding protein A-FITC (a gift from Thomas Bächi from our Institute) to air dried and acetone fixed hepatocyte cultures established on glass cover slips coated with collagen (Calbiochem Corp, San Diego, Calif.).

Mouse β interferon (IFN-β), purified to 10^7 ref units/mg protein, and a sheep anti-mouse interferon globulin preparation (AIFN), both gifts of Ion Gresser, Institut de Recherches Scientifiques sur le Cancer, Villejuif, France, were those previously described (7). AIFN was routinely used to neutralize interferon occurring spontaneously in hepatocyte cultures (7).

RESULTS

Influence of the host cell genotype on MHV_3 replication in hepatocytes in culture

Cultured hepatocytes were infected with MHV_3 at multiplicities of 0.1 to 0.001. With C57BL/6 hepatocytes, infection caused a marked cytopathic effect. Cell fusion, first detectable after 7 hours, finally resulted in formation of a giant syncytium over the whole culture plate. With hepatocytes from resistant A/J or semiresistant A/Sn or C3H/HeJ mice, syncytium formation was only detected after high multiplicity infection. It was delayed as compared to C57BL/6 cultures and was restricted to foci containing no more than 50 cell nuclei at the end of a 4 day incubation period (Fig. 1).

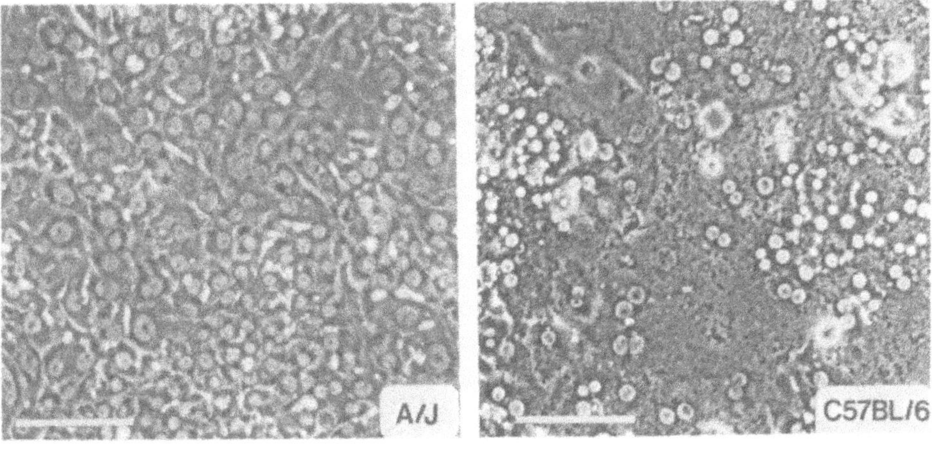

Fig. 1. Hepatocytes obtained from resistant A/J and susceptible C57BL/6 mice were cultured for 24 hrs and were then infected with MHV_3 at a multiplicity of 0.01. The micrographs were taken 24 hrs after infection. Phase contrast microscopy. Bars represent 50 µm.

Virus growth curves also revealed differences between the 2 types of hepatocyte cultures: at the moment of maximal virus production in C57BL/6 cells, the titers were 10^2 to 10^3 fold lower in resistant cells and never exceeded 10^5 plaque forming units (pfu)/ml thereafter (Fig. 2).

Replication of unrelated viruses in hepatocytes is independent of the host cell genotype influencing MHV_3 multiplication

A/J, C3H/HeJ and C57BL/6 mice are equally susceptible to influenza A virus infection (including the hepatotropic M-TUR variant) and to VSV (9, and unpublished observations), but differ with respect to MHV_3 (where A/J are resistant, C3H/HeJ are partially resistant, and C57BL/6 are susceptible) and HSV-1 (where C57BL/6 and C3H/HeJ are relatively resistant and A/J are susceptible) (10,11).

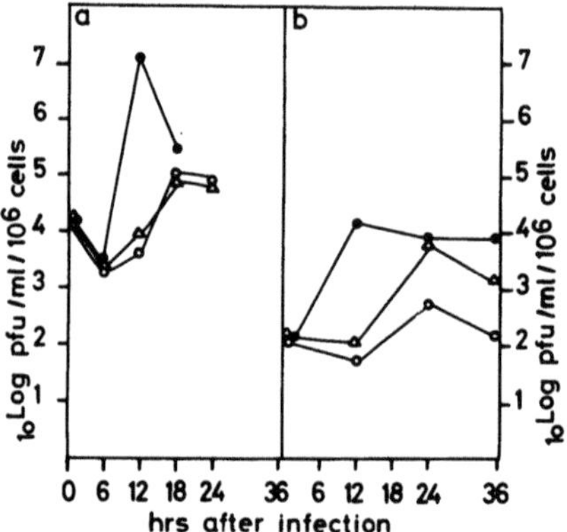

Fig. 2. Hepatocyte cultures established from adult A/J (o——o), C3H/HeJ (△——△) and C57BL/6 (●——●) mice were cultured for 48 hrs and were then infected with MHV_3 at a multiplicity of 0.1 (a) or 0.001 (b). Infectivity (plaque forming units,pfu) of cultures frozen and thawed 3 times at the end of the incubation period indicated was assayed in mouse DBT cells. In C57BL/6 hepatocytes, cytopathic effect was complete at 18 hrs (high multiplicity) and 36 hrs (low multiplicity) after infection.

A difference in permissiveness between hepatocytes prepared from these 3 strains was only seen with respect to MHV_3 (Table 1).

Study of MHV_3 replication of cultured liver cells by immunofluorescence and electron microscopy

Delayed production of infectious virus as seen in hepatocytes of resistant mice might be the result of improper morphogenesis or impaired excretion of viral particles, a phenomenon which would lead to intracellular accumulation of viral proteins. C57BL/6 cultures, labelled at 3 hour intervals after infection at a multiplicity of 0.1, showed a continuous increase of fluorescent cells from 5% at 6 hours to 100% at 12 hours. Spotty fluorescence was spread over the whole cytoplasma. Labelled nuclei could not be detected. In cultures from resistant A/J mice, a remarkebly different picture emerged: the percentage of fluorescent cells (themselves not distinguishable from those in the susceptible cultures) was 5% at 6 hours as in C57BL/6 cells, but even 48 hours after infection there were still large areas devoid of fluorescent cells. Labelled foci contained no more than 30 cells.

By transmission electron microscopy, cell fusion was first detected 7 hours after infection in C57BL/6 but not in A/J hepatocytes. At 12 hours, viral particles were found only in susceptible cultures.

Table 1. Susceptibility of hepatocytes from different mouse strains for various viruses

Mouse strain	MHV_3	M-TUR	VSV	HSV-1
A/J	$0.5x10^4$	$3.2x10^7$	$2.0x10^7$	$1.0x10^7$
C3H/HeJ	$1.0x10^4$	$4.0x10^7$	$1.0x10^7$	$6.5x10^7$
C57BL/6	$2.0x10^6$	$2.5x10^7$	$1.6x10^7$	$0.5x10^7$

Hepatocyte cultures were established from adult mice and were given AIFN from 0-24 hours. They were then infected with MHV_3 or herpes simplex type 1 virus (HSV-1) at a multiplicity of 0.1 or influenza A (M-TUR) or vesicular stomatitis virus (VSV) at a multiplicity of 10. 12 hour yields of MHV_3 are given as pfu/ml/10^6 cells. 24 hour yields of the other viruses are given as 50% tissue culture infective doses/ml, assayed in chicken embryo cells (M-TUR and VSV) or Vero cells (HSV-1).

Expression of the resistant phenotype in cultured hepatocytes: a role for interferon?

The striking observation that neutralization of endogenous interferon by specific antibodies enhanced the susceptibility of mice to MHV3 infection and could even abrogate the partial resistance of adult C3H/HeJ mice (12) suggested that interferon was at least partially responsible for resistance in vivo. But would interferon also account for resistance at the cellular level?

Hepatocytes spontaneously release interferon during the first 24 hours after being put in culture independently of their genotype (7, and unpublished observations). They were therefore exposed to anti-IFN-antibodies for a first culture period. These antibodies could be washed out thereafter, i.e. no detectable IFN neutralizing activity remained in the supernatant fluids. After MHV3 infection, small amounts of IFN became detectable but were difficult to interpret. To test indirectly whether IFN induced by the infection would have any effect on the course of virus growth, we added AIFN after infection. There was no enhancement of MHV3 yield in either A/J or C57BL/6 hepatocytes, just as previously observed for VSV and HSV-1 (7, and unpublished observations).

We then tested hepatocyte cultures for their sensitivity to the anti-viral effect of IFN. Mouse IFN-β was added at graded doses to A/J and C57BL/6 hepatocyte cultures for 18 hours. The cells were then infected with either MHV3, VSV or HSV-1. Yield reductions observed after exposure to 1000 ref units/ml of IFN are given in Table 2. The capacity of IFN to inhibit MHV3 was similar in A/J and C57BL/6 cultures, as was its inhibitory activity against VSV or HSV-1. No effect of the resistance phenotype on interferon action was discernible.

DISCUSSION

Liver parenchymal cells isolated from mice with inborn resistance to MHV3 infection were able to express a certain degree of virus specific resistance in vitro. Rather than being totally non-permissive for MHV3, such cultures showed a delay in production of infectious virus as compared to their susceptible counterparts. This delay correlated well with the absence of widespread cell fusion, the scarcity of budding virions and the limitation of spread of viral antigens.

Macrophage cultures prepared from resistant A/J mice have been reported to be either totally resistant to MHV3 (5) or to show a delay in onset of cytopathic effect (13). Hence, the course of MHV3 infection in hepatocytes resembled that in macrophages of the same

Table 2. Inhibition of virus replication in hepatocytes of C57BL/6 and A/J mice by exogenous interferon

Virus	$_{10}$Log yield reduction after treatment with 1000 ref units/ml of mouse IFN-β	
	A/J	C57BL/6
MHV_3	1.3[a]	1.2
VSV	2.1	2.2
HSV-1	1.5	1.4

Legend to Table 2: Hepatocyte cultures, virus infections and titrations were as indicated in Table 1. Mouse IFN-β was given from 24-42 hours after cell harvest. Thereafter, the cultures were washed 3 times and were infected in presence of AIFN sufficient to neutralize 10,000 ref units of IFN. Yield reductions were calculated as $_{10}$log (yield without IFN/yield with IFN).
[a]The comparative value for A/Sn hepatocytes was 1.1.

genotype. It is therefore tempting to speculate that, at the molecular level, the same mechanisms act in the 2 cell types.

Of the various factors known to modulate acute infection, interferon appears to be very important (14). Its neutralization has been shown to abrogate the partial resistance of mice to MHV_3 (12). The growth curve of MHV_3 as seen in cells from resistant mice could be mimicked by treating susceptible cells with interferon, and this both in hepatocyte and macrophage cultures (data not shown). Furthermore, interferon is a prerequisite for expression of resistance against orthomyxoviruses, both in the living mouse and in its isolated cells (7,15,16). In contrast, IFN was obviously not required for expression of innate resistance to MHV_3 at the cellular level: its neutralization after infection was without effect and it protected susceptible and resistant cultures to the same extent. That other types of IFN or lymphokines might exert a differential effect is however still conceivable.

We assume that hepatocytes of resistant animals behave in vivo as they do in culture: they are intrinsically less permissive for MHV_3 than those from susceptible strains. A temporal delay in virus growth would be sufficient to enable the host specific and unspecific immune system to cope with the infection. The immune system of susceptible hosts, even if similarly effective in principle, would start too late to limit the rapid virus growth in the main target cells. When the immune system of a resistant host is substantially disturbed, delayed virus growth in its target cells cannot protect the animal from death. This would explain why various immunosuppressive treatments, impairment of macrophage function or the neutralization of endogenous interferon may fully or partly abrogate resistance in vivo. We conclude that cellular resistance, even of cells not usually involved in antiviral defence, is a necessary but by far not sufficient condition for protection in vivo.

ACKNOWLEDGEMENT

We are grateful to Drs. Ion Gresser for his generous gift of interferon and anti-interferon antibodies, Kathrin Holmes for her anti-JHMV antiserum, and A. Kirn for providing us the DBT cell line We thank J. Lindenmann for constant interest and critically reading the manuscript, C. Kaufmann and L. Schmutz for excellent technical and R. Leemann for expert secretarial assistance. This work was supported by the Swiss National Science Foundation, grant no. 3.393.078.

REFERENCES

1. C. Le Prévost, J.L. Virelizier, and J.M. Dupuy, Immunopathology of mouse hepatitis virus type 3 infection. III. Clinical and virologic observation of a persistent viral infection. J. Immunol. 115:640 (1975).
2. E. Lévy-Leblond, D. Oth and J.M. Dupuy, Genetic study of mouse sensitivity to MHV_3 infection: influence of the H-2 complex. J. Immunol. 122:1359 (1979).
3. J.L. Virelizier, A.D. Dayan and A.C. Allison, Neuropathological effects of persistent infection of mice by mouse hepatitis virus. Infect. Immun. 12:1127 (1975).
4. S.M. Sabesin and R.S. Koff, Pathogenesis of experimental viral hepatitis. New Engl. J.Med. 290:944 (1974).
5. J.L. Virelizier and A.C. Allison, Correlation of persistent mouse hepatitis virus (MHV-3) infection with its effect on mouse macrophage cultures. Arch. Virol. 50:279 (1976).
6. H. Arnheiter, Primary monolayer culture of adult mouse hepatocytes - A model for the study of hepatotropic viruses. Arch. Virol. 63:11 (1980).
7. H. Arnheiter, O. Haller and J. Lindenmann, Host gene influence on interferon action in adult mouse hepatocytes: specificity for influenza virus. Virology 103:11 (1989).
8. N. Takayama and A. Kirn, An improved method for titration of mouse hepatitis virus type 3 in a mouse cell culture. Arch.

10. H. Kirchner, H.M. Hirt, D.L. Rosenstreich and S.E. Mergenhagen, Resistance of C3H/HeJ mice to lethal challenge with herpes simplex virus (39983). Proc. Soc. Exp. Biol. Med. 157:29 (1978).
11. C. Lopez, Genetics of natural resistance to herpesvirus infections in mice. Nature 258:152 (1975).
12. J.L. Virelizier and I. Gresser, Role of interferon in the pathogenesis of viral diseases of mice as demonstrated by the use of anti-interferon serum. V. Protective role in mouse hepatitis virus type 3 infection of susceptible and resistant strains of mice. J. Immunol. 120:1616 (1978).
13. M.R. Macnaughton and S. Patterson, Mouse hepatitis virus strain 3 infection of C57, A/Sn and A/J strain mice and their macrophages. Arch. Virol. 66:71 (1980).
14. I. Gresser, M.G. Tovey, C. Maury and M.T. Bandu, Role of interferon in the pathogenesis of virus diseases in mice as demonstrated by the use of anti-interferon serum. II. Studies with herpes simplex, Moloney sarcoma, vesicular stomatitis, Newcastle disease, and influenza viruses. J. Exp. Med. 144:1316 (1976).
15. O. Haller, H. Arnheiter, I. Gresser and J.Lindenmann, Genetically determined, interferon-dependent resistance to influenza virus in mice. J. Exp. Med. 149:601 (1979).
16. O. Haller, H. Arnheiter, J. Lindenmann and I. Gresser, Host gene influences sensitivity to interferon action selectively for influenza virus. Nature 283:660 (1980).

BIOLOGY OF CORONAVIRUSES 1980

D.A.J. Tyrrell

Clinical Research Center

Harrow, England

INTRODUCTION

It is well established that the large group of coronavirus induce, in a variety of hosts, a spectrum of acute diseases. As summarized in Table 1, it is shown that both murine and feline coronaviruses induce infection in several different organs of the host, when for example these agents lead in man, cattle, dogs or rats only to single disease manifestation . Current interest in the biology of coronaviruses centers around the mechanism of the pathogenesis as well as virus-host interactions which lead to subacute or chronic diseases.

CORONAVIRUS PERSISTENT INFECTION IN TISSUE CULTURE

This meeting provided an opportunity to review the characteristics of several different systems in which it has been established that persistent coronavirus infections can be induced in tissue cultures of one sort or another. Some of the main characteristics are set out in Table 2. It is not certain whether the systems described are really homogeneous and comparable. In other words, even when cloned cells and cloned viruses are used it is possible that there is more than one interaction that can take place and lead to the interaction for which we select, namely that the cells survive and divide and virus is shed. It is clear for instance that there may be only 1-20 % cells producing

Table 1. Spectrum of Diseases Caused by Different Coronavirus Groups

Virus :	MHV*	RCV	TBDV	TGEV	HEV	NCDCV	IBV	CCV	FCV	HCV	HECV
Host :	mouse	rat	turkey	pig	pig	bovine	chicken	dog	cat	man	man
TYPE OF DISEASE											
encephalitis	+				+				+		
enteritis	+		+	+	+	+		+	+		+
hepatitis	+								+		
adenitis	+										
nephritis	+			+			+		+		
pancreatitis	+										
peritonitis	+								+		
respiratory infections	+	+	+	+	+		+		+	+	

*Abbreviations according to Tyrrell et al., Intervirology, 5, 76, 1975.

virus antigens as judged by immunofluorescence; in some instances the other cells which are resistant have been cloned and found to be uninfected and susceptible and the system represents the outcome of some sort of cell coronaviruses and may indeed shed virus either on further culture or by fusion with susceptible cells. It is therefore important that in future the cultures are analysed at the cellular level by obtaining clones and studying them individually.

The viruses recovered from persistently infected cells seem very variable. The common idea that such cultures select <u>ts</u> viruses was not supported, though some showed small plaques, and in some, virulence for the animal host was also reduced. Nevertheless in one case there was increased virulence for the original host cells. There seems to be a need to look in more detail at the growth of these cells and to examine at the molecular level how cloned cells achieve an equilibrium with the virus. This will allow further biological investigation, but it cannot substitute for a study of experimental diseases in animals.

CORONAVIRUS INFECTION in vivo

A number of different model diseases have been described and particular attention directed to the subacute or chronic conditions, the implication being that we understand fairly well how acute infections occur and are dealt with. I found these interesting but I was concerned that so often experiments were evaluated solely as to whether an animal lived or died. This is a clear cut "all or none" phenomenon and can be readily determined without using special equipment, but death has a very important qualitative aspect too. We should know how the animal died. Pathological examination showed there were at least three different sorts of subacute disease of mice and rats, the demyelinating syndrome, meningo-ependymitis and generalised vasculitis (Virelizier, this volume). It is good that workers are trying to provide defined and reproducible models in this field too, and the use of cloned virus and mutants and of inbred strains of animals is valuable.

I am however rather unhappy with the references to genetic factors as though these were a separate

Table 2. Persistent Infections by Coronaviruses in Tissue Cultures

	Investigators (see this volume)				
	Chaloner-Larsson Johnson-Lussenburg	Hirano et al.	Holmes Behnke	Sorensen et al.	Stohlman-Frelinger (personal communication)
ESTABLISHMENT					
virus	229E	JHM	A 59	JHM/MHV3	JHM
host cell	L132	DBT	17 Cl1	RN 2-2	N_2A
reproducibility	15 %	100 %	100 %	100 %	100 %
time of appearance (passage No.)	3	15	1	1	3
PROPERTIES OF PERSISTENT CELL LINES					
percentage of cells expressing viral antigen (FA)	N.D.*	10-15 %	10-20 %	1 %	20 %
presence of infectious virus	+	+	+	+	+
resistence to					
superinfection by					
corona virus	+	+	+	+	+
other virus	-	-	-	-	-
PROPERTIES OF THE VIRUS					
temp. sensitive	-	-	+	-	-
altered plaque morphology	-	+	+	-	-
alteration in virulence	increased	reduced	reduced	N.D.	N.D.

* N.D. not done

aspect of biology. Both the host and the parasite are totally the expression of genes and gene products, and what we are talking about is genetic factors which are identifiable or genetically controllable situations that can be exploited in one way or another. It was mentioned for instance (Klenk) that avirulent influenza viruses in the chick embryo infect the endoderm because the haemagglutinin is cleaved by a trypsin-like enzyme in these cells and as a result particles become infectious, whereas in mesoderm or ectoderm the haemagglutinin is not cleaved and the virus particle may be formed but does not become infectious. The pathogenetic virus on the other hand, is cleaved in all three types of cells.

This is the best example of how a minor difference in the structure of a virus polypeptide modifies its interaction with host enzymes and thus reveals genetic and structural facts which we should otherwise know nothing about. This is a particular example of a general principle referred to by Dr. Bang and enunciated by plant pathologists to the effect that one can only recognize and study changes in virulence if there is a susceptible host to study and that corresponding to the genes in the pathogen that determine its pathogenicity are corresponding genes in the host that determine its susceptibility and resistance.

A virus produces a disease by performing a long series of functions, including entry into the host, absorption, replication, cytopathogenicity etc. and it is important to remember this. I am against using loose phrases such as saying a virus is "virulent". It is better to try to describe what it does or does not do, e.g. initiate infection, multiply or kill cells. The presentation by Andries (this volume) was a fine example of how exactly the course of a disease may be mapped out, so that one can trace a complete series of links of a causal chain from the death from malnutrition, via the loss of gastric motility back to the neurotoxic effect of a virus and its original entry into the animal. Compared with this the course of events in many experimental diseases is not well worked out and it is therefore difficult, if not impossible, to postulate the likely key stages in the disease process.

INDICATION FOR FUTURE RESEARCH

It seems to me that one should consider using the philosophy of the "T club" who under the guidance of Hershey in the early days of the exploitation of the bacteriophages decided to concentrate work on phage T2. Thus they were able to concentrate a wide range of special skills and difficult investigations on a limited but still very complicated problem, and to make more progress, in the sense of answering important questions, than by doing as much work on a number of different and less well defined experimental systems. There are dangers of course - one may miss something by narrowing one's view - but I hope workers will consider it seriously. It is important to consider not only the immediate experiments, but also the possibilities for the future -for example whether inbred strains of animals are available with a good background of information on genetic characteristics, transplantation antigens and so on and a wide range of immunological reagents. The mouse is an obvious suggestion, but the rat might be satisfactory. It would also be desirable to mimic a significant human or veterinary disease as closely as possible.

The communications provided a number of warnings against being too easily persuaded by "neat" single experiments on isolated cells or with single so-called specific immunological reagents. Dr. Bang admitted that all the conclusions he drew from the early experiments on MHV in mouse peritoneal macrophages had to be changed in the light of further experiments. The results may only show "significant" results if the conditions such as the dose of virus or the type of culture medium are tightly controlled. In vitro results may nevertheless be significant, for example in showing differences in the susceptibility of hepatocytes to hepatotropic viruses. In the subacute and chronic conditions it is important to assess fully the functioning of the immune system and there are many gaps in our knowledge. Antibody is found in the demyelinated brain tissue, but against what antigen is it directed and is it pathogenic or merely an epiphenomenon ? The general MHV vasculitis is apparently due to circulatory immune complexes, but what is the antigen, and what type of antibody do they contain ?

In conclusion it seems to me that this is a particularly valuable meeting in which molecular biologists, virologists and experimental pathologists have sat down together to hear the latest results and to see things from each other's point of view.

I think all involved are most grateful to Professor ter Meulen and his staff for arranging it and running it so well. There is no doubt that we have all benefited and that our future research will be improved by the new ideas we are taking away and the personal contacts we have made.

PARTICIPANTS

Andries, K., Rijksuniversiteit Gent, Faculteit van de Diergeneeskunde, Laboratory of Virology, B -9000 Gent, Belgium

Arnheiter, H., Institut für Immunologie und Virologie der Universität, CH-8028 Zürich, Switzerland

Bachmayer, H., Sandoz-Forschungsinstitut, A - 1235 Wien, Austria

Bang, F.B., Department of Pathobiology, School of Hygiene and Public Health, Johns Hopkins University, School of Medicine, Baltimore, Md. 21205, USA

Billeter, M., Universität Zürich, Institut für Molekularbiologie I, CH - 8093 Zürich, Switzerland

Bond, C.W., Dept. of Microbiology, University of Montana, Bozeman, Montana, 59715, USA

Brian, D.A., Dept. of Microbiology, The University of Tennessee, Knoxville, Tenn. 37916, USA

Burks, J.S., University of Colorado, Health Sciences Center, Denver, Co. 80262, USA

Cereda, P.M., Virus Laboratory, Institute of Infectious Diseases, Policlinico S. Matteo, Universita degli Studi di Pavia, I - 27100 Pavia, Italy

Chaloner-Larsson, G., University of Ottawa, Faculty of Health Sciences, Micróbiology and Immunology, School of Medicine, Ottawa, Ontario, K1N 9A9, Canada

Chu, H.P., Department of Veterinary Medicine, University of Cambridge, Cambridge CB2 2QQ, United Kingdom

Dauvergne, M., IFFA Merieux, Laboratoire de microbiologie vétérinaire, F - 69007 Lyon, France

Dales, S., Cytobiological Group, Department of Microbiology and Immunology, University of Western Ontario, London, Ontario, N6A5C1, Canada

Fleischer, B., Institut für Virologie und Immunbiologie, D -8700 Würzburg, FRG

Frisch-Niggemeyer, W., Institut für Virologie der Universität Wien, A - 1095 Wien, Austria

Fujiwara, K., The Institute of Medical Science, The University of Tokyo, Japan

Garwes, D.J., Institute for Research on Animal Diseases, Compton, Nr. Newbury, Berkshire, RG16 0NN, United Kingdom

Gerdes, J.C., University of Colorado, Health Sciences Center, Denver, Co. 80262, USA

Goto, N., Veterinary School, Yamaguchi University, Yamaguchi, Japan

Habermehl, K.O., Institut für Virologie, Freie Universität, D -1000 Berlin, FRG

Hierholzer, J.C., Respiratory Virology Branch, Center for Diseases Control, Atlanta, Ga. 30333, USA

Hirano, N., Department of Veterinary Microbiology, Faculty of Agriculture, Iwate University, Morioka 020, Japan

Holmes, K., Department of Pathology, Uniformed Services, University of Health Sciences, Bethesda, Maryland 20014, USA

Johnson-Lussenburg, D.M., University of Ottawa, Faculty of Health Sciences, Microbiology and Immunology, School of Medicine, Ottawa, Ontario K1N 9A9, Canada

Kennedy, S.I.T., Dept. of Biology, University of California San Diego, La Jolla, Ca., USA

Klenk, H.D., Institut für Virologie der Universität Giessen, D -6300 Giessen, FRG

Knobler, R.L., Scripps Clinic and Research Foundation, La Jolla, Ca. 92037, USA

Kraft, V., Zentralinstitut für Versuchstiere -Virologie - D -3000 Hannover, FRG

Koga, M., Institut für Virologie und Immunbiologie, Universität Würzburg, D - 8700 Würzburg, FRG

Koolon, M., Fakulteit der Diergeneeskunde, Rijksuniversiteit te Utrecht, Vakgroep Virologie, Utrecht-de Uithof, The Netherlands

Kung, F., Cetus Corporation, Berkeley, Ca., 94710, USA

Kurth, H., Paul-Ehrlich-Institut, D - 6000 Frankfurt, FRG

Lai, M.C., Dept. of Neurology, University of Southern California, School of Medicine, Los Angeles, Ca. 90033, USA

Laude, H., Institut National de la Recherche Agronomique, Station de Recheches de Virologie et d'Immunologie, F -78850 Thiverval-Grignon, France

Laporte, J.,Institut National de la Recherche Agronomique, Station de Recheches de Virologie et d'Immunologie, F - 78850 Thiverval-Grignon, France

Leibowitz, J.L., University of California San Diego, School of Medicine, Dept. of Pathology, La Jolla, Ca. 92093, USA

Leinikki, P.O., Institute for Biomedical Sciences, University of Tampere, SF - 33101 Tampere, Finland

Lomnicizi, B., Veterinary Medical Research Institute, Hungarian Academy of Sciences, H - 1581 Budapest, Hungary

Ludwig, H., Institut für Virologie, Freie Universität, D-1000 Berlin, FRG

Macnaughton, M., Division of Communicable Diseases, Clinical Research Centre, Harrow, Middlesex HA 13UJ, United Kingdom

Mahy, B.W.J., Department of Pathology, Division of Virology, Laboratories Block, Addenbrooke's Hospital, Cambridge CB2 2 OQ, United Kingdom

Martin, S., Department of Biochemistry, Medical Biology Centre, The Queen's University of Belfast, Belfast BT9 7BL, Northern Ireland

ter **Meulen,** V., Institut für Virologie und Immunbiologie, Universität Würzburg, D - 8700 Würzburg, FRG

Monreal, G., Institut für Geflügelkrankheiten, D - 1000 Berlin, FRG

Niemann, H., Institut für Virologie, Universität Giessen, D -6300 Giessen, FRG

Pickel, K., Institut für Virologie und Immunbiologie, Universität Würzburg, D - 8700 Würzburg, FRG

Rott, R. Institut für Virologie der Vet.-Med. Fakultät, Universität Giessen, D - 6300 Giessen, FRG

Rottier, P.J.M., Fakulteit der Diergeneeskunde, Rijksuniversiteit te Utrecht, Vakgroep Virologie, Utrecht-de Uithof, The Netherlands

Schmidt, O.W., University of Washington, School of Medicine, Dept. of Laboratory Medicine, Seattle, Washington 98185, USA

Siddell, S.G., Institut für Virologie und Immunbiologie, Universität Würzburg, D - 8700 Würzburg, FRG

Soula, A., Laboratoire de microbiologie vétérinaire, F -69007 Lyon, France

Spaan, W.J.M., Fakulteit der Diergeneeskunde, Rijksuniversiteit te Utrecht, Vakgroep Virologie, Utrecht-de Uithof, The Netherlands

Stephenson, J.R., Public Health Laboratory Service, Centre for Applied Microbiology and Research, Vaccine Research and Production Laboratory, Porton Down, Salisbury, Wilshire SP4 0JG, United Kingdom

Stohlman, S.A., Deptartment of Neurology, University of Southern California, School of Medicine, 2025 Zonal Avenue, Los Angeles, Ca. 90033, USA

Sturman, L., Division of Laboratories and Research, New York State Department of Health, Albany, New York, 12201, USA

Tamura, T., Institut für Virologie, Universität Giessen, D -6300 Giessen, FRG

Tyrrell, D.A.J., Clinical Research Centre, Division of Communicable Diseases, Warford Road, Harrow, Middlesex, United Kingdom

Verhagen, W., Medizinische Hochschule, Institut für Virologie und Seuchenhygiene, D - 3000 Hannover, FRG

Virelizier, J.L., Unité d'Immunpathologie et de Rhumatologie Pediatrique, Hopital Necker-Enfants Malades, Paris, 15, France

Wecker, E., Institut für Virologie und Immunbiologie, Universität Würzburg, D - 8700 Würzburg, FRG

Wege, H., Institut für Virologie und Immunbiologie, Universität Würzburg, D - 8700 Würzburg, FRG

Weiss, S.R., Dept. of Microbiology, School of Medicine, University of California, Medical Center, San Francisco, Ca. 94143, USA

van der **Zeijst,** B.A.M., Fakulteit der Diergeneeskunde, Rijksuniversiteit te Utrecht, Vakgroep Virologie, Utrecht-de Uithof, The Netherlands

INDEX

GPSR Compliance
The European Union's (EU) General Product Safety Regulation (GPSR) is a set of rules that requires consumer products to be safe and our obligations to ensure this.

If you have any concerns about our products, you can contact us on

ProductSafety@springernature.com

In case Publisher is established outside the EU, the EU authorized representative is:

Springer Nature Customer Service Center GmbH
Europaplatz 3
69115 Heidelberg, Germany

www.ingramcontent.com/pod-product-compliance
Ingram Content Group UK Ltd.
Pitfield, Milton Keynes, MK11 3LW, UK
UKHW051131260726
13967UKWH00010B/2981

* 9 7 8 1 4 7 5 7 0 4 5 7 0 *